Neuromodulation Techniques for Pain Treatment

Tiago da Silva Freitas
Bernardo Assumpcao de Monaco
Stanley Golovac
Editors

Neuromodulation Techniques for Pain Treatment

A Step-by-Step Guide to Interventional Procedures and Managing Complications

Springer

Editors
Tiago da Silva Freitas
Department of Functional Neurosurgery
Hospital de Base and Brasília Pain Institute
Brasília
Brazil

Bernardo Assumpcao de Monaco
Department of Neurosurgery
University of Sao Paulo
São Paulo
Brazil

Stanley Golovac
Florida Pain
Coral Gables, FL
USA

ISBN 978-3-030-84777-7 ISBN 978-3-030-84778-4 (eBook)
https://doi.org/10.1007/978-3-030-84778-4

This Springer imprint is published by the registered company Springer Nature Switzerland AG
The registered company address is: Gewerbestrasse 11, 6330 Cham, Switzerland

Preface

Chronic pain is a global public health problem, and the education and improvement of professionals dedicated to interventional pain treatment is one of the factors that make a difference in the treatment of patients. With that in mind, 6 years ago, we created a course to improve the technique of invasive neuromodulation for pain treatment in Brasília, the capital of Brazil.

INDOR's Invasive Neuromodulation Course was born out of the interest in disseminating neuromodulation correctly and appropriately in the treatment of patients with chronic pain and, from the beginning, had the participation of the three authors of this book: Tiago Freitas, Bernardo de Monaco, and Stanley Golovac.

Over the years, we realized that there was a gap in the literature that involved technical aspects of implants in the treatment of these patients, and that's how the idea for this book was born. It would not have materialized without the persistence and commitment of all the authors and especially the leadership of Dr. Stanley Golovac in always supporting and encouraging us.

A book is like a child, we try to produce it in the best possible way and we hope to always see the need to update it, since neuromodulation is an exciting field and each day brings new technologies to help us in pain management of our patients.

We would like to thank all colleagues, from different parts of the world, who shared their experience, their time, and their commitment to our project. This is priceless for us. Thank you very much!

Finally, we would like to thank our families for their resilience, support, and patience during the preparation of this work.

Finally, we would like to thank the patients, for their confidence in our work and for the encouragement to always evolve in the search for an improvement in their quality of life.

Brasília, Brazil — Tiago da Silva Freitas
São Paulo, Brazil — Bernardo Assumpcao de Monaco
Coral Gables, FL, USA — Stanley Golovac

Contents

Contributors

Eduardo Joaquim Lopes Alho Division of Functional Neurosurgery, Clinics Hospital, School of Medicine, University of São Paulo, São Paulo, Brazil

Functional Neurosurgery, Disabled Children Assistance Association (AACD), São Paulo, Brazil

Department of Neurology, School of Medicine, University of São Paulo, São Paulo, Brazil

Daniel Benzecry Almeida Department of Neurosurgery, Instituto de Neurologia de Curitiba, Curitiba, Brazil

Charles Amaral Singular, Campinas, Brazil

João Henrique Araújo Centro de Dor Criciúma, Criciúma, Brazil

Fabricio Assis Singular, Campinas, Brazil

César Araújo Britto Department of Urology, Onofre Lopes University Hospital, Natal, Brazil

José Luis de Campos Anaesthesiology and Pain Management Hospital Vera Cruz and Clinica Adora em, Campinas, SP, Brazil

Physician Responsible for the Teaching and Training Center for Specialization in Pain, CET/SBA, Hospital Vera Cruz, Campinas, SP, Brazil

Joacir Graciolli Cordeiro Division of Functional Neurosurgery – University of Miami/Jackson Memorial Hospital, Miami, FL, USA

Tiago da Silva Freitas Functional Neurosurgery/Pain Ttreatment, Brasilia Pain Institute (INDOR), Brasília, Distrito Federal, Brazil

Neurosurgery Department Hospital de Base de Brasília (HBDF), Brasília, Distrito Federal, Brazil

Functional Neurosurgery Department Hospital Sírio Libanês, Brasília, Distrito Federal, Brazil

Brasilia Pain Institute(INDOR), Neurosurgery Department Hospital de Base de Brasília(HBDF), Functional Neurosurgery Department Hospital Sírio Libanês, Brasília, Distrito Federal, Brazil

Brasilia Pain Institute(INDOR), Neurosurgery department Hospital de Base de Brasília (HBDF), Functional Neurosurgery department Hospital Sírio Libanês, Brasília, Brasília, Distrito Federal, Brazil

Sérgio Adrian Fernandes Dantas Department of Neurosurgery, Onofre Lopes University Hospital, Natal, Brazil

Gilberto de Almeida Fonseca Filho Functional Neurosurgery Department, Madre Teresa Hospital, Belo Horizonte, Brazil

Functional Neurosurgery Department, Biocor Institute, Nova Lima, Brazil

Kleber Carlos de Azevedo Junior Department of Neurology, School of Medicine, University of São Paulo, São Paulo, Brazil

Bernardo Assumpcao de Monaco Division of Functional Neurosurgery, Clinics Hospital, University of Sao Paulo Medicine School, São Paulo, Brazil

Functional Neurosurgery – Association of Assistance to Disabled Children [AACD], São Paulo, Brazil

Division of Functional Neurosurgery, Clinics Hospital, School of Medicine, University of São Paulo, São Paulo, Brazil

Functional Neurosurgery, Disabled Children Assistance Association (AACD), São Paulo, Brazil

Antônio Jorge Barbosa de Oliveira Functional Neurosurgery/Pain treatment; Brasilia Pain Institute (INDOR), Brasilia, Brazil

Functional Neurosurgery Department, Hospital Sirio Libanes, Brasilia, Brazil

Neurosurgery Department, Associação de Assistência à Criança Deficiente – AACD, Sao Paulo, Brazil

Timothy R. Deer The Spine and Nerve Center of The Virginias, Charleston, WV, USA

Pavli S. Demian The Pain Management Center, Hamilton Township, NJ, USA

Simran Dua Chronic Pain Research Institute, Winston-Salem, NC, USA

Steven Falowski Neurosurgical Associates of Lancaster, Lancaster, PA, USA

Claudio A. Feler Carbondale, CO, USA

Joshua Feler Neurosurgery Resident, Brown University, Providence, RI, USA

Erich Talamoni Fonoff Department of Neurology, School of Medicine, University of São Paulo, São Paulo, Brazil

Stanley Golovac Space Coast Pain Institute, Merritt Island, FL, USA

Florida Pain, Melbourne, FL, USA

Golovac Consulting, Coral Gables, FL, USA

Surgery Partners, Merritt Island, FL, USA

Physician Partners of America, Tampa, FL, USA

Clement Hamani Sunnybrook Research Institute, Toronto, ON, Canada

Harquail Centre for Neuromodulation, Sunnybrook Health Sciences Centre, Toronto, ON, Canada

Division of Neurosurgery, Sunnybrook Health Sciences Centre, University of Toronto, Toronto, ON, Canada

Corey Hunter Ainsworth Institute of Pain Management, New York, NY, USA

Jonathan Russell Jagid Neurology, Orthopedics and Rehabilitation, University of Miami/ Jackson Memorial Hospital, Functional and Epilepsy Neurosurgery, Functional and Epilepsy, Neurotrauma, Miami, FL, USA

Leonardo Kapural Chronic Pain Research Institute, Winston-Salem, NC, USA

Ryan B. Kochanski Department of Neurosurgery, University of California, San Francisco, CA, USA

Paul J. Lynch Arizona Pain, Scottsdale, AZ, USA

Mostafa Maita UT Health San Antonio, San Antonio, TX, USA

Brandon May UT Health San Antonio, San Antonio, TX, USA

Tory L. McJunkin Arizona Pain, Scottsdale, AZ, USA

Plinio Duarte Mendes Functional Neurosurgery Department, Madre Teresa Hospital, Belo Horizonte, Brazil

Functional Neurosurgery Department, Biocor Institute, Nova Lima, Brazil

Daniel Lee Neuman Resident Physician, Department of Anesthesiology, The University of Kansas Health System, Kansas City, Kansas, USA

Thiago Frederico Nouer Singular Pain Clinic, Campinas, São Paulo, Brazil

Fabian C. Piedimonte Functional Neurosurgery, Fellow of Interventional Pain Procedures (FIPP/WIP), Buenos Aires, Argentina

Francisco Irochima Pinheiro Department of Oftalmology, Onofre Lopes University Hospital, Natal, Brazil

Priodarshi Roychoudhury Department of Anesthesia and Pain, Toronto General Hospital, University of Toronto, Toronto, ON, Canada

Dawood Sayed The American Society of Pain and Neuroscience, Pain Medicine, Interventional Pain, The Marc Asher Comprehensive Spine Center, The Center of Neuromodulation, Kansas City, Kansas, USA

Keith-Austin Scarfo Department of Neurosurgery, Warren Alpert Medical School of Brown University, Providence, RI, USA

Rhode Island Hospital, Norman Prince Spine Insititue, Providence, RI, USA

Konstantin V. Slavin Department of Neurosurgery, University of Illinois at Chicago, Chicago, IL, USA

Natalie Strand Mayo Clinic Arizona, Phoenix, AZ, USA

Introduction and History of Neuromodulation for Pain

Eduardo Joaquim Lopes Alho, Joacir Graciolli Cordeiro, Bernardo Assumpcao de Monaco, and Jonathan Russell Jagid

Introduction

Neuromodulation has several definitions, but it can be accurately described as the process of "inhibition, stimulation, modification, regulation or therapeutic alteration of activity, electrically or chemically, in the central, peripheral, or autonomic nervous system" [1]. At first glance, it might seem a very broad definition, but it solely reflects the use of electrical or chemical stimuli to modify the nervous system's activity with therapeutical purposes. The first observations that electricity could be applied in the treatment of painful conditions date from ancient Rome [2], but it was only in the twentieth century that knowledge of neurophysiology associated with technology allowed a more organized use of electricity or intrathecal drug delivery to modulate the human nervous system with defined therapeutic purposes, based on scientific understanding. In this chapter, we divide the evolution of neuromodulation into three parts. In the first, we describe the early applications of neuromodulation principles in the treatment of pain. The second part of the chapter is

E. J. Lopes Alho · B. Assumpcao de Monaco (✉)
Division of Functional Neurosurgery, Clinics Hospital, School of Medicine, University of São Paulo, São Paulo, Brazil

Functional Neurosurgery, Disabled Children Assistance Association (AACD), São Paulo, Brazil
e-mail: bernardo.monaco@usp.br

J. Graciolli Cordeiro
Division of Functional Neurosurgery – University of Miami/Jackson Memorial Hospital, Miami, FL, USA

J. Russell Jagid
University of Miami/Jackson Memorial Hospital, Miami, FL, USA

T. d. S. Freitas et al. (eds.), *Neuromodulation Techniques for Pain Treatment*,
https://doi.org/10.1007/978-3-030-84778-4_1

dedicated to the times when physiological and technological achievements led to the development of the neuromodulation systems that we use nowadays. The third part is dedicated to the state of the art of neuromodulation for pain.

Part I: From Electrical Fishes to Faradic Currents

The first known depiction of an electric Nile catfish (*M. electricus*) is displayed on the famous palette of the predynastic Egyptian ruler Na'rmer, ca 3100 BC [3]. The catfish appears at the top, as a hieroglyph as the phonetic representation of Na'rmer's name through the symbols *n'r* (catfish) and *mr* (chisel) (Fig. 1). Although this

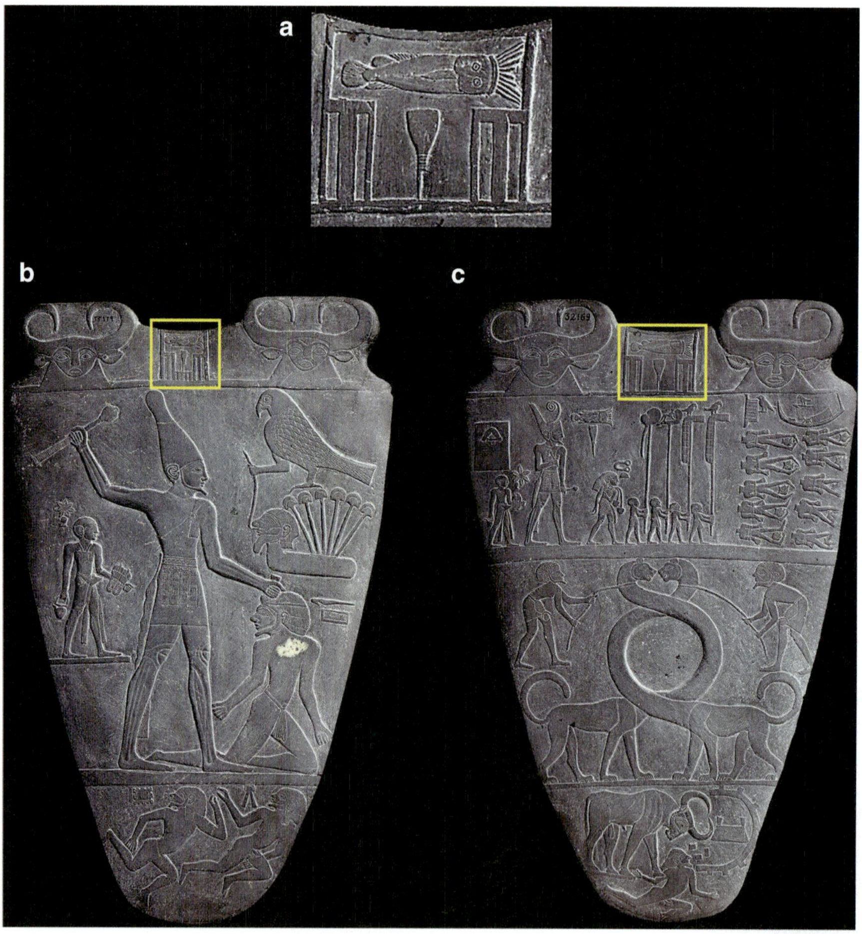

Fig. 1 Na'rmer's palette, ca 3100 BC. (**a**) Detail of the hieroglyph magnified from the yellow squares at the palettes. It is possible to see the catfish and the chisel used as phonetic symbols meaning Na'rmer's name (**b**) recto side and (**c**) verso side

appearance led to some speculation that ancient Egyptians would treat painful conditions using Nile catfish's electrical properties, the Greeks were the first to provide written records of neurological effects of the torpedo fish (*T. torpedo*). Aristotle stated that the torpedo causes numbness in human beings [4]. The precise use of these fishes for therapeutic purposes was only inferred until approximately 46 AD, when Scribonius Largus described in his book *Compositiones Medicae* [5], a detailed description of how to use the torpedo fish to treat inferior limb pain and migraine (among several other treatments for various diseases). *Compositiones Medicae* was published in 1655.

Anteros, who was a freeman of Tiberius Claudius (Roman emperor from 37 to 54 AD), was affected by gout and consequently intense pain in his feet. While walking by Sicily's coast, Anteros stepped on a torpedo fish and felt a shock, which was surprisingly followed by pain relief. Anteros reported this effect to Scribonius, who further investigated this therapy on Anteros himself, with good pain relief. In his book, he then recommended that "For both kinds of gout (hot and cold), a live black torpedo should, when pain begins, be placed under the feet. The patient must stand on a moist shore washed by the sea and should stay like this until his whole foot and leg, up to the knee, is numb. This takes away the present pain and prevents pain from coming on, if has not already arisen." Tiberius Claudius, who suffered from chronic migraine, was also treated with black torpedos prescribed by Scribonius Largus. The original descriptions in Latin with English translations [4] can be found in Fig. 2. It should be noted that the concept described by Scribonius is still valid, as

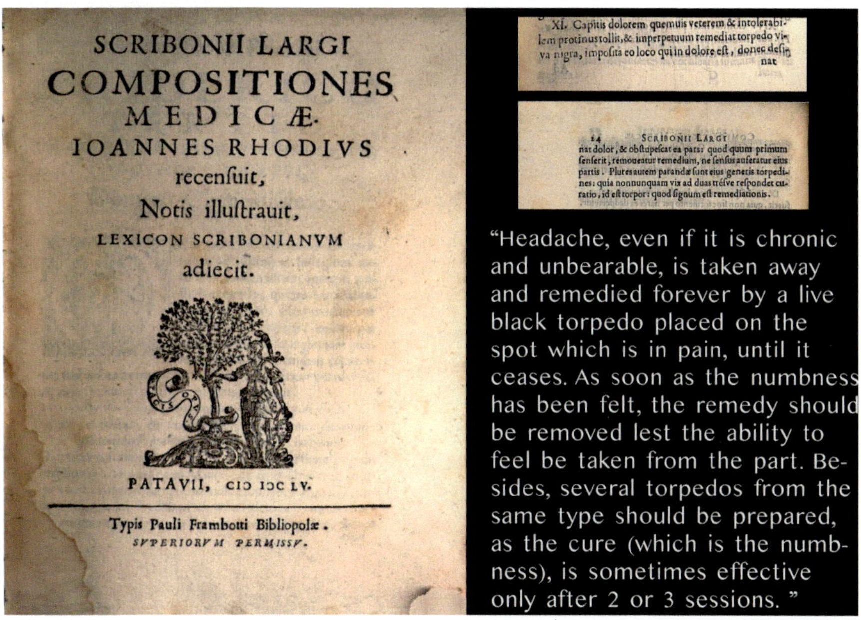

Fig. 2 Front page of the 1655 publication of Compositiones Medicae (47 AD). On the upper right side, original descriptions of torpedo fish use for headache and its translation to English

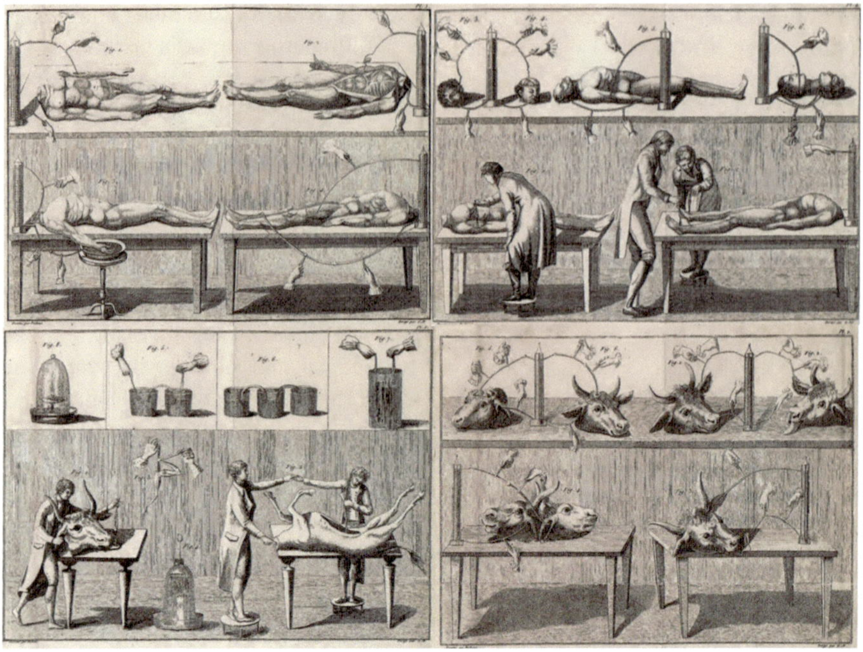

Fig. 3 Giovani Aldini's experiments with electricity and nervous system in decapitated humans (upper half) and bulls (lower half). (Illustrations from Aldini's 1804 book [7])

occipital nerve stimulation is a current state-of-the-art treatment for chronic migraine, and peripheral nerve stimulation, causing numbness, is also an effective recommendation almost 2000 years after.

The effects of electricity in biological systems were not enthusiastically explored until electricity itself could be mastered. Luigi Galvani, in 1791, published his discovery of bioelectricity [6], while demonstrating that electricity is the mean to transfer commands from the nervous system to the muscles (*De Viribus Electricitatis in Motu Musculari Commentarius)*. His nephew, Giovanni Aldini, performed electrical stimulations on exposed animal brains and also the human cortex of recently decapitated prisoners (Fig. 3), reporting in 1804 that these stimuli evoked horrible facial grimaces [7, 8]. These experiments showed that the nervous system was excitable by electricity. This concept led to investigations in the next years, regarding understanding the functions of the nervous system (neurophysiology) and the use of electric stimulation for therapeutic purposes. Sixty-six years later, in 1870, Fritsch and Hitzig demonstrated that limb movements could be elicited by stimulating the motor cortex in a dog [9]. Neurosciences had an important development during the nineteenth century, and a few competing (and controversial) theories of localization of brain functions emerged in that period [10]. In 1874, Dr. Roberts Bartholow was the first to electrically stimulate the parietal cortex of a living human brain. The cortex of a 30-year-old woman was exposed due to a purulent ulcer of the scalp, diagnosed as basal cell carcinoma. After several attempts of treatment, Dr. Bartholow proposed the experiments of stimulating her brain with galvanic and faradic currents, which she agreed. A detailed description of the procedure can be found elsewhere [11]. Dr. Bartholow published his findings in April 1874 [12].

This procedure was only possible due to the current status of the so-called "electrotherapy." The use of electricity in medicine reached its apogee in the second half of the nineteenth century, and it was so important that to be considered properly equipped, a hospital should own an electrical apparatus [11]. One of the best electrotherapy rooms in the United States of America was conceived and developed by Dr. Robert Bartholow. Multiple applications for electricity in medicine were suggested, either using galvanic or faradic currents. The main idea was to profit from local changes in the tissues produced by electric currents, as increase of blood flow and relieve from local congestion by muscle contraction, forcing the fluids in direction of the lymphatic system [13]. The effects on the brain and spinal cord were just postulated, and several concerns about electricity interactions with nervous tissue were raised in the early 1900s [13]. Placebo effect was already discussed, or whether electricity can influence directly the brain and cord with a safe current strength. If so, would it be of therapeutic value? The indications at the time were neurological diseases (treatment of motor paralysis, tabes dorsalis, spasticity and pain, including ciatica and headaches, epilepsy, and psychiatric diseases), arthritis and myalgia, visceral diseases (tuberculosis and stomach problems), arterial hypertension, and genitourinary and pelvic diseases. The Electreat was a portable electrical stimulator patented in 1919 and resembled the later developed transcutaneous electrical nerve stimulation (TENS). Even major amputations were carried out with local application of currents, instead of general anesthesia. With electrodes placed at appropriate nerves in the leg, using 40 V, 40 mA, and pulse widths of 10 msec, several major lower limb amputations were preceded at St Francis Hospital in 1910 [4]. The technological knowledge to build batteries and electrical stimulators acquired at this time associated with a deeper understanding of neuroscience was important to the next steps in neuromodulation history. The first modern therapeutic application of brain stimulation came in 1938, introduced by Ugo Cerletti, the electroconvulsotherapy [8].

Part II: Neuromodulation as a Long-Term Treatment

The surgical treatment for pain in the late 1800s and the first half of the twentieth century was centered on ablative techniques. Lesions have been produced in the past with wire loops, alcohol injections, cryoprobes, or probes that heat tissue with a radiofrequency current while maintaining constant temperatures [14]. Proposed ablative procedures included trigeminal rhizotomy (Cushing, 1896), cordotomy (Spiller and Martin, 1912), median myelotomy (Armour, 1926), mesenchephalotomy (Wycsis, 1947), cingulotomy (Foltz and White, 1962), and DREZotomy (Sindou, 1972).

Neuromodulation techniques can be subdivided into electrical and chemical neuromodulation. Electrical neuromodulation comprises deep brain stimulation (DBS), spinal cord stimulation (SCS), motor cortex stimulation (MCS), and peripheral nerve stimulation (PNS). Chemical neuromodulation is represented mainly by intrathecal drug infusion through pumps. Each of these techniques had its own history and development, and therefore, they will be discussed in separate topics.

Deep Brain Stimulation

In 1908, Sir Victor Horsley and R. H. Clarke published a comprehensive paper about the structure and functions of the cerebellum. They aimed to investigate the anatomical relations of the cerebellar cortex to its nuclei and peduncles and to the rest of the brain and spinal cord [15]. The method for these investigations included electrolytic lesions (application of an electrical current to the nuclei by means of needles) placed precisely in cerebellar nuclei, with a stereotaxic apparatus described also in this paper for the first time. They also discussed in detail the methods of electrical stimulation of the cerebellum (excitation) and how to produce different kinds of lesions (electrolysis). Several electrical parameters were experimented in monkeys (constant currents, faradic excitation, sparks form high tension currents, anodal x cathodal, unipolar needle x bipolar needles), with postmortem macroscopical and microscopical analysis of the lesions produced. The different types of stimulation of cerebellar structures are also discussed in detail.

This knowledge was only applied to humans in 1947 when Spiegel and Wycis adapted the Horsley's stereotaxic apparatus to use in humans [16]. Although stereotactic procedures were at that time, ablative, surgeons would first stimulate the target to assure that the needle's tip was not in the internal capsule before producing the lesion [2]. The first to insert permanent electrodes in the human brain for purposes of stimulation was Pool, in 1948 [17]. An induction-coil system was used to activate the caudate nucleus in a depressed cachectic woman suffering from advanced Parkinson's disease. This data was not published in 1948, but only in his 1954 paper. He carried stimulation almost daily for 8 weeks, as the patient and her family said it made her "feel better." The coil and wires remained in place for over 3 years, but one of them finally broke, and the stimulation was discontinued. Permanent electrodes were implanted by either direct operative approach or stereotactic apparatus. Wires could be connected to a miniature induction coil set permanently in an opening in the skull or connected to fine insulated wires led out through the scalp for purposes of direct stimulation and recording. Since 1950, Heath also developed a technique of deep focal stimulation, with good results for pain relief. As reported by Pool [17], a 61-year-old woman with severe pain in both shoulders and arms was submitted by deep brain stimulation for pain. The patient had a diagnosis of multiple myeloma, with increasing pain, progressive cachexia, requiring high doses of meperidine to relieve the symptoms. A deep frontal stimulation with two electrodes placed in the right frontal lobe was carried out by stereotaxy. One electrode was inserted close to the midline, anterior to the hypothalamus in the horizontal plane of the anterior commissure (septal region). The other lay in a more lateral, anterior, and dorsal position. Stimulation was carried out for 60 seconds, at

3 mA, with square waves of 5 ms pulse duration. No response was elicited below 3 mA, but Pool reports that at 3 mA, the patient exclaimed, "Oh, doctor, I feel so fine! My pains have all gone away." Simultaneously piloerection, slight pupil dilatation, and deeper and rapid breath occurred. The same phenomena occurred in a second stimulation of 120 s, 10 minutes later. In the next 4 weeks, meperidine daily doses dropped from 650 to 50 mg. A mild degree of euphoria was reported. As early as 1954, Pool already considered that as Heath had shown, deep brain stimulation could be an even more satisfactory procedure for alleviating cancer pain than ablative procedures.

In 1952, José Delgado described the technique of intracranial electrode placement for recording, stimulation, and verification of possible therapeutic value in psychotic patients [18]. He placed the electrodes under direct visualization through a trephine opening, placing two plate electrodes on the orbital surface of one frontal lobe and one needle electrode in the white matter of the superior frontal quadrant. He recorded spontaneous and evoked electrical brain activity and use mono or bipolar stimulation. Some of his later research is controversial, as he implanted electrode arrays equipped with radio wave transmission, showing that he could control subject's minds (including animals and humans) with a remote control. There is classical footage of a Spanish bullfight where Delgado stops the bull (with such electrodes implanted) from attacking the "toreador" by remote control.

After these initial developments of the technique, other authors started using deep brain implants to treat other neurological conditions. Bekthereva in 1963 implanted electrodes to treat hyperkinetic disorders [19], and Sem-Jacobsen in 1965 used depth electrodes to record and stimulate patients with Parkinson's disease [20], aiming to perform lesion of the basal ganglia. In this paper, he describes already the insertion effect: "The introduction of the electrodes alone frequently abolishes or alters the patient's symptoms from six hours up to a week or more." Electrophysiological mapping of the trajectory was performed, eliciting sensory, visual, speech, and vegetative symptoms. He concludes that with intracerebral stimulation, it is possible to localize the target and avoid undesirable side effects, predicting the result of the lesion.

Besides the already discussed targets to treat chronic pain (septal region and caudate nucleus), Hosobuchi proposed in 1973 the stimulation of the nucleus posterior ventralis medialis (PVM) to treat facial anesthesia dolorosa following trigeminal rhizotomy [21]. Stimulation of the sensory thalamus was also performed by Mazars [22], but several other targets were later proposed to treat chronic pain as periaqueductal gray area [23], anterior cingulate cortex [24, 25], and nucleus accumbens [26]. Limbic stimulation for pain aims to target the affective component of pain. The possible targets for DBS in chronic pain will be discussed further in separate chapters. Evolution in engineering also allowed better electrodes and implantable pulse generators (IPGs), with better results. The modern DBS era started with Alim-Louis-Benabid's preliminary report in 1987 on stimulation of the nucleus ventralis intermedius (V.i.m.) thalamic nucleus to treat tremors related to Parkinson's disease [27]. In the 30th anniversary of this seminal publication, the long-term (21 years) outcomes of thalamic

DBS implanted in 159 patients treated at the Grenoble University Hospital for tremor in PD, essential tremor, and dystonia were published, and we proudly co-authored this important publication [28].

Spinal Cord Stimulation and Peripheral Nerve Stimulation

Understanding the physiopathology of pain was crucial for the development of neuromodulation strategies to treat it. An important theory of pain mechanisms was presented by Melzack and Wall in 1965. In this paper [29], they debate the current pain theories (specificity theory and pattern theory) and propose a new theory called gate control theory of pain.

In this theory, they propose that the substantia gelatinosa in the dorsal horn functions as a gate control system that modulates the afferent patterns before they influence the first central transmission cells. The afferent patterns (large and small fibers) in the dorsal column act as a central control trigger which activates selective brain processes that influence the modulating properties of the gate control system. The gate can be opened or closed depending on the balance of the afferent large (touch) and small (pain) caliber fibers. This means that a touch sensation could close the gate for pain, decreasing the painful sensation. The simulation of a touch sensation could be elicited by applying small currents in skin electrodes, the transcutaneous stimulation, today renamed as TENS [2].

One of the predictions of the gate control was that stimulating large-diameter cutaneous afferent nerve fibers might reduce the pain. So, 2 years after proposing the theory, Wall and Sweet stimulated eight patients with intense chronic cutaneous pain [30] in sensory nerves or roots supplying the painful area. The voltage was raised until the patient reported tingling in the area. They reported good results in pain reduction, introducing the peripheral nerve stimulation concept.

Norman Shealy confirmed these results in ten patients with peripheral nerve stimulation. However, in cases of diffuse pain, he did not achieve good results, because stimulation was very selective. Soon after, in the same year of 1967, he proposed to stimulate the large afferent fibers not in their peripheral fields, but just before they entered into the dorsal columns of the spinal cord. He first experimented with his idea in 35 adult cats, with good results [31].On March 24, 1967, a 70-year-old man with severe diffuse pain in the right lower part of the abdomen with an inoperable bronchogenic carcinoma (probably metastatic to pleura and liver) was submitted to the first spinal cord stimulation [32]. Thoracic laminectomy at D2-D3 levels was performed, and a chromium-nickel-molybdenum alloy (Vitallium) electrode with 3 by 4 mm was approximated to the dorsal columns at D3 by suturing to the dura mater. This electrode and the stimulator used were adaptations of Medtronic's cardiovascular stimulating systems (Barostat and Angiostat) developed to treat hypertension and angina by carotid sinus stimulation. Subcutaneous jacks were placed inferior to the wound for later external plug-in and stimulation. At 6 p.m. on the same day, stimulation started, and the patient felt a "buzzing" sensation in his back, extending around and throughout his chest, but not into his legs. Both incisional and original pain were immediately abolished. After 5–15 minutes, pain recurred, but a simple change in stimulation frequency promptly alleviated it. For 1 hour, the pain was controlled. The next day, stimulation continued for almost 12 hours, and the pain was controlled with success. The day after, he became confused, aphasic, and with right hemiplegia and died on March 30. Autopsy revealed subacute bacterial endocarditis with embolism to the left hemisphere. These results were encouraging, and soon in 1968, Medtronic made SCS commercially available. The stimulators at that time consisted of an electrode connected to a circular antenna implanted in subcutaneous tissue. The stimulation occurred through an external part, with a battery power supply connected to an external antenna. A fully implantable device was presented only in 1981.

Spinal cord stimulation was applied then not only for pain, but in 1971, Gildenberg used to treat spasmodic torticollis [2], and others recognized improvement in spasticity (Cook and Dooley) and peripheral vascular disease. In 1977, a symposium on the safety and clinical efficacy of implanted neuroaugmentative devices discussed DBS, chronic cerebellar stimulation, SCS, PNS, and neuroaugmentation. SCS was considered to be both safe and effective for pain, but not for other indications (including conus medullaris stimulation for neurogenic bladder) [33]. Later, other conditions as angina pectoris, failed back surgery syndrome, and complex regional pain syndrome were considered indications for SCS and will be further discussed elsewhere.

Motor Cortex Stimulation

Deafferentation pain secondary to central nervous system (CNS) lesions is challenging, even with all accumulated technology that we afford in the twenty-first century. In 1991, Tsubokawa estimated that any forms of therapies, including DBS, would provide satisfactory control of the pain in only one-third of such cases [34]. In order to develop more effective treatments to deafferentation pain due to CNS lesions, Tsubokawa and his co-workers had been exploring the effects of stimulation of various brain regions in the previous years. Surprisingly, they recognized that motor cortex stimulation could provide good results in such patients. In his 1991 casuistic treatment, a total of 12 patients were treated, being 6 thalamic lesions, 3 small lesions at the posterior limb of the internal capsule, 1 pontine hemorrhage, 1 multiple sclerosis, and 1 postrhizotomy pain. The 4-contact electrode was placed at the epidural space, and the locations were confirmed by neurophysiological monitoring. The electrode was placed in the region where the muscle twitch of the painful area could be observed at the lowest threshold. In the same 1991 year, Tsubokawa and his co-workers published another series of seven cases, but this time only with thalamic pain [35].

The authors hypothesized that thalamic hyperactivity is observed following transection of the spinothalamic tract (in cats) and such hyperactivity can be inhibited more efficiently by stimulation of the motor cortex rather than the sensory cortex. This neuromodulation technique has been reproduced by others since then, and it is reserved for such difficult cases.

Intrathecal Infusion Pumps

The history of chemical modulation of the CNS is confounded with the history of anesthesia and regional blocks for pain. The first description of a neuraxial blockade is attributed to James Leonard Corning in 1885, who injected cocaine between the spinous processes of the lower lumbar vertebrae (first in a dog, then in a healthy man). Cocaine was employed as an anesthetic since 1884, when Karl Koller described its properties.

The first reports of major surgeries under spinal blockade date from 1899, when August Bier describes six cases of cocaine injection into subdural lumbar space to perform limb amputations due to infections (tuberculosis and necrosis by osteomyelitis). He used the puncture technique described by Quincke in 1891 [36]. On the 16th August 1898, a 34-year-old worker with hopeless tuberculosis was submitted to his ankle's resection after "spinal cord cocainization" with a 0.5% cocaine solution [37]. The surgery started 20 minutes after the puncture, and the patient reported feeling pressure and awareness of the procedure, but not pain. After 2 hours, he started feeling pain in the left leg and back and intense headache. The leg pain was relieved within a short time, but the headache remained important until the next day. Committed to understanding the effects of "cocainization of the spinal cord," on the 24th August 1898, Bier submitted himself to injection of a cocaine solution into his lumbar spine, through the hands of his colleague, Dr. Hildebrandt. He describes in his 1899 paper [37] the sensory and motor effects minute after minute. They tested pain in several (and unbelievable for our days) ways, such as applying a burning cigar on the legs (13 minutes after the injection) and strong pushing and pulling his testicles (after 25 minutes). Rudolph Matas, among others, was concerned about the effects of general anesthetics (especially cocaine) and described several regional and local anesthesia, not only with cocaine but also with other analgesic drugs, as morphine [38].

The short duration of opioid effects in the epidural space led to the development of continuous catheter infusion and, later, implantable delivery systems. Dr. Grafton Love was a neurosurgeon with great experience in treating patients with meningitis. He used ureteral catheters placed into the lateral ventricles to treat those patients and in 1935 proposed the same technique to introduce catheters in the lumbar space [39]. The first application of continuous anesthetics delivered by a catheter implanted in the lumbar spine was performed in 1940 by Dr. William Leonard, who administered procaine to approximately 200 patients. The technique for delivering anesthetic drugs in the lumbar spine was improved in the next years by several authors. Dr. Samuel Manalan, Edward Tuohy, Yaksh, and Rudy are important contributors to the development of spinal analgesia.

The first attempt to control cancer pain with intrathecal (IT) infusion of morphine was performed in 1979 by Wang and his colleagues [40]. Onofrio and collaborators also described in 1981 the continuous infusion of morphine in the subarachnoid space to treat a 73-year-old man with pelvic chordoma [41]. In 1983, Coombs adapted a heparin infusion pump to deliver intraspinal morphine via an implanted reservoir in ten patients with intractable pain patients (five cancer and five nonmalignant pain), discouraging further use in nonmalignant pain, but with satisfactory results in the cancer group.

Implantable pumps have reservoirs of varying capacities (generally 10–50 ml), which can be refilled by injection through a self-sealing septum. Different systems can be classified in terms of programmability, ranging from simple pulsatile pumps (purely mechanical hand-operated systems), to continuous flow pumps (powered by Freon gas), to fully programmable remote-controlled battery-powered electromechanical pumps [42]. The programmable pumps are particularly beneficial when the therapeutic window is small or fine-tuning is required.

Part III: State-of-the-Art of Neuromodulation for Pain

Neuromodulation for pain is an ever-expanding field. There have been numerous technical advances leading to a wide variety of surgical techniques to manage chronic pain. A multitude of surgical targets have been described, including the central and peripheral nervous system, including the motor cortex, thalamus, periventricular/periaqueductal gray area, dorsal spinal cord, dorsal root ganglia (DRG), nerve roots, peripheral nerves, as well as subcutaneous peripheral field stimulation. Covering all these paradigms is beyond the scope of this chapter; hence, we will focus on the most recent advances and indications.

State of the Art in Spinal Cord Stimulation for Pain

Spinal cord stimulation (SCS) is the mainstay of neuromodulation for pain as it is the most frequently targeted site. Therapy is based on the gate theory of pain originally described by Melzack and Wall in 1965 [29]. This theory suggests that excitation of sensory pathways peripherally mitigates the cortical perception of pain. The surgical device delivers tonic low-frequency square wave stimulation to the dorsal column inducing paresthesia in the painful dermatome. Indications for tonic SCS were classically neuropathic pain secondary to chronic regional pain syndromes (CRPS), failed back syndrome, diabetic neuropathy, as well as vascular disease including peripheral arterial disease and refractory heart angina due to its vasorelaxant properties [43–46]. A common unwanted result was erratic stimulation producing either inconsistency in the paresthetic field or, worse, unpleasant dysesthesias. This side effect was felt to be due to changes in the stimulation field induced by the

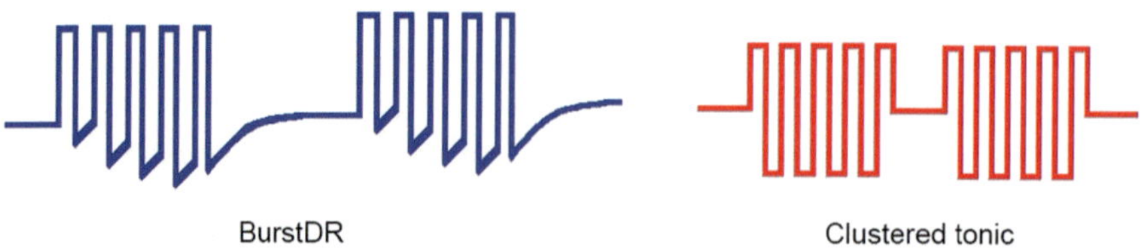

Fig. 4 Illustration comparing BurstDR stimulation with nonlinear charge accumulation and Burst stimulation modalities resembling a clustered tonic stimulation

positional movement of the leads during common activities. As the patient moves and the spinal canal diameter narrows, the electrodes are in closer contact with the spinal cord causing enlargement of the stimulated field including the sensory rootlets and vice-versa. To compensate for these changes, stimulation systems coupled to accelerometers were designed to automatically adjust the stimulation intensity according to the patient's position [47].

During the last decade, an explosion of new technologies in SCS occurred. In 2010, the concept of "burst" stimulation started to gain more acceptance. The use of trains of high-frequency pulses (500 Hz) of increasing charges in the form of "bursts" is referred to as BurstDR spinal cord stimulation (Abbott, Illinois, USA) [48]. The underlying concept involves the attempt to resemble a physiological firing pattern to better modulate pathways involved in pain generation and maintenance [49]. This approach produces a nonlinear charge accumulation, contrary to the classic tonic stimulation. It is important to mention that there are different SCS systems available to deliver burst stimulation. However, BurstDR is provided only by a single system. Other systems use burst stimulation with biphasic square waves with a linear charge accumulation resembling a clustered tonic stimulation (Fig. 4).

Furthermore, one should bear in mind that different types of burst stimulation are associated with different patterns of neurophysiological response. The BurstDR paradigm is able to induce a more intense single afterdischarge in the thalamic projections, while the burst pattern resembling clustered tonic stimulation induces multiple small afterdischarges in its suprasegmental projections [50]. Source-localized EEG performed in patients undergoing BurstDR SCS revealed the activation of ascending projections to the anterior cingulate cortex and the right dorsolateral prefrontal cortex pointing to a co-stimulation of the lateral (somatosensory) and medial pathways in the brain [51]. It seems meaningful to modulate the medial pathways to effect the emotional component of chronic pain [52].

Burst stimulation has been used clinically for approximately 9 years in more than 670 patients. At least six studies with level I evidence including one randomized clinical trial have been completed. Multiple studies demonstrated a therapeutic advantage of burst stimulation compared to standard tonic stimulation [48, 51–61]. The SUNBURST study compared the effect of burst vs. tonic stimulation delivered from the same SCS system. This unblinded study randomly assigned 100 patients, deemed eligible for an implant after a successful tonic SCS trial, into two groups. Each group was initially treated for 12 weeks with either tonic or burst stimulation.

For tonic stimulation, the pulse width was programmed in the range of 100–500 msec with frequencies typically between 30 and 100 Hz and at amplitudes producing comfortable paresthesia according to each individual patient's perception. For burst programming, 500 Hz stimulation was delivered in groups of five pulses with a 1 msec pulse width, with the five pulses repeated at a frequency of 40 Hz. After a period of 12 weeks, the groups underwent a crossover maintaining the interval to exclude any carryover effect. Results showed that burst stimulation was not only noninferior ($p < 0.001$) but superior ($p < 0.017$) to tonic stimulation. More patients (70.8%) preferred burst stimulation over tonic stimulation ($p < 0.001$). This preference was maintained after 1 year in 68.2% of the cases [48].

Innovative paradigms using very high-frequency SCS have shown remarkable clinical efficacy. In 2015, the SENZA trial was performed with pulses delivered up to 10 kHz, referred to as high-frequency SCS (HF10) [62]. The underlying theory is that, instead of targeting the dorsal columns with low-frequency SCS, HF10 would encompass the wide dynamic range neurons in the posterior horns. In order to assess the efficacy of HF10 SCS, a randomized controlled trial was conducted in 10 centers including 171 patients with both back and leg pain. From the total, 90 were implanted with the Senza® System for HF10 (Nevro Corp., USA) and the rest with the commercially available SCS system for conventional tonic stimulation (Precision Plus System; Boston Scientific, USA). The patients were assessed for pain response to the SCS and deemed remitters if they achieved a visual analog scale (VAS) of 2.5 or less. At 12 months' follow-up, approximately 80% of the HF10 patients were responders compared with 50% for traditional SCS. Leg pain response showed the same trend, favoring HF10. Remarkably, around 67% of the HF10 patients were back and leg pain remitters versus approximately 35% for back pain and 40% for leg pain with traditional SCS, respectively. The superiority of the HF10 effect was sustained over the long term. At 2-year follow-up, HF10 responder rates were 76% for back pain and 73% for leg pain vs. around 49% for both leg and back pain with traditional SCS. Likewise, remission rates were also significantly better for HF10 (back pain: 65.9% vs 31.0 and leg pain: 65.9% vs 39.4%) [62, 63].

In 2016, Sweet et al. published a study using paresthesia-free high-density (HD) SCS (Medtronic, MN, USA). This study included 15 patients with response to conventional SCS (60 Hz/350 μsec) and a trial with subthreshold HD SCS (1200 Hz/200 μsec/amplitude 90% paresthesia threshold). Subsequently, they were randomized into two groups and treated with four two-week periods of conventional, subthreshold HD, and sham stimulation in a randomized crossover design. The study concluded that paresthesia is not necessary for pain relief and subthreshold HD SCS could be an alternative to conventional stimulation in selected patients [64].

One year later, in 2017, Berg et al. reported on the use of multiple stimulation waveforms and field shapes with the goal of potential avoidance of habituation. The study enrolled 250 patients with chronic pain. The breakdown of stimulation paradigms was 72.8% of patients used standard rate, 34.8% anode intensification, 23.2% higher rate, and 8.4% burst stimulation waveforms. Collectively, 60% used 1 or more advanced waveforms. A trend showed patients continuing to use up to three programs one-year post-implant. Those findings suggested that patients continually benefit from the use of multiple waveforms and field shapes, customizing the therapy and possibly overcoming or delaying habituation phenomena [65].

In parallel during 2017, a key study focused on peripheral neuromodulation for chronic refractory pain was published. Distinctly different from previous neuromodulatory strategies in the spinal cord, this new approach aimed at modulating the hyperexcitation observed in the dorsal root ganglia (DRG) of patients with neuropathic pain. This was accomplished using a midline percutaneous approach to the spinal canal and deploying leads through the spinal foramina over the involved DRG.

This pivotal trial for DRG stimulation (Abbott, Spinal Modulation; LLC, Menlo Park, CA) named ACCURATE was a prospective study performed at 22 U.S. sites. A group of 152 patients with CRPS in the lower extremities was randomized into DRG stimulation vs. SCS. The primary end point was safety and efficacy at 3 and 12 months. Responders were defined as those with a 50% or greater decrease in VAS scores. At 3 months, the response rate was greater in the DRG arm (81.2%) compared to the SCS (55.7%, $P < 0.001$). After 12 months, the response in the DRG arm (74.2%) was again greater than that in the SCS (53.0%), which demonstrated both noninferiority ($p < 0.0001$) and superiority ($p < 0.0004$) at long-term follow-up. Greater improvements in quality of life and psychological disposition were observed with DRG stimulation. As expected, DRG stimulated patients reported less postural variation in paresthesia ($p < 0.001$) and less stimulation effect in non-involved areas ($p = 0.014$). Device-related and serious adverse events were similar in both groups [66].

Recently, in 2019, the concept of closed-loop SCS based on sensing of evoked potentials underwent a more detailed clinical evaluation. Evoked compound action potentials (ECAPs) are the sum of multiple action potentials that result from the activation of multiple nerve fibers by an electrical stimulus. In other words, ECAPs represent a way to directly measure the degree of axonal activation during SCS. ECAPs can be coupled to a closed-loop system to adjust SCS intensity. Currently, a closed-loop system (Evoke SystemTM, Saluda Medical, Sydney, Australia) is under evaluation with aim of gaining FDA approval. All commercially available SCS systems deliver continuous energy in a constant pattern irrespective of the underlying neural response. Closed-loop stimulation, if approved, will be the first modality to tailor stimulation according to in vivo, real-time, continuous objective measure of spinal cord activation via recorded ECAPs to maintain a steadier state of activation of the spinal cord. Initial results from smaller studies produced encouraging data to warrant a larger better-controlled study. The AVALON study, as an example, was a prospective, multicenter, single-arm study in which 36 out of 51 patients with back and/or leg pain were implanted after an external trial. At least a 50% reduction in pain was achieved in 85.7% (back) and 82.6% (leg) of subjects at 6 months' follow-up. At 6 months, 80% reduction of pain was achieved in 64.3% (back) and 60.9% (leg) of subjects [67].

The EVOKE trial (clinical trials.gov NCT02924129) involved 134 participants naïve from any form of neuromodulation presenting with pain of the trunk and/or limbs, which was deemed refractory to conservative therapy. The primary outcome was reduction of 50% or more in the overall back and leg pain (i.e., responders). The participants were randomly assigned to two groups, open-loop or closed-loop stimulation using ECAPs. Both groups were implanted with the same system. Two thoracic percutaneous leads were implanted, and conventional stimulation parameters were used for trial and therapy. ECAP-controlled closed-loop stimulation provided statistically significant greater pain relief than the open-loop spinal cord stimulation. At 12-month follow-up, responders were on the order of 83% in closed-loop vs 61% in open loop. Additionally, the reduction of pain intensity in the leg was significantly higher in the closed-loop group (i.e., 72% vs. 62%). Safety profile appeared to be equivalent in both groups with the most common adverse events being lead migration in 7%, IPG pocket pain in 4%, and muscle spasm in 2% [68, 69]. It's worth noting that the validity of the results from the EVOKE study was controversial due to possible issues with participant blinding and the lack of a control group with sham stimulation [70].

Currently, the aforementioned studies suggest that SCS is effective for the improvement and management of the neuropathic pain component of chronic pain syndromes. Unfortunately, this leaves out a large number of patients with refractory chronic back pain, in which the predominant component of the pain is nociceptive. This is the case in patients with nonspecific chronic low back pain (NSCLBP) syndromes, in which the pain is postural, unrelated to specific spine anomalies. To date, there is no level I evidence that SCS is highly effective for NSCLBP, and the European guidelines on NSCLBP state that "spinal cord stimulation cannot be recommended for nonspecific CLBP" [71, 72]. Furthermore, the Neuromodulation Appropriateness Consensus Committee (NACC) from the International Neuromodulation Society recommends SCS for neuropathic pain but found insufficient, low-quality, or contradictory evidence for SCS use (including high-frequency SCS) in patients with predominant low back pain [73]. It was hypothesized that motor neurostimulation to induce repeated contractions of the lumbar multifidus could be helpful to manage chronic mechanical low back pain (CMLBP). This hypothesis was based on the underlying theory that dysfunction of the lumbar multifidus would allow vertebral segments to move outside their pain-free zone increasing the risk of being reinjured, resulting in potential further motor control impairment and arthrogenic muscle inhibition leading to a chronic pain state [74, 75]. This innovative approach was called restorative neuromodulation. ReActiv8-A (Mainstay Medical, Dublin, Ireland) was an international multicenter study, in which, 53 patients were implanted with bilateral electrodes close to the medial branch of the L2 dorsal ramus nerve. The average duration of CMLBP in the study population was 14 years, and the average 10-point numerical rating scale was 7. The study concluded that this restorative approach is a new treatment option for CMLBP with clinically important, statistically significant, and lasting improvement in pain, disability, and QoL and is currently FDA approved [72].

State of the Art in Deep Brain Stimulation (DBS) for Pain

DBS is routinely performed for movement disorders, epilepsy, and OCD. Its use for pain is not FDA approved due to previous trials showing limited efficacy. With the recent concept that affective and cognitive aspects of pain play a major role in pain perception, there is a renewed interest in the therapy [76]. A systematic review of the literature from 2020 included 22 articles [77]. A total of 228 patients were included in the review. The most common targets used were periaqueductal/periventricular gray matter region (PAG/PVG), ventral posterior lateral/posterior medial thalamus (VPL/VPM), or both. Poststroke pain was the most common indication followed by phantom limb pain and brachial plexus injury.

Sensory thalamus and PAG/PVG or both were the targets selected for stimulation for poststroke pain. One of the largest series was comprised of 12 patients implanted in the PAG/PVG or sensory thalamus. In this series, 70% of the patients responded with an average pain relief of around 40–50% [78]. Another group reported a different surgical approach. The electrode was first placed in the PAG/PVG, and intraoperative testing was performed. If the patient didn't report analgesia or pleasant warmth, the electrode would be moved to the sensory thalamus [79].

For phantom limb pain, authors targeted either PAG/PVG and sensory thalamus or the latter only. Among the largest series, 8 of 9 patients responded to stimulation. In another series, 8 of 11 patients responded with an average VAS pain reduction of 60% [80].

DBS for pain after brachial plexus injury (BPI) is associated with poor outcome. The largest series for BPI included nine patients with DBS targeting the sensory thalamus with poor outcome. Moreover, targeting PAG/PVH and/or the sensory thalamus did not improve pain control for this indication [81].

Noteworthy is the frequent observation that isolated pain control does not necessarily equate to improved quality of life. According to the neuromatrix theory, the cognitive, affective, and sensory-discriminative spheres would play equally important roles in pain perception [82]. For this reason, different targets were investigated with the idea of improving the affective component of pain including the anterior cingulate cortex (ACC) and the ventral striatum and the anterior limb of the internal capsule (VS/ALIC). Results in the literature are heterogeneous and do not meet the criteria for adequate pain response in many cases. However, for poststroke pain, despite pain persistence, significant improvements in quality of life, depression, and anxiety were observed. Improvements were sustained at two-year follow-up, and half of the patients stated they would undergo the procedure again for the same result [81, 83]. Those findings reinforce the theory of addressing both the somatosensory and the affective component of pain together when planning DBS.

Pain as a result of spinal cord injury (SCI) can be classified as neuropathic or nociceptive, affecting 34% and 64% of long-term survivors, respectively. Aberrant neurotransmission coming from the injured spinal cord and abnormal cortical reorganization have been implicated as underlying mechanisms [84]. A systematic review identified a group of 36 SCI patients, out of which 19 had a successful trial and were implanted in the sensory thalamus ± central gray. Unfortunately, only three patients experienced long-term success [85]. Stimulation paradigms may have an impact on outcome in addition to the target, as reports have shown that very low-frequency stimulation (<0.67 Hz) may be more effective. Furthermore, time may be a factor such that stimulation parameter changes may take time to manifest (hours to days) [86]. Successful pain relief was reported within a case of DBS to the rostral ACC and another one with bilateral PAG DBS also improving associated autonomic dysfunction [24, 87]. Despite scarce and heterogeneous findings in the literature, it is suggested that motor cortex stimulation might be more effective than DBS for SCI, as it provided long-term success in four out of seven patients in a review paper [85].

This chapter provides an overview of the history of neuromodulation for pain, culminating in a state-of-the-art review of procedures using both peripherally and centrally targeted therapy. It describes how the technology has changed over the course of time ultimately producing better outcomes for peripheral stimulation. Additionally, it illustrates how different targets may produce different results suggesting the importance and further research needed to better understand the neurocircuitry involved in pain and its perception. Ultimately, surgical therapy of pain is a necessity given the abundance of medication for refractory pain syndromes.

References

1. Krames E, Peckham PH, Rezai AR. Neuromodulation. Amsterdam; Boston; San Diego, CA: Elsevier; Academic Press; 2009.
2. Gildenberg PL. History of electrical neuromodulation for chronic pain. Pain Med. 2006;7(suppl_1):S7–13.
3. Howes GJ. The phylogenetic relationships of the electric catfish family Malapteruridae (Teleostei: Siluroidei). J Nat Hist. 1985;19(1):37–67.
4. Kane K, Taub A. A history of local electrical analgesia. Pain. 1975;1(2):125–38.
5. Scribonius (Largus). Compositiones medicae. 1655. 696 p.
6. Galvani A. De Viribus Electricitatis In Motu Musculari Comentarius Cum Joannis Aldini Dissertatione Et Notis; Accesserunt Epistolae ad animalis electricitatis theoriam pertinentes. Apud Societatem Typographicam; 1792. 128 p.
7. Aldini G (1762–1834) A du texte. Essai théorique et expérimental sur le galvanisme, avec une série d'expériences faites en présence des commissaires de l'Institut national de France, et en divers amphithéâtres de Londres, par Jean Aldini,... Avec planches [Internet]. 1804 [cited 2020 Jul 30]. Available from: https://gallica.bnf.fr/ark:/12148/bpt6k61162023.
8. Sironi VA. Origin and evolution of deep brain stimulation. Front Integr Neurosci [Internet]. 2011 Aug 18 [cited 2020 Jul 30];5. Available from: https://www.ncbi.nlm.nih.gov/pmc/articles/PMC3157831/.
9. Fritsch G, Hitzig E. Über die elektrische Erregbarkeit des Grosshirns. Leipzig: Veit; 1870. (Archiv für Anatomie, Physiologie und wissenschaftliche Medicin).
10. de Almeida AN, Alho EJ, Teixeira MJ. Models of functional cerebral localization at the dawning of modern neurosurgery. World Neurosurg. 2014;81(2):436–40.
11. Morgan JP. The first reported case of electrical stimulation of the human brain. J Hist Med Allied Sci. 1982;XXXVII(1):51–64.

12. Bartholow R. Experimental investigations into the functions of the human brain. Am J Med Sci. 1874;66:305–13.
13. Potts CS. The practical uses of electricity in medicine. J Am Med Assoc. 1910;55(11):936–40.
14. Giller CA. The neurosurgical treatment of pain. Arch Neurol. 2003;60(11):1537–40.
15. Horsley V, Clarke RH. The structure and functions of the cerebellum examined by a new method. Brain. 1908;31(1):45–124.
16. Spiegel EA, Wycis HT, Marks M, Lee AJ. Stereotaxic apparatus for operations on the human brain. Science. 1947;106(2754):349–50.
17. Pool JL. Psychosurgery in older people. J Am Geriatr Soc. 1954;2(7):456–66.
18. Delgado JMR, Hamlin H, Chapman WP. Technique of intracranial electrode implacement for recording and stimulation and its possible therapeutic value in psychotic patients. Confin Neurol. 1952;12(5–6):315–9.
19. Bekhtereva N, Grachev K, Orlova A, IATSUKSL. Utilization of multiple electrodes implanted in the subcortical structure of the human brain for the treatment of hyperkinesis. Zhurnal Nevropatol Psikhiatrii Im SS Korsakova Mosc Russ 1952. 1963;63:3–8.
20. Sem-Jacobsen CW. Depth electrographic stimulation and treatment of patients with Parkinson's disease including neurosurgical technique. Acta Neurol Scand. 1965;41(S13):365–76.
21. Hosobuchi Y, Adams JE, Rutkin B. Chronic thalamic stimulation for the control of facial anesthesia dolorosa. Arch Neurol. 1973;29(3):158–61.
22. Mazars G, Mérienne L, Ciolocca C. [Intermittent analgesic thalamic stimulation. Preliminary note]. Rev Neurol (Paris). 1973;128(4):273–9.
23. Adams JE. Naloxone reversal of analgesia produced by brain stimulation in the human. Pain. 1976;2(2):161–6.
24. Spooner J, Yu H, Kao C, Sillay K, Konrad P. Neuromodulation of the cingulum for neuropathic pain after spinal cord injury: case report. J Neurosurg. 2007;107(1):169–72.
25. Boccard SGJ, Fitzgerald JJ, Pereira EAC, Moir L, Van Hartevelt TJ, Kringelbach ML, et al. Targeting the affective component of chronic pain. Neurosurgery. 2014;74(6):628–37.
26. Mallory GW, Abulseoud O, Hwang S-C, Gorman DA, Stead SM, Klassen BT, et al. The nucleus accumbens as a potential target for central poststroke pain. Mayo Clin Proc. 2012;87(10):1025–31.
27. Benabid AL, Pollak P, Louveau A, Henry S, de Rougemont J. Combined (thalamotomy and stimulation) stereotactic surgery of the VIM thalamic nucleus for bilateral Parkinson disease. Appl Neurophysiol. 1987;50(1–6):344–6.
28. Cury RG, Fraix V, Castrioto A, Pérez Fernández MA, Krack P, Chabardes S, et al. Thalamic deep brain stimulation for tremor in Parkinson disease, essential tremor, and dystonia. Neurology. 2017;89(13):1416–23.
29. Melzack R, Wall PD. Pain mechanisms: a new theory. Science. 1965;150(3699):971–9.
30. Wall PD, Sweet WH. Temporary abolition of pain in man. Science. 1967;155(3758):108–9.
31. Shealy CN, Taslitz N, Mortimer JT, Becker DP. Electrical inhibition of pain: experimental evaluation*. Anesth Analg. 1967;46(3):299–305.
32. Shealy CN, Mortimer JT, Reswick JB. Electrical inhibition of pain by stimulation of the dorsal columns: preliminary clinical report. Anesth Analg. 1967;46(4):489–91.
33. Burton CV, Ray CD, Nashold BS. Symposium on the safety and clinical efficacy of implanted neuroaugmentive devices. Neurosurgery. 1977;1(2):185–232.
34. Tsubokawa T, Katayama Y, Yamamoto T, Hirayama T, Koyama S. Chronic motor cortex stimulation for the treatment of central pain. Acta Neurochir Suppl (Wien). 1991;52:137–9.
35. Tsubokawa T, Katayama Y, Yamamoto T, Hirayama T, Koyama S. Treatment of thalamic pain by chronic motor cortex stimulation. Pacing Clin Electrophysiol PACE. 1991;14(1):131–4.
36. Bechter K, Benveniste H. Quinckes' pioneering 19th centuries CSF studies may inform 21th centuries research. Neurol Psychiatry Brain Res. 2015;21(2):79–81.
37. Bier A. Versuche über Cocainisirung des Rückenmarkes. Dtsch Z Für Chir. 1899;51(3):361–9.
38. Matas R. Local and regional anesthesia with cocain and other analgesic drugs, including the subarachnoid method, as applied in general surgical practice. Philadelph Med J. 1900;6:820–43.

39. Deer TR, Pope JE. Atlas of implantable therapies for pain management. Springer-Verlag, New York. 2015. 310 p.
40. Wang J, Nauss L, Thomas J. Pain relief by intrathecally applied morphine in man. Anesthesiology. 1979;50:149–51.
41. Onofrio BM, Yaksh TL, Arnold PG. Continuous low-dose intrathecal morphine administration in the treatment of chronic pain of malignant origin. Mayo Clin Proc. 1981;56(8):516–20.
42. Lazorthes Y, Sallerin-Caute B, Verdie JC, Bastide R. Advances in drug delivery systems and applications in neurosurgery. In: Symon L, Calliauw L, Cohadon F, Antunes JL, Loew F, Nornes H, et al., editors. Advances and technical standards in neurosurgery [Internet]. Vienna: Springer; 1991 [cited 2020 Aug 10]. p. 143–92. (Advances and technical standards in neurosurgery). Available from: https://doi.org/10.1007/978-3-7091-6697-0_5.
43. Ubbink DT, Vermeulen H. Spinal cord stimulation for non-reconstructable chronic critical leg ischaemia. Cochrane Database Syst Rev. 2013;(2):CD004001.
44. Buchser E, Durrer A, Albrecht E. Spinal cord stimulation for the management of refractory angina pectoris. J Pain Symptom Manag. 2006;31(4 Suppl):S36–42.
45. Tykocki T, Guzek K, Mandat T. [Spinal cord stimulation for the treatment of refractory angina pectoris]. Kardiol Pol. 2011;69(4):383–7.
46. Cruccu G, Garcia-Larrea L, Hansson P, Keindl M, Lefaucheur J-P, Paulus W, et al. EAN guidelines on central neurostimulation therapy in chronic pain conditions. Eur J Neurol. 2016;23(10):1489–99.
47. Schultz DM, Webster L, Kosek P, Dar U, Tan Y, Sun M. Sensor-driven position-adaptive spinal cord stimulation for chronic pain. Pain Physician. 2012;15(1):1–12.
48. Deer T, Slavin KV, Amirdelfan K, North RB, Burton AW, Yearwood TL, et al. Success using neuromodulation with BURST (SUNBURST) study: results from a prospective, randomized controlled trial using a novel burst waveform. Neuromodulation J Int Neuromodulation Soc. 2018;21(1):56–66.
49. De Ridder D, Vanneste S, Plazier M, Vancamp T. Mimicking the brain: evaluation of St Jude medical's prodigy chronic pain system with burst technology. Expert Rev Med Devices. 2015;12(2):143–50.
50. De Ridder D, Vancamp T, Falowski SM, Vanneste S. All bursts are equal, but some are more equal (to burst firing): burstDR stimulation versus Boston burst stimulation. Expert Rev Med Devices. 2020;17(4):289–95.
51. De Ridder D, Plazier M, Kamerling N, Menovsky T, Vanneste S. Burst spinal cord stimulation for limb and back pain. World Neurosurg. 2013;80(5):642–649.e1.
52. De Ridder D, Vanneste S, Plazier M, Loo E, Menovsky T. Burst spinal cord stimulation: toward paresthesia-free pain suppression. Neurosurgery. 2010;66(5):986–90.
53. Courtney P, Espinet A, Mitchell B, Russo M, Muir A, Verrills P, et al. Improved pain relief with burst spinal cord stimulation for two weeks in patients using tonic stimulation: results from a small clinical study. Neuromodulation J Int Neuromodulation Soc. 2015;18(5):361–6.
54. Schu S, Slotty PJ, Bara G, Knop M, Edgar D, Vesper J. A prospective, randomised, double-blind, placebo-controlled study to examine the effectiveness of burst spinal cord stimulation patterns for the treatment of failed back surgery syndrome. Neuromodulation J Int Neuromodulation Soc. 2014;17(5):443–50.
55. Tjepkema-Cloostermans MC, Vos CC, Wolters R, Dijkstra-Scholten C, Lenders MWPM. Effect of burst stimulation evaluated in patients familiar with spinal cord stimulation. Neuromodulation J Int Neuromodulation Soc. 2016;19(5):492–7.
56. Vos CC, Bom MJ, Vanneste S, Lenders MWPM, Ridder D. Burst spinal cord stimulation evaluated in patients with failed back surgery syndrome and painful diabetic neuropathy. Neuromodulation J Int Neuromodulation Soc. 2014;17(2):152–9.
57. Kriek N, Groeneweg JG, Stronks DL, Ridder D, Huygen FJPM. Preferred frequencies and waveforms for spinal cord stimulation in patients with complex regional pain syndrome: a

multicentre, double-blind, randomized and placebo-controlled crossover trial. Eur J Pain. 2017;21(3):507–19.
58. De Ridder D, Lenders MWPM, De Vos CC, Dijkstra-Scholten C, Wolters R, Vancamp T, et al. A 2-center comparative study on tonic versus burst spinal cord stimulation: amount of responders and amount of pain suppression. Clin J Pain. 2015;31(5):433–7.
59. Kinfe TM, Muhammad S, Link C, Roeske S, Chaudhry SR, Yearwood TL. Burst spinal cord stimulation increases peripheral antineuroinflammatory interleukin 10 levels in failed back surgery syndrome patients with predominant back pain. Neuromodulation J Int Neuromodulation Soc. 2017;20(4):322–30.
60. Muhammad S, Roeske S, Chaudhry SR, Kinfe TM. Burst or high-frequency (10 kHz) spinal cord stimulation in failed back surgery syndrome patients with predominant back pain: one year comparative data. Neuromodulation J Int Neuromodulation Soc. 2017;20(7):661–7.
61. Falowski SM, Moore GA, Cornidez EG, Hutcheson JK, Candido K, Peña I, et al. Improved psychosocial and functional outcomes and reduced opioid usage following burst spinal cord stimulation. Neuromodulation J Int Neuromodulation Soc. 2021;24(3):581–90.
62. Kapural L, Yu C, Doust MW, Gliner BE, Vallejo R, Sitzman BT, et al. Novel 10-kHz high-frequency therapy (HF10 therapy) is superior to traditional low-frequency spinal cord stimulation for the treatment of chronic back and leg pain: the SENZA-RCT randomized controlled trial. Anesthesiology. 2015;123(4):851–60.
63. Kapural L, Yu C, Doust MW, Gliner BE, Vallejo R, Sitzman BT, et al. Comparison of 10-kHz high-frequency and traditional low-frequency spinal cord stimulation for the treatment of chronic back and leg pain: 24-month results from a multicenter, randomized, controlled pivotal trial. Neurosurgery. 2016;79(5):667–77.
64. Sweet J, Badjatiya A, Tan D, Miller J. Paresthesia-free high-density spinal cord stimulation for postlaminectomy syndrome in a prescreened population: a prospective case series. Neuromodulation J Int Neuromodulation Soc. 2016;19(3):260–7.
65. Berg AP, Mekel-Bobrov N, Goldberg E, Huynh D, Jain R. Utilization of multiple spinal cord stimulation (SCS) waveforms in chronic pain patients. Expert Rev Med Devices. 2017;14(8):663–8.
66. Deer TR, Levy RM, Kramer J, Poree L, Amirdelfan K, Grigsby E, et al. Dorsal root ganglion stimulation yielded higher treatment success rate for complex regional pain syndrome and causalgia at 3 and 12 months: a randomized comparative trial. Pain. 2017;158(4):669–81.
67. Russo M, Cousins MJ, Brooker C, Taylor N, Boesel T, Sullivan R, et al. Effective relief of pain and associated symptoms with closed-loop spinal cord stimulation system: preliminary results of the Avalon study. Neuromodulation J Int Neuromodulation Soc. 2018;21(1):38–47.
68. Levy R, Deer TR, Poree L, Rosen SM, Kapural L, Amirdelfan K, et al. Multicenter, randomized, double-blind study protocol using human spinal cord recording comparing safety, efficacy, and neurophysiological responses between patients being treated with evoked compound action potential-controlled closed-loop spinal cord stimulation or open-loop spinal cord stimulation (the Evoke study). Neuromodulation J Int Neuromodulation Soc. 2019;22(3):317–26.
69. Mekhail N, Levy RM, Deer TR, Kapural L, Li S, Amirdelfan K, et al. Long-term safety and efficacy of closed-loop spinal cord stimulation to treat chronic back and leg pain (Evoke): a double-blind, randomised, controlled trial. Lancet Neurol. 2020;19(2):123–34.
70. Maher C, Littlewood C. Unanswered questions from the Evoke trial. Lancet Neurol. 2020;19(5):380.
71. Airaksinen O, Brox JI, Cedraschi C, Hildebrandt J, Klaber-Moffett J, Kovacs F, et al. Chapter 4. European guidelines for the management of chronic nonspecific low back pain. Eur Spine J Off Publ Eur Spine Soc Eur Spinal Deform Soc Eur Sect Cerv Spine Res Soc. 2006;15 Suppl 2:S192–300.
72. Deckers K, De Smedt K, Mitchell B, Vivian D, Russo M, Georgius P, et al. New therapy for refractory chronic mechanical low back pain—restorative neurostimulation to activate the lumbar multifidus: one year results of a prospective multicenter clinical trial. Neuromodulation. 2018;21(1):48–55.

73. Deer TR, Mekhail N, Provenzano D, Pope J, Krames E, Leong M, et al. The appropriate use of neurostimulation of the spinal cord and peripheral nervous system for the treatment of chronic pain and ischemic diseases: the Neuromodulation Appropriateness Consensus Committee. Neuromodulation J Int Neuromodulation Soc. 2014;17(6):515–50; discussion 550.
74. O'Sullivan P. Diagnosis and classification of chronic low back pain disorders: maladaptive movement and motor control impairments as underlying mechanism. Man Ther. 2005;10(4):242–55.
75. Panjabi MM. Clinical spinal instability and low back pain. J Electromyogr Kinesiol Off J Int Soc Electrophysiol Kinesiol. 2003;13(4):371–9.
76. Machado AG, Baker KB, Plow E, Malone DA. Cerebral stimulation for the affective component of neuropathic pain. Neuromodulation J Int Neuromodulation Soc. 2013;16(6):514–8.
77. Frizon LA, Yamamoto EA, Nagel SJ, Simonson MT, Hogue O, Machado AG. Deep brain stimulation for pain in the modern era: a systematic review. Neurosurgery [Internet]. 2019 Feb 25 [cited 2020 Aug 8]; Available from: https://academic.oup.com/neurosurgery/advance-article/doi/10.1093/neuros/nyy552/5364269.
78. Owen SLF, Green AL, Stein JF, Aziz TZ. Deep brain stimulation for the alleviation of post-stroke neuropathic pain. Pain. 2006;120(1–2):202–6.
79. Levy R, Deer TR, Henderson J. Intracranial neurostimulation for pain control: a review. Pain Physician. 2010;13(2):157–65.
80. Yamamoto T, Katayama Y, Obuchi T, Kano T, Kobayashi K, Oshima H, et al. Thalamic sensory relay nucleus stimulation for the treatment of peripheral deafferentation pain. Stereotact Funct Neurosurg. 2006;84(4):180–3.
81. Boccard SGJ, Pereira EAC, Moir L, Aziz TZ, Green AL. Long-term outcomes of deep brain stimulation for neuropathic pain. Neurosurgery. 2013;72(2):221–30; discussion 231.
82. Melzack R. From the gate to the neuromatrix. Pain. 1999;Suppl 6:S121–6.
83. Lempka SF, Malone DA, Hu B, Baker KB, Wyant A, Ozinga JG, et al. Randomized clinical trial of deep brain stimulation for poststroke pain. Ann Neurol. 2017;81(5):653–63.
84. Chari A, Hentall I, Papadopoulos M, Pereira E. Surgical neurostimulation for spinal cord injury. Brain Sci. 2017;7(12):18.
85. Prévinaire J-G, Nguyen JP, Perrouin-Verbe B, Fattal C. Chronic neuropathic pain in spinal cord injury: efficiency of deep brain and motor cortex stimulation therapies for neuropathic pain in spinal cord injury patients. Ann Phys Rehabil Med. 2009;52(2):188–93.
86. Hentall ID, Luca CC, Widerstrom-Noga E, Vitores A, Fisher LD, Martinez-Arizala A, et al. The midbrain central gray best suppresses chronic pain with electrical stimulation at very low pulse rates in two human cases. Brain Res. 2016;1632:119–26.
87. Jermakowicz WJ, Hentall ID, Jagid JR, Luca CC, Adcock J, Martinez-Arizala A, et al. Deep brain stimulation improves the symptoms and sensory signs of persistent central neuropathic pain from spinal cord injury: a case report. Front Hum Neurosci. 2017;11:177.

Spinal Cord Stimulation: Percutaneous Technique

Fabricio Assis, Charles Amaral, and João Henrique Araújo

Introduction to the Technique

Chronic pain is one of the most common and challenging medical problems facing our society. The strategy of modulating neural transmission with an electrical stimulus dates to ancient Rome with Scribonius' observation that the pain of gout could be alleviated through accidental contact with a torpedo fish [1]. Acceptance of the gate theory of pain in the 1960s led to renewed interest in electrical stimulation spinal cord stimulation (SCS). It is an adjustable, reversible, and nondestructive treatment for a variety of chronic pain syndromes [1].

In spinal cord stimulation, an electrode is positioned posteriorly in the epidural space to the dorsal column at the level of the nerve roots that transmit the nociceptive information from the painful area. The epidural lead is connected to a battery producing an electrical current, which induces paresthesia, a sensation that suppresses the pain according to the gate control theory [2]. Patients can reduce or increase the intensity of the electric current by means of a device that uses radio frequency transmission.

The development of percutaneous electrodes in 1975 has facilitated a wider application of spinal cord stimulation. With the most recent advancements including high-frequency stimulation, burst stimulation, and precise dorsal root ganglion stimulation, spinal cord stimulation is a rapidly growing modality for pain management [3]. Before implantation of a permanent system, patients first undergo a spinal cord stimulation trial to determine if full implantation is appropriate. The trial involves the placement of flexible catheter-type leads into the posterior epidural

F. Assis (✉) · C. Amaral
Singular, Campinas, Brazil
e-mail: charles@singular.med.br

J. H. Araújo
Centro de Dor Criciúma, Criciúma, Brazil

T. d. S. Freitas et al. (eds.), *Neuromodulation Techniques for Pain Treatment*,
https://doi.org/10.1007/978-3-030-84778-4_2

space under fluoroscopic guidance, and this period offers the unique opportunity for the patient to experience what life is like with the implant before deciding to have it permanently [4].

Indications [5]

- Angina pectoris
- Ischemic pain due to peripheral vascular disease
- Complex regional pain syndromes
- Phantom pain
- Diabetic neuropathy
- Postherpetic neuralgia
- Deafferentation pain
- Cerebral palsy
- Multiple sclerosis
- Radicular neuropathic pain
- Failed back surgery syndrome
- Whiplash injury
- Post-thoracotomy syndrome (PTS)
- Arachnoiditis
- Deafferentation pain

Contraindications [5]

- Any contraindication for regional anesthesia
- Psychopathologies
- Drug dependence, with behavioral abnormalities
- Pregnancy
- Lack of ability to cooperate (e.g., due to active psychosis or cognitive impairment)
- Severe central canal stenosis

Strategies for Prevention of Spinal Cord Stimulator Infection

Preoperative [6, 7]

- MSSA/MRSA screening and decolonization (IA)
- Nasal decontamination using 2% mupirocin twice a day for 5 days
- Optimize glucose control (IB)
- Hemoglobin A1c <8.0% within 30 days trial/ implant

- Smoking cessation (IB)
- Preoperative chlorhexidine baths (IA)
- Global assessment of other known risk factors (IB)
- Revision surgery
- Chronic immunosuppression
- Steroid therapy
- Obesity

Intraoperative [6, 7]

- Weight-based antibiotic selection (IA)
- Cefazolin (within 60 minutes before incision)
- 1 g for a patient weighing <80 kg, 2 g for a patient weighing 81–160 kg of vancomycin (within 2 hours before incision), 20 mg/kg single dose of clindamycin (within 60 minutes before incision): 600–900 mg (for a patient with severe β-lactam allergy)
- Chlorhexidine-alcohol–based skin preparation (IA)
- Incise drape (Ioban) (IB)
- Antibacterial-impregnated enveloped in select patients (II)
- Layered closure
- Operating room personnel, number, and movement in and out of the operating room during the surgery should be minimized (III)

Postoperative [6, 7]

- Occlusive dressing for 24–48 hours (IB)
- Surgical site monitoring (IB)

Before the Procedure

- Informed consent
- ASRA guidelines need to be followed for SCS procedures in anticoagulated patients [8]
- Obtain an intravenous access
- Administer oxygen by nasal cannula and monitor the vital signs noninvasively
- Check any allergies or dermatological diseases
- Prepare equipment and medications
- Sterile techniques are followed throughout

Technical Details of Procedure (Trial)

The patient is brought to the fluoroscopy suite and placed on the fluoroscopic table in prone position (face down). One or two pillows are placed under the abdomen, which opens access to the epidural space between the lumbar vertebrae (Fig. 1).

The fluoroscope is placed in the anteroposterior (AP) position, then tilted if necessary, in a cephalad to caudad motion to "square up" the endplates of the vertebral bodies.

Identify the medial aspect of the ipsilateral pedicle at the level below the desired interlaminar entry level. This will be the skin entry point and may be marked with a sterile marker. Skin entry commonly is marked along a line joining the L2, L3, or L4 pedicles. Entry into the epidural space should occur between one to two vertebral body levels cephalad to the skin entry point. Needle entry into the epidural space between the laminae of T12 and L1 is optimal (Figs. 2, 3, and 4).

The needle is then ideally placed at an angle of 30–45° and advanced until it contacts the lamina just lateral to the spinous process of the vertebral body caudal to the planed interlaminar space entry. Once the lamina is contacted, the needle is

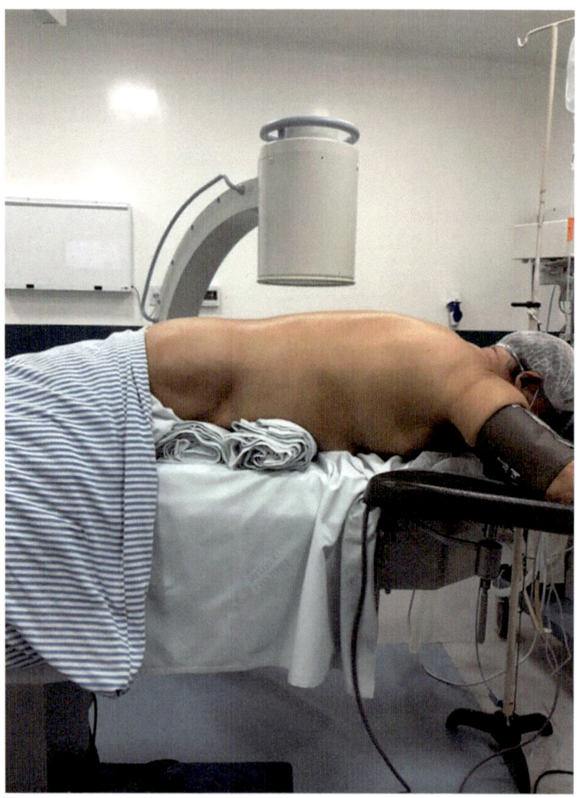

Fig. 1 Patient position

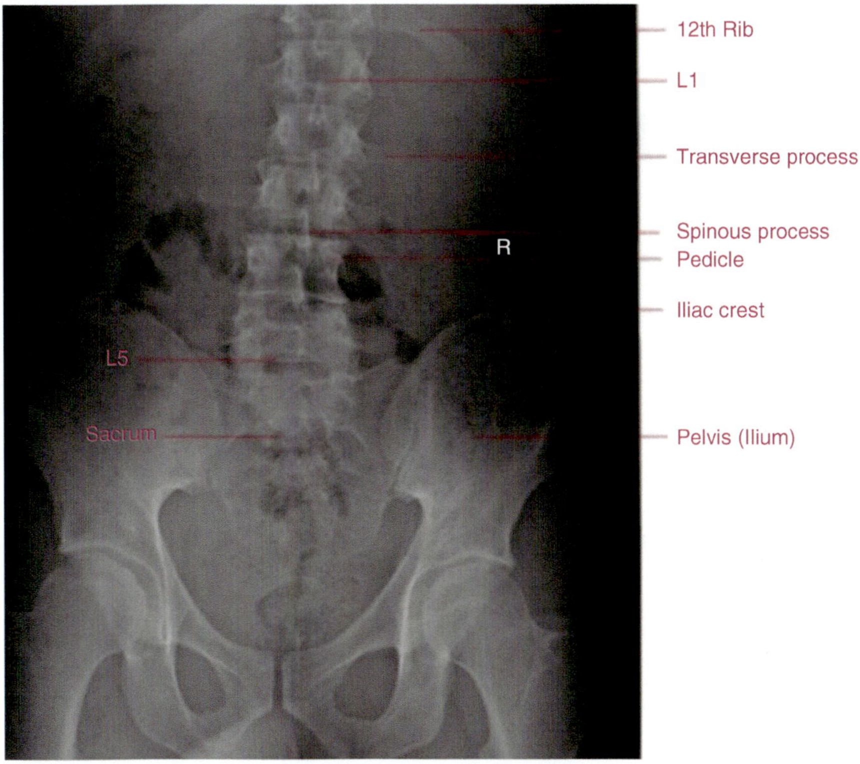

Fig. 2 AP view

Fig. 3 Needle position

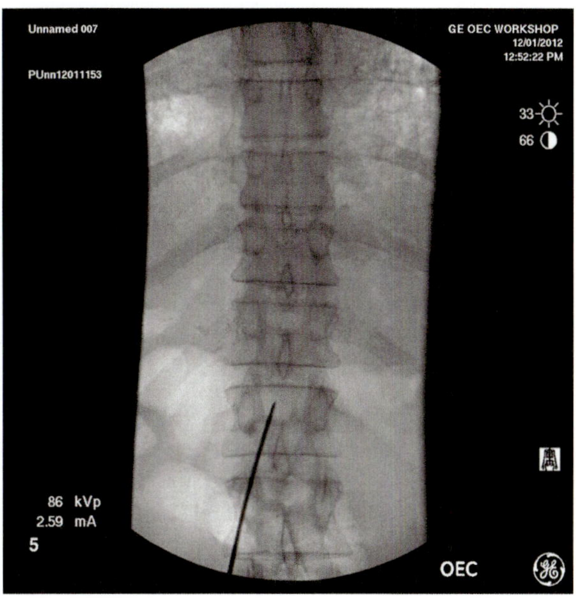

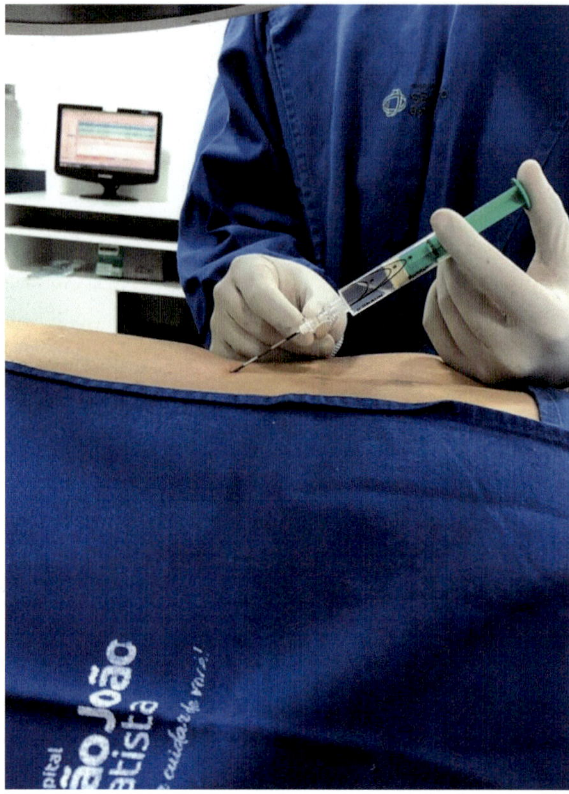

Fig. 4 Needle angle during procedure

slightly retracted and advanced superiorly and medially toward the center of desired epidural space.

Then position the C-arm laterally and advance the needle with the loss of resistance technique. Lateral view confirms needle positioning on the posterior epidural space (Figs. 5, 6, 7, and 8).

Aspiration is performed, which should be negative for blood and cerebrospinal fluid. When all these checkpoints are confirmed, a spinal cord stimulator lead is fed through the Tuohy needle into the epidural space under live fluoroscopy. If the needle is properly positioned, the lead will travel cephalad without resistance as it is advanced. Lead steering is performed in PA view (Fig. 9).

Once the lead is driven to the desired target, handheld computer screening can be used to ensure that the patient has the desired response. When the clinician is satisfied with the placement, a fluoroscopic image should be taken on lateral and anteroposterior views and saved for future comparisons if there are any concerns about lead migration.

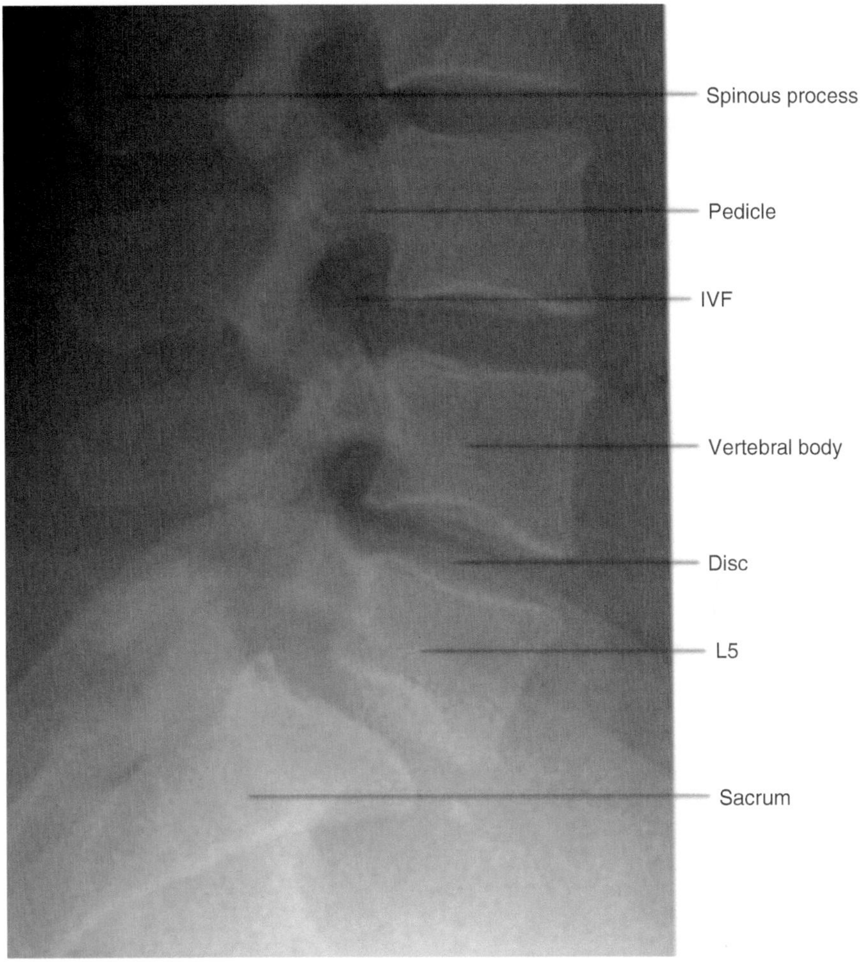

Fig. 5 Lateral view

Choose your target according to the test to ensure appropriate lead placement. Barolat map can help for the initial test location [9]

After the position of the electrode is confirmed, slightly withdraw the epidural needle to the fascia. Make a 5 cm incision, dissect down to the supraspinous ligament, withdraw the needle, and check the position of the electrode under fluoroscopy. Lead anchoring is then performed, either to the supraspinous ligament or fascia in permanent implants or to skin in trials.

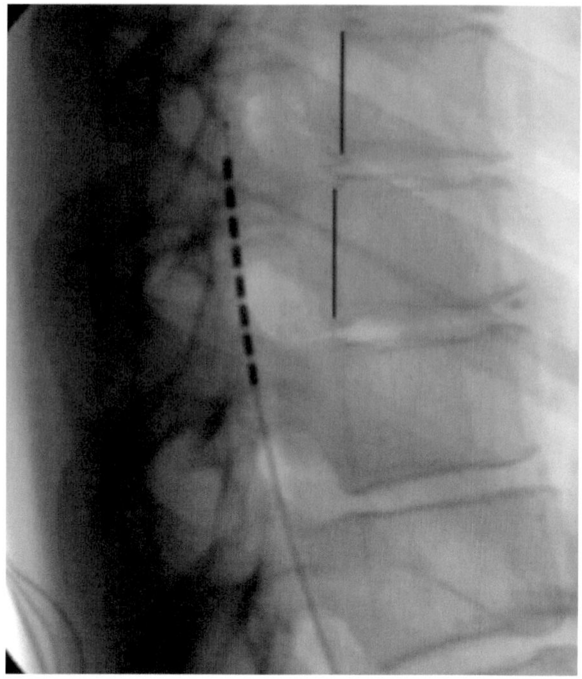

Fig. 6 Lead position on the posterior epidural space. (Adapted from Boston Scientific)

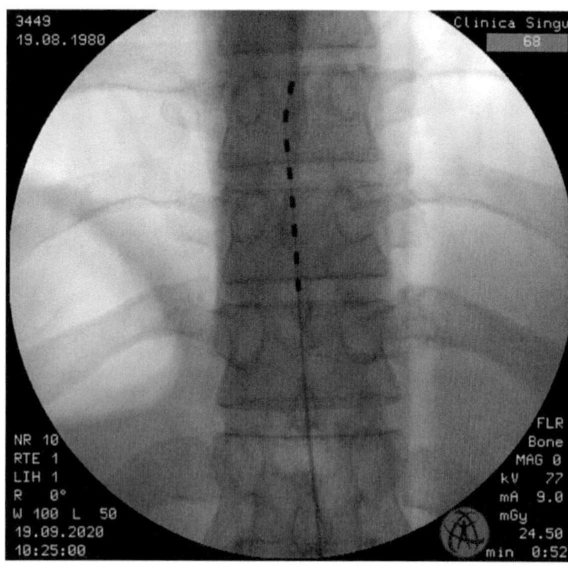

Fig. 7 Central progression. (Provided from Fabricio Assis)

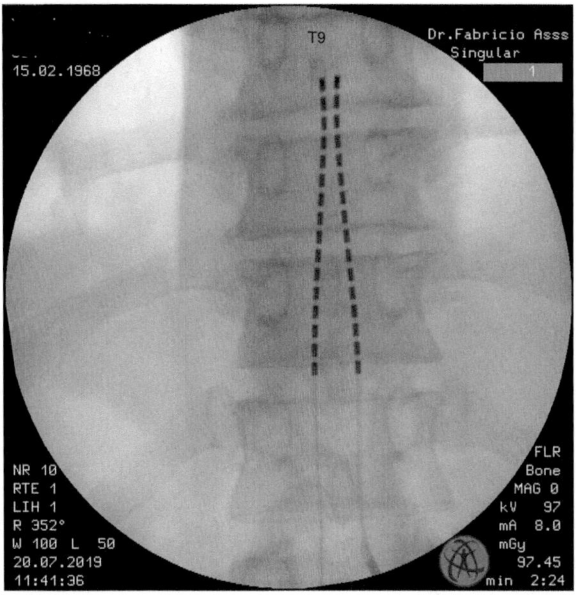

Fig. 8 PA view. (Adapted from Boston Scientific)

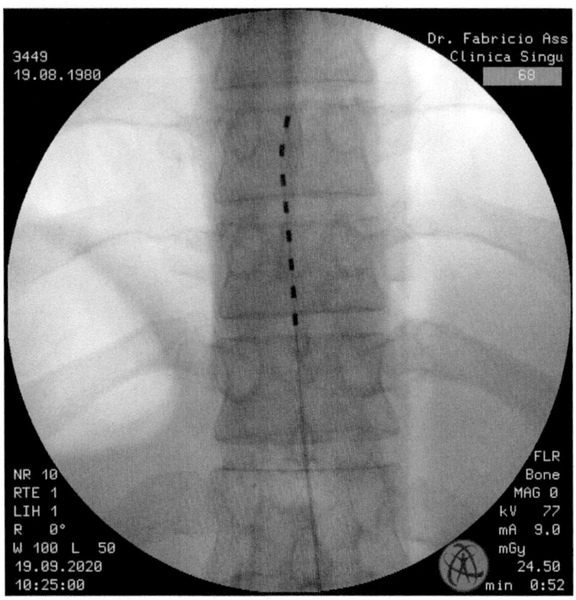

Fig. 9 Lead steering performed in PA view. (Provided by Dr. Fabricio Assis)

Then carefully close the incisions. A 2.0 absorbable sutures sufficient. Then oppose the skin edges with sterile strips (Table 1).

Trial Period

A successful trial is measured by an average pain intensity reduction of 50% and paresthesia overlap with 80% of the somatotopic pain distribution (Figs. 10 and 11).

Table 1 Barolat paresthesia mapping

Level	Typical paresthesia coverage
C2-C3	Occipital
C3-C4	Shoulder
C4-C5	Radial
C5-C6	Median
C6-C7	Ulnar
T1-T4	Angina
T4-T6	Abdomen/viscera
T6-T8	Low back
T8-T11	Low extremities
T11-L1	Foot

C cervical, *T* thoracic, *L* lumbar

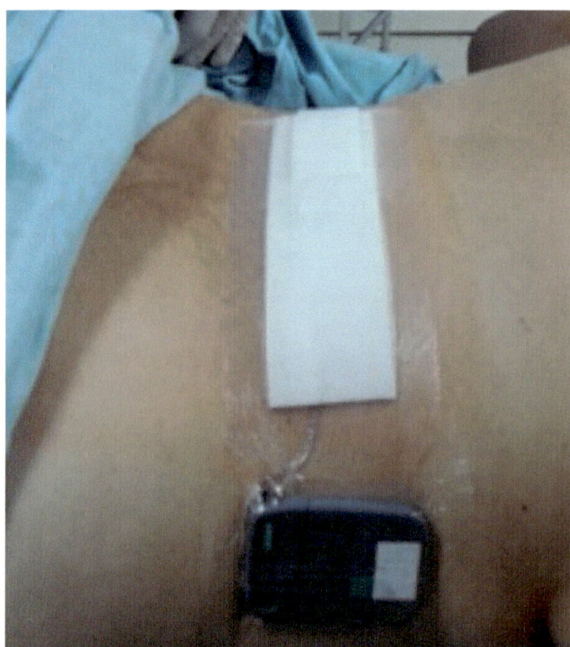

Fig. 10 Trial period. (Provided by Dr. Angel Juarez)

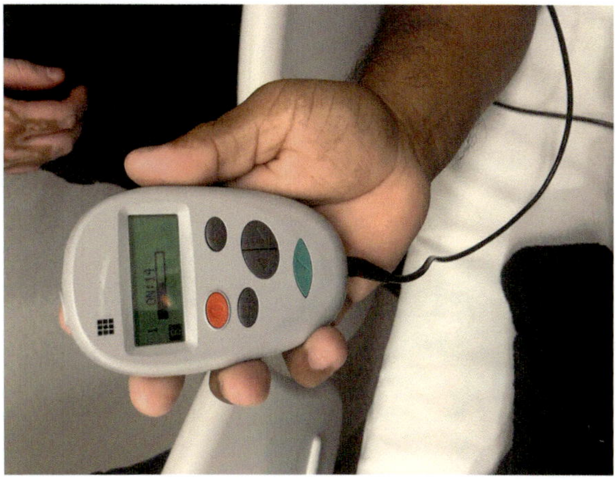

Fig. 11 Control. (Provided by Dr. Angel Juarez)

Permanent Implant

A permanent implant generally follows an SCS trial. It is presented below:

1. The skin at the predetermined incision site is anesthetized.
2. A midline incision of approximately 2 cm is then made. The skin is then dissected down to the level of the supraspinal ligament using both sharp and blunt dissections. Through the incision, the same steps that were performed for the trial are used to place the leads into the posterior epidural space. Hemostasis is achieved with electrocautery carefully, as the probe should not come in contact with the needle;
3. Anchors are used to stabilize the leads to the fascia or the supraspinous ligament. Nonabsorbable sutures should be placed into deep fascial planes or around the supraspinous ligament that will hold the anchor in place through its suture sleeves. Good anchoring technique plays a major role in the prevention of lead migration – the most common etiology for future treatment failure and surgical revision. Anchoring can be a challenge in some patients who tend to be more technically difficult. Patients in this category may include those with uncontrolled diabetes, morbid obesity, a history of multiple spine surgeries, or poor tissue health secondary to cachexia. Attention to detail will be critical in this patient group (Figs. 12, 13, and 14).

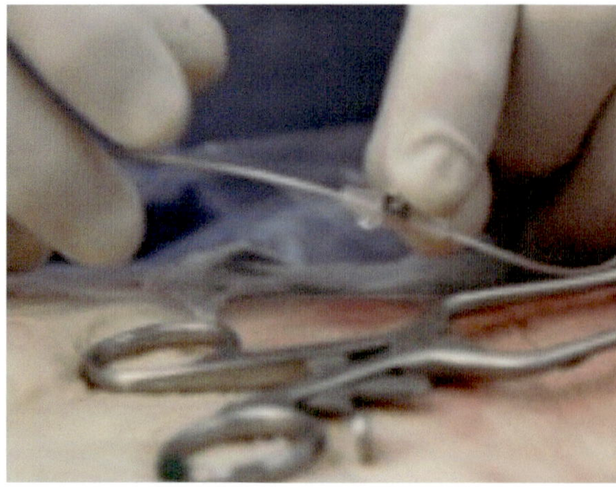

Fig. 12 The anchor is slid down the lead to the desired location

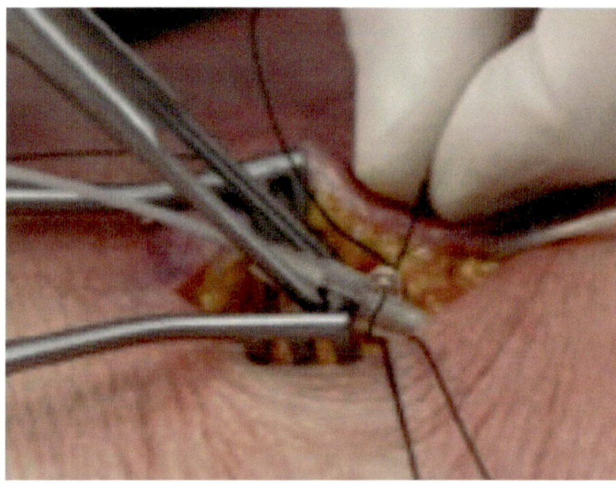

Fig. 13 The anchor is sutured to the patient

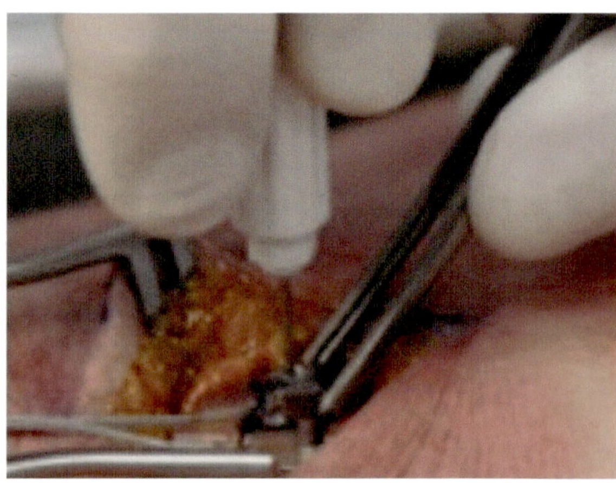

Fig. 14 The hex wrench is turned to lock the anchor to the lead

Implantable Pulse Generator Placement

4. Before the implantation, one should decide on the side and the location of the pulse generator. The pocket is an equally important part of the procedure that deserves special attention. New devices are becoming smaller, and the choice of pocketing sites may continue to evolve, providing less impact on body contours and greater comfort. Typical locations are usually the superior gluteal region or the low back, with the side determined by patient preference.
5. A subcutaneous pocket is created in the buttock area for an implantable pulse generator (IPG). The ideal pocket size should be 120–130% of the generator volume. The extra room will allow tissue slack, to avoid wound dehiscence and to decrease pain. If the pocket is larger than the recommended size, the patient may be prone to generator flipping, which can lead to a need for surgical revision (Figs. 15 and 16).

Fig. 15 Pocket

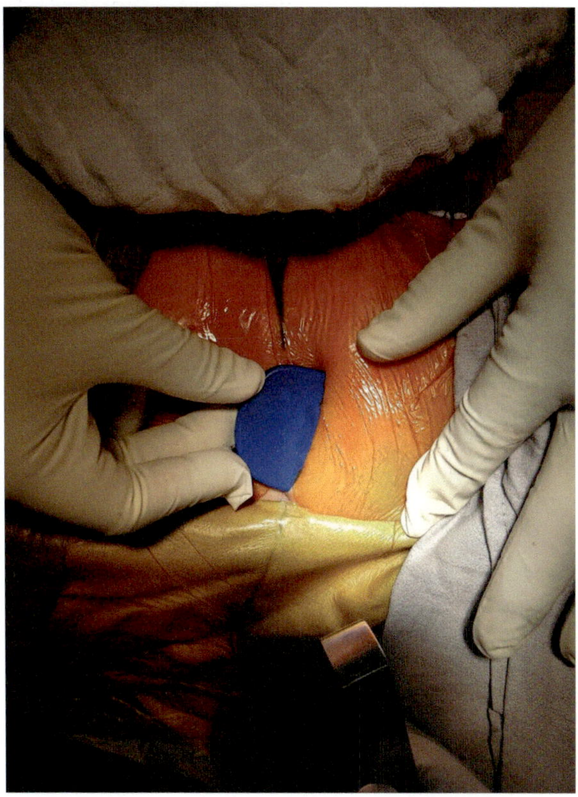

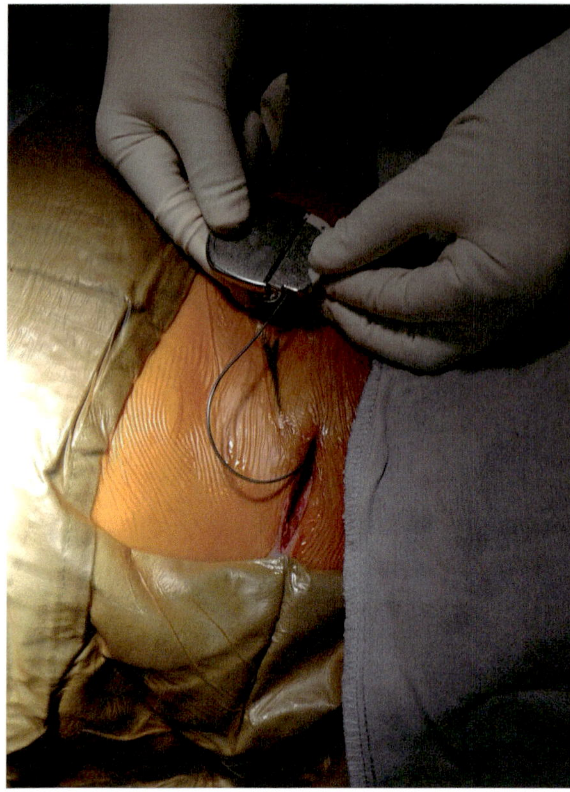

Fig. 16 Pulse generator

A tunneling device is used to advance the lead in the subcutaneous tissue to the pocket, and then the lead is connected to the IPG (Figs. 17 and 18).

6. Wound closure should be another critical point in the implant process. It is important to use a two-layer to three-layer closure technique, to ensure proper skin alignment, and to avoid the tension of the tissue, which can lead to necrosis.

Complications

- Epidural fibrosis
- Epidural hematoma
- Epidural abscess
- Post-dural puncture headache
- Unacceptable programming
- Lead migration
- Current leak
- Generator failure
- Wound infection
- Seroma
- Hematoma
- Pain at a generator

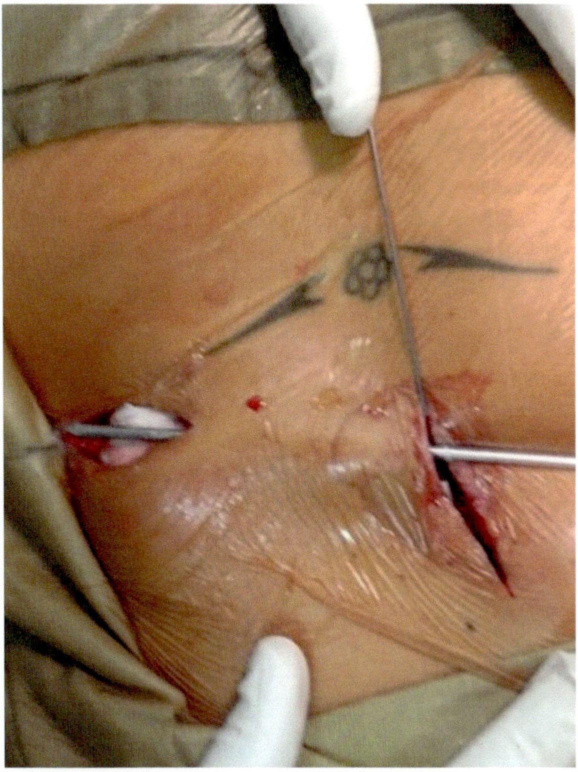

Fig. 17 Tunneling

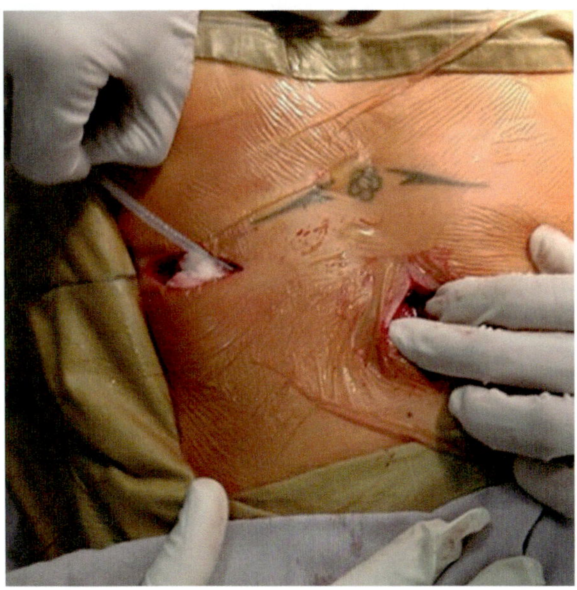

Fig. 18 Wound closure

Dorsal Root Ganglion Stimulation

Dorsal root ganglion (DRG) stimulation, in which the electrodes are placed adjacent to relatively immobile spinal structures and activate highly specific sensory neurons, allows more precise targeting of stimulation and likely a higher degree of pain control [10–13]. Even in some conditions, such as complex regional pain syndrome, DGR stimulation has shown superiority and can be used even in patients who have not had relief with spinal cord stimulation [14]. An understanding of the relationship between dermatomal distributions and that sensory afferents arrive at the spinal cord is key to successful DRG lead implantation. As for conventional SCS, the needle is placed epidurally under fluoroscopy, and we recommend a contralateral one-level or two-level approach for the targeted DRG. The ability to have another approach for DRG-S lead insertion may expand the realm in which we can apply DRG-S technology. In cases of thoracic access, the transforaminal or retrograde technique may be more appropriate; below are pictures. The target is in a consistent location anatomically; thus, lead position can accurately reflect the ability to stimulate the ganglion (Figs. 19, 20, 21, and 22).

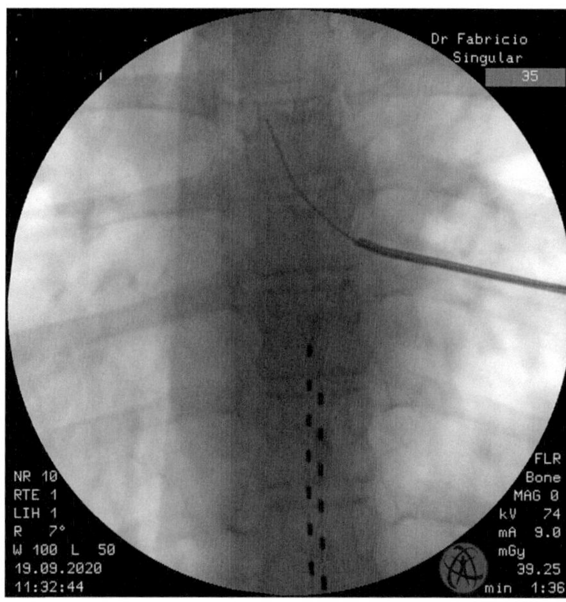

Fig. 19 DRG lead insertion. (Provided by Charles Amaral and Fabricio Assis)

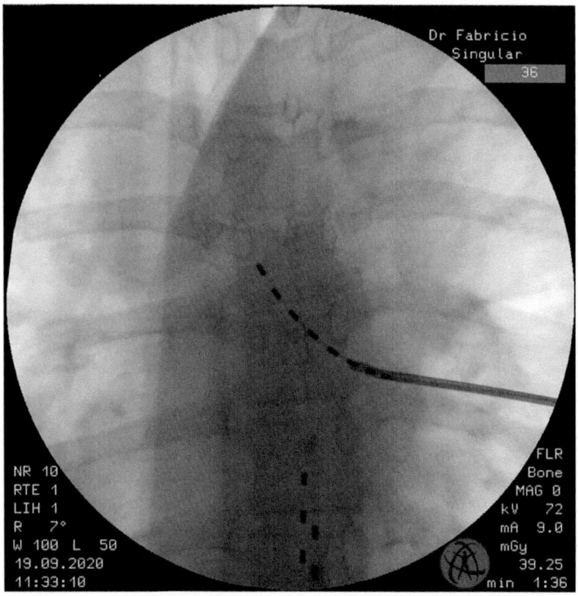

Fig. 20 DRG lead progression. (Provided by Charles Amaral and Fabricio Assis)

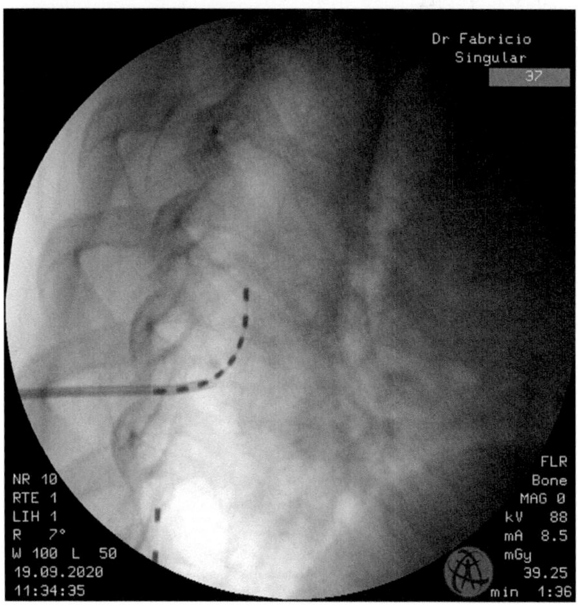

Fig. 21 DRG lateral view. (Provided by Charles Amaral and Fabricio Assis)

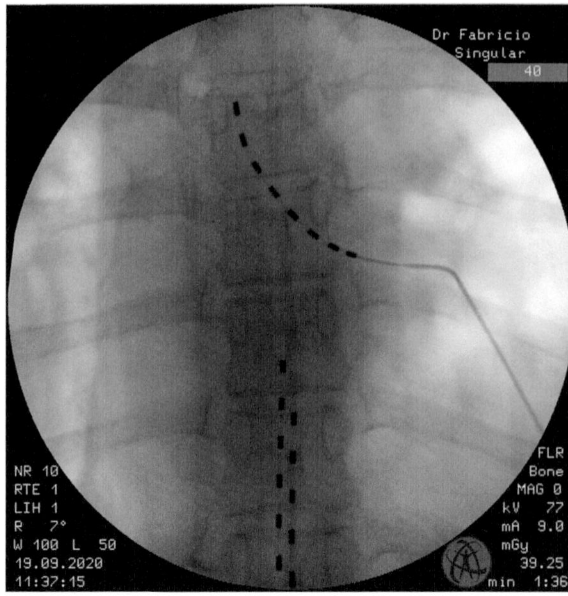

Fig. 22 Final position. (Provided by Charles Amaral and Fabricio Assis)

References

1. Stillings D. A survey of the history of electrical stimulation for pain to 1900. Med Instrum. 1975;9:255–9.
2. Petraglia FW, Farber SH, Gramer R, Verla T, Wang F, Thomas S, et al. The incidence of spinal cord injury in implantation of percutaneous and paddle electrodes for spinal cord stimulation. Neuromodulation. 2016;19(1):85–90. https://doi.org/10.1111/ner.12370.
3. Melzack R, Wall PD. Pain mechanisms: a new theory. Science. 1965;150:971–9.
4. Kumar K, Hunter G, Demeria D. Spinal cord stimulation in treatment of chronic benign pain: challenges in treatment planning and present status, a 22-year experience. Neurosurgery. 2006;58:481–96. https://doi.org/10.1227/01.neu.0000192162.99567.96.
5. Meier K. Spinal cord stimulation: background and clinical application. Scand J Pain. 2014;5(3):175–81. https://doi.org/10.1016/j.sjpain.2014.03.001.
6. Esquer Garrigos Z, Farid S, Bendel MA, Sohail MR. Spinal cord stimulator infection: approach to diagnosis, management, and prevention. Clin Infect Dis. 2020;70(12):2727–35. https://doi.org/10.1093/cid/ciz994.
7. Alexander JW, Solomkin JS, Edwards MJ. Updated recommendations for control of surgical site infections. Ann Surg. 2011;253:1082–93. https://doi.org/10.1097/SLA.0b013e31821175f8.
8. Narouze S, Benzon HT, Provenzano D, Buvanendran A, de Andrés J, Deer T, et al. Interventional spine and pain procedures in patients on antiplatelet and anticoagulant medications (Second edition): guidelines from the American Society of Regional Anesthesia and Pain Medicine, the European Society of Regional Anaesthesia and Pain Therapy, the American Academy of Pain Medicine, the International Neuromodulation Society, the North American Neuromodulation Society, and the World Institute of Pain. Reg Anesth Pain Med. 2018;43(3):225–62. https://doi.org/10.1097/AAP.0000000000000700.
9. Barolat G, Massaro F, He J, Zeme S, Ketcik B. Mapping of sensory responses to epidural stimulation of the intraspinal neural structures in man. J Neurosurg. 1993;78(2):233–9. https://doi.org/10.3171/jns.1993.78.2.0233.
10. Haque R, Winfree CJ. Spinal nerve root stimulation. Neurosurg Focus. 2006;21:E4–E10. https://doi.org/10.3171/foc.2006.21.6.7.

11. Lynch PJ, McJunkin T, Eross E, Gooch S, Maloney J. Case report: successful epiradicular peripheral nerve stimulation of the C2 dorsal root ganglion for postherpetic neuralgia. Neuromodulation. 2011;14:58–61. https://doi.org/10.1111/j.1525-1403.2010.00307.x.
12. Deer TR, Grigsby E, Weiner RL, Wilcosky B, Kramer JM. A prospective study of dorsal root ganglion stimulation for the relief of chronic pain. Neuromodulation. 2013;16:67–72. https://doi.org/10.1111/ner.12013.
13. Liem L, Russo M, Huygen FJPM, VanBuyten JP, Smet I, Verrilis P, et al. A multicenter, prospective trial to assess the safety and performance of the Spinal Modulation dorsal root ganglia neurostimulator system in the treatment of chronic pain. Neuromodulation. 2013;16:471–82. https://doi.org/10.1111/ner.12072.
14. Deer TR, Levy RM, Kramer J, Poree L, Amirdelfan K, Grigsby E, et al. Comparison of paresthesia coverage of patient'spain: dorsal root ganglion vs. spinal cord stimulation. An ACCURATE Study Sub-Analysis. Neuromodulation. 2019;22:8. https://doi.org/10.1111/ner.12920.

Suggested Reading

Augustinsson LE. Spinal cord electrical stimulation in severe angina pectoris: surgical technique, intraoperative physiology, complications and side effects. Pacing Clin Electrophysiol. 1989;12:693–4. https://doi.org/10.1111/j.1540-8159.1989.tb02716.x.

Cheng J, Rosenquist RW. Fundamentals of pain medicine; 2018. https://doi.org/10.1007/978-3-319-64922-1.

Chivukula S, Tempel ZJ, Weiner GM, Gande AV, Chen CJ, Ding D, Moossy JJ. Cervical and cervicomedullary spinal cord stimulation for chronic pain: efficacy and outcomes. Clin Neurol Neurosurg. 2014;127:33–41. https://doi.org/10.1016/j.clineuro.2014.09.023.

Deer TRS, Pope JE. Atlas of implantable therapies for pain management; 2016. https://doi.org/10.1007/978-1-4939-2110-2.

Deer TR, Mekhail N, Provenzano D. The appropriate use of neurostimulation of the spinal cord and peripheral nervous system for the treatment of chronic pain and ischemic diseases: the Neuromodulation Appropriateness Consensus Committee (NACC). Neuromodulation. 2014;17:515–50. https://doi.org/10.1111/ner.12208.

Diwan S, Deer TRS. Advanced procedures for pain management: a step-by-step atlas; 2018. https://doi.org/10.1007/978-3-319-68841-1.

Kemler MA, Barendse GA, van Kleef M, de Vet HC, Rijks CP, Furnée CA, et al. Spinal cord stimulation in patients with chronic reflex sympathetic dystrophy. N Engl J Med. 2000;343:618–24. https://doi.org/10.1056/NEJM200008313430904.

Kumar K, Toth C, Nath RK. Spinal cord stimulation for chronic pain in peripheral neuropathy. Surg Neurol. 1996;46:363–9. https://doi.org/10.1016/s0090-3019(96)00191-7.

Manchikanti L, Kaye AD, FJE F, Hirsch JA. Essentials of interventional techniques in managing chronic pain; 2018. https://doi.org/10.1007/978-3-319-60361-2.

Pope J, Deer JE, Timothy R. Treatment of chronic pain conditions: a comprehensive handbook; 2017. 358p. https://doi.org/10.1007/978-1-4939-6976-0.

Raj PP, Erdine S. Pain-relieving procedures: the illustrated guide. Pain-relieving procedures: the illustrated guide; 2012. 460p. https://doi.org/10.1002/9781118300480.

Raso LJ, Deer TR, Schocket SM, Chapman JA, Duarte LE, Justiz R, et al. Use of a newly developed delivery device for percutaneous introduction of multiple lead configurations for spinal cord stimulation. Neuromodulation. 2014;17(5):465–71. https://doi.org/10.1111/ner.12138.

Simpson EL, Duenas A, Holmes MW, Papaioannou D, Chilcott J. Spinal cord stimulation for chronic pain of neuropathic or ischaemic origin: systematic review and economic evaluation. Health Technol Assess. 2009;13:iii, ix–x, 1–154. https://doi.org/10.3310/hta13170.

Taylor RS, Van Buyten JP, Buchser E. Spinal cord stimulation for complex regional pain syndrome: a systematic review of clinical and cost-effectiveness literature and assessment of prognosticfactors. Eur J Pain. 2006;10:91–101. https://doi.org/10.1016/j.ejpain.2005.02.004.

Spinal Cord Stimulation: Surgical (Paddle) Technique

Daniel Benzecry Almeida

Introduction

Patients with chronic pain syndromes impose a great challenge for health professionals all around the world. Despite many advances in the understanding, diagnosis, and treatment of those individuals, the rate of unsuccess is high, even with the increased use of health care services, with many consultations and procedures. Therefore, at least 40% of sufferers will be unsatisfied with the treatment results [1].

Spinal cord stimulation is a technique described since 1967 which has gained acceptance, indicated mainly to the treatment of refractory neuropathic pain syndromes. It uses an electrical pulse generator that delivers energy to one or more electrodes implanted epidurally.

Electrodes have different configurations, depending on the implanting technique, spinal area to be covered, and complexity of the pain symptoms. Classically, they can be divided into percutaneous leads (cylindrical) or paddle leads (surgical).

Paddle leads have the advantage of a lower incidence of migration and higher spinal area of stimulation, causing a more predictable pattern of tonic stimulation. On the other hand, it needs a more experienced surgical team, and the rate of complications such as spinal compression and neurological deficits is higher.

History

The idea of stimulation of the spinal cord was derived soon after the classical paper by Melzack and Wall in 1965 describing the gate theory [2]. At that time, they theorized that while the application of a simple painful stimulation generated an action

D. Benzecry Almeida (✉)
Department of Neurosurgery, Instituto de Neurologia de Curitiba, Curitiba, Brazil

T. d. S. Freitas et al. (eds.), *Neuromodulation Techniques for Pain Treatment*,
https://doi.org/10.1007/978-3-030-84778-4_3

potential towards the spine and brain, the simultaneous application of both tactile (non-nociceptive) and painful stimuli at the nearby region would inhibit the transmission of pain. In their point of view, interneurons located at the posterior horn of the spinal cord would "close the gate" to the propagation of pain (transmitted through smaller fibers) when a concurrent non-painful stimulus (transmitted through gross fibers) was applied.

Two years later, based on these assumptions, Norman Shealy, a neurosurgeon from Western Reserve Medical School (late Case Western Reserve) contacted two engineers (Thomas Mortimer and Norm Hagfors) to develop a special electrode to be implanted in the subdural space, connected initially into a cardiovascular stimulator [3]. Soon, he published good results in the pain alleviation from the first implant in a cancer patient [4].

In the beginning, the implantable electrode was connected to a circular wound antenna at the subcutaneous tissue. An external battery was placed over the antenna to generate an appropriate stimulus [5].

Several developments have occurred since that publication, which contributed to better results and comfort to the patient and medical team, including improvements in (a) the electrode, (b) the pulse generator, and (c) the configuration of the electrical stimulation.

The first change in the electrodes has been the change from an intradural stimulator to an epidural electrode. Moreover, in the beginning, electrodes had only two points of contacts, while further development allowed the possibility of a progressive increase in the number of contacts to 4, 8, 16, and even more, while the diameter of the percutaneous electrodes decreased.

Surgical electrodes using paddle leads were improved, either with an increased number of contact points as well as with a thinner and more adjustable silicon implanted plate. The arrangement in rows with an appropriate interspace has been studied in order to provide a wider area of stimulation to the spinal cord (Fig. 1).

The pulse generator has also progressed, mainly with new batteries. Historically, the external generator has been changed to an internal generator that was used judiciously, including the smallest possible amount of energy and cyclic and

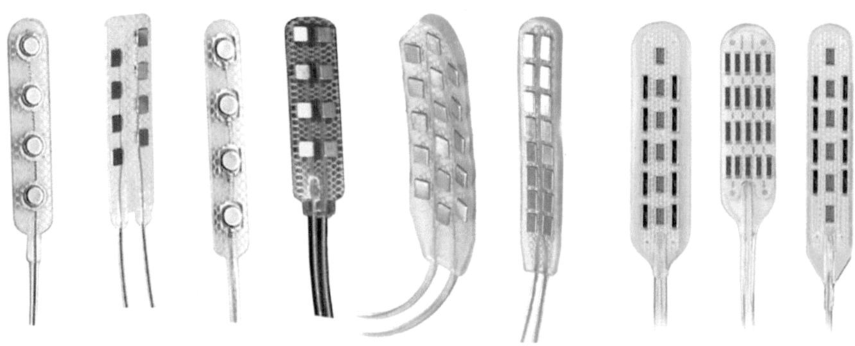

Fig. 1 Paddle lead models

intermittent delivery of pulses. The advent of rechargeable batteries allowed a generation of smaller batteries that could work for up to 10–15 years with a more constant delivery of energy.

The configuration of the electrical stimulation has evolved with studies showing the role of appropriate frequency and pulse width in most pain patients, despite that an individual scenario must always be pursued. The combination of different simultaneous stimulation allowed a more complex adjustment in patients.

Recently, newer stimulation parameters such as burst stimulation, high frequency, high density, and differential target multiplexed have shown encouraging results [6].

Rationale

Since its beginning, SCS has gained medical acceptance, and now, thousands of patients worldwide have had benefits due to this technique. The mechanism of action is obtained after an electric charge is delivered to the posterior spinal cord structures, generating a local electric field. At first, nervous structures such as neuronal bodies, synapses, and axons at the region of the stimulation may be modulated [7], but further studies have shown that glial cells also play a significant role in the pain suppression mechanism [8, 9].

Further studies have shown different concurrent mechanisms involved in analgesia. They include decreased transmission of painful stimuli through the spinothalamic and medial lemniscus tracts, activation of descending inhibitory control, increased release of neurotransmitters (such as serotonin, GABA, noradrenaline, dopamine, and acetylcholine), release of endogenous opioids, decreased glial activation, and modulation of cytokines and neurotrophic factors [10].

Indications and Results

Spinal cord stimulation is a well-known treatment modality indicated to patients with chronic pain that are refractory to conservative therapy, which includes especially a combination of medications, intensive rehabilitation program, and psychological interventions.

But not all chronic pain patients are amenable to this kind of technology. Traditionally, better results have been found in neuropathic pain patients [11] despite that some specific cases of nociceptive pain have also been related to good results.

Actually, the two most common indications that are supported by high-level studies are failed-back surgery syndrome and complex regional pain syndrome (types I and II).

Failed-back surgery syndrome (FBSS) is a term used to refer to a subset of patients who have new or persistent pain after spinal surgery for back or leg pain [12]. FBSS has a high incidence with the increasing number of patients operated, including older and more complex cases [13], even though this does not mean that a medical problem occurred during the surgery.

FBSS has a high incidence and spine surgery failure rates vary from 10% to 40% (mostly assumed as 20%) [14]. It is related to a multiplicity of factors such as poor indication, wrong level surgery, insufficient decompression, infection (discitis and superficial tissue infection), instability, pseudarthrosis, malpositioning of arthrodesis materials (screws and cages), fibrosis, facet pain, muscle trigger points, or new spinal canal and nerve compressions.

Notably, in some patients where an adjacent cause can be treated, such as infections and muscle pain, the treatment should be focused on the origin of the problem, but one should keep in mind that in most patients there is no anatomical cause of pain and the origin of the symptoms are related to the dysfunctional status, including central sensitization.

North et al., in 2005, conducted a prospective randomized controlled trial in patients selected for reoperation where they were randomized for either reoperation or spinal cord stimulation. Forty-five patients were available for follow-up. They found that SCS was related to a better outcome (9 out of 19 patients – 53%) when compared with reoperation (good results in 3 out of 26–11.5%). The group submitted to SCS was less likely to cross over to the other group and needed a significant lower dose of opioids [15].

The same main author showed that a successful outcome (improvement higher than 50% and patient satisfaction) was present in 47% of patients in a 5-year follow-up [16].

A similar study was published by Kumar et al. [17] when they randomized 100 patients with neuropathic failed back syndrome with predominant leg pain to receive either spinal cord stimulation plus conventional medical management or conventional medical management (CMM) alone. At 6-month follow-up, 48% of patients with SCS achieved good results (50% or more pain relief), while in the CMM group, only 9% of them had good results. Furthermore, the SCS group had a significant improvement in both leg and back pain, as well as in the quality of life, functional capacity, and treatment satisfaction.

Additionally, further randomized controlled trials (RCT) showed a superior benefit with SCS versus sham with different waveforms [18–21] in such a way that there is a 1B+ level of evidence for pain relief, functional status, quality of life, utilization of analgesics, and patient satisfaction [22].

The second indication with a higher level of evidence for SCS is complex regional pain syndrome (CRPS). This yet poorly understood clinical entity is characterized by a continuous limb pain, usually starting after an injury, but with duration and intensity disproportionate to the inciting event. Other clinical signs and symptoms in CRPS have been organized according to the Budapest criteria which include (a) sensory changes (hyperesthesia, hyperalgesia, allodynia), (b) vasomotor changes (temperature asymmetry, changes in skin color), (c) sudomotor/edema signs and symptoms (edema, sweating changes, and asymmetry), and (d) motor and trophic changes (decreased range of motion, trophic changes, weakness, tremor, and dystonia) [23].

Kemler et al. analyzed a total of 54 patients, which were assigned to undergo SCS plus physical therapy (total of 36 patients) versus physical therapy alone (a total of 18 patients). Only two-thirds of those that underwent a trial with SCS obtained a significant relief and had a permanent implant. The results showed that the SCS group had a significant improvement in pain intensity, with a decrease in 2.4 cm in the Verbal Analog Scale (VAS) score versus an increase of 0.2 cm in the control group. There was a significant improvement in quality of life only when comparing those with permanent implant over the control group [24].

An additional prospective randomized controlled trial named ACCURATE compared the results of SCS versus dorsal root ganglion (DRG) stimulation for complex regional pain syndrome in the lower limbs [25]. The analysis at 3 months showed that 81.2% of patients that were randomized to receive DRG stimulation had an improvement of at least 50%, while 55.7% of patients randomized to receive SCS had the same result. At the 12-month follow-up, the results had only mild changes. The DRG stimulation group had also a better quality of life and psychological disposition at follow-up.

Other indications for SCS are peripheral diabetic neuropathy [26, 27], critical limb ischemia [28, 29], and refractory angina pectoris [30]. Other less studied indications that need further studies to recognize possible good candidates are phantom limb pain, post-thoracotomy syndrome, chronic abdominal pain, and neck pain [31–33]. The evidence of efficacy of SCS in cancer-related pain is limited, due to the small number of trials, all of which were small and non-randomized [34].

All patients undergoing SCS should have an adequate psychological evaluation by experienced specialists. Important factors should be recognized such as the existence of major psychiatric disorders; an evaluation on how the patient may deal with a new device and the impact of a possible failure in pain alleviation. If a major psychiatric disorder or drug addiction is found, the patient should be discouraged to undergo the implant [35–37].

The major tool for psychological evaluation in the literature has been the Minnesota Multiphasic Personality Inventory. Depression has been related to poorer outcomes in most articles, while hypochondriasis and hysteria had conflicting results [38, 39].

Likewise, patients with major cognitive abnormalities should be carefully analyzed, and as a rule, the implant is performed only if a good result is predicted. In mild cognitive affected patients, a nonrechargeable SCS generator should be preferred.

At last, obesity has been related to a poorer outcome, and a negative relationship between body mass index and SCS effectivity has been found [40]. Therefore, patients should be oriented to undergo strategies for weight loss before and after SCS.

Percutaneous Leads Versus Paddle Leads

Before any consideration about advantages and disadvantages of each technique, it is relevant to explain that the final decision of which kind of lead should be implanted depends on the interventionist pain physician and should be settled based on the surgeon personal experience and skill, the location of the pain, and the anatomical conditions of the patient. It is noteworthy that both techniques have good results when correctly indicated.

Percutaneous or cylindrical leads have the advantages of the possibility of being implanted by most pain interventionists, usually under local anesthesia, with lower risks of procedure related to adverse events, with less risk of hardware or lead malfunction or breakage. The risk of initial adverse event is lower.

As opposed to it, paddle leads have the advantage of a more predictable electrical current directed to the spinal cord (with no stimulation of the ligamentum flavum), with a constant distance between the contacts, usually increasing the coverage of the pain zone. Beyond that, they are involved with less migration and a lower rate of reoperations and related with less adverse events in the long-term [41].

Since percutaneous leads are performed under local anesthesia, some surgical and anesthetic risks are minimized. Paddle leads, on the other hand, are usually performed under general or spinal anesthesia. Additionally, paddle lead implantation is related to a higher incidence of postoperative pain in the first weeks [42].

North et al., in 2005, published the results of a prospective randomized controlled trial comparing the results of percutaneous leads versus paddle leads (through laminectomy). After a mean follow-up of 1.9 years, 83% of patients with paddle leads had a good result (improvement of at least 50%) versus 41% for those with percutaneous leads [15]. Additionally, more patients in the paddle lead group had a decrease in analgesic intake.

An additional study reviewed 27 patients, comparing patients with laminectomy or percutaneous leads after a median follow-up of 34 months. Paddle leads showed a significant improvement in the Verbal Analog Scale of Pain (decrease of 4.6 points in the laminectomy group versus 3.1 in the percutaneous group). Moreover, the paddle lead group had a greater long-term pain relief [43].

A study cohort of 13,774 patients evaluated by the MarketScan database compared laminectomy versus percutaneous lead implantation. They found that the paddle lead group had a higher incidence of short-term postoperative complications (3.4% vs 2.2%). However, the rate of reoperation at long-term was higher in the percutaneous lead group. No significant difference was found in long-term health cost of both procedures [42].

In our service, the choice of which electrode should be implanted is extensively discussed with the patient, but as a rule, percutaneous leads are preferred when the pain is limited to smaller territories (for example one or two limbs), while paddle leads are chosen when a more complex configuration of the pain zone needs to be treated (for example, when the lumbar, buttocks, and limbs regions are affected or cervical, dorsal, and upper limbs symptoms occur).

Technical Aspects

Most pain physicians advocate that the implant of SCS should be done in two steps, despite that a cost impact analysis in the United Kingdom has shown that an implantation strategy without a screening trial could be cost saving [44].

In the first part, an epidural installation is done as a trial, and the patient and the physician evaluate the rate of improvement. In our service, this trial period varies from 4 to 14 days. The second procedure corresponds to the implant of the pulse generator itself and is done only if the patient had an improvement of at least 50%.

Due to the complexity of the spine and spinal cord, a neurosurgeon or an orthopedic surgeon is needed in most cases. In a large retrospective analysis using the Truven MarketScan database, percutaneous implants have been done predominantly by anesthesiologists, while neurosurgeons and orthopedic surgeons performed a significantly greater number of paddle implants [45]. This study also showed that among patients undergoing a trial of SCS, neurosurgeons had a higher rate of conversion rate to the permanent implant, followed respectively by orthopedic surgeons, anesthesiologists, and physical medicine and rehabilitation.

Some authors propose that in the first step, a percutaneous implant should be performed, while the laminectomy lead is done only after a positive response. However, authors as Pahapill and Lee et al. showed that a paddle lead insertion can be done in the first trial procedure and then connected to the pulse generator in a second surgery if the patient had a significant improvement [46, 47].

Currently, we perform the implant of a paddle lead since the first procedure, in a way that the patient may have a real preview of how the stimulation will work. Thereafter, our further description will show a paddle lead implant in a trial period. For details of a percutaneous lead implant as a trial, please proceed to the proper chapter.

Before the operation, the patient should have a magnetic resonance imaging of the implant site, with special attention to the epidural space and to the spinal canal. The surgeon must analyze any previous constriction or stenosis that could produce further spinal cord compression in the postoperative period after the placement of the paddle electrode. If this risk is predicted, a percutaneous lead implant should be elected.

Trial Procedure

First of all, the involved surgical team should carry out a checklist, confirming important topics for a safe and correct surgery. Many items should be verified, such as the correct identification of the patient, inquiry of past surgical problems and allergies, revision of preoperative tests, and the confirmation that all surgical supplies and the medical staff are available and in place. The consent form should always be signed, expressing that the patient is aware of any possible benefit and risk of the operation.

In most services worldwide, general anesthesia is used, with the patient in ventral decubitus using surgical cushion in the hip plus one or two cushions in the thorax, avoiding compression of the anterior chest. The thoracic pressure should be kept as low as possible, in order to decrease the incidence of venous enlargement in the epidural space and consequently decreasing the incidence of epidural hematomas. The patient should be positioned in a radiotransparent surgical table in order to remain possible to have radiographic images in anteroposterior and lateral views.

A special attention should be kept to the patient's face, avoiding compressions to the eyes, anterior neck, or the endotracheal tube.

Some authors have advocated the safety and feasibility of regional anesthesia with epidural blocks [48].

A right-handed surgeon usually should be located on the left side of the patient so that it becomes easier to open the vertebral bone and ligaments and to introduce the electrode towards the superior region of the epidural space. On the opposite side remains the medical assistant as well as the image intensifier (C-arm) and monitor.

The medical team should follow strict sterile and aseptic care, including degermation, application of antiseptic solutions (such as chlorhexidine), and the placement of sterile drapes. We strongly recommend the use of a double glove to decrease the patient's rate of infection as demonstrated by some authors [49].

The use of electrocautery is not recommended while the electrode or the pulse generator has been placed and should be used only in the surgical access before any material has been positioned. On the other hand, bipolar coagulators are safer, since the delivery of energy is mostly located around the two forceps and they can be used with little risk when the electrode or the generator is not around the coagulation zone [50].

The first step is to locate the surgical level of the laminectomy. In most cases, a T10-T11 or T11-T12 laminectomy is used. Factors such as previous surgeries or compressions should be anticipated. A small incision of 4 cm is usually enough to expose all the anatomical structures. The aponeurosis should be opened in the midline (when a midline laminectomy is predicted) or slightly lateral to the midline (when a hemilaminectomy is indicated). The paravertebral muscles are dissected, exposing the vertebral lamina and the spinous process.

The next step is the opening of the superior part of the lamina and a small part of the spinous process, exposing the ligamentum flavum. In some cases, a high-speed drill can be used. The ligamentum flavum is then opened, exposing the dura mater. The surgeon should be aware of where the midline is located for a correct positioning of the electrode.

Most companies have a plastic model similar to the electrode that should be placed before the electrode itself to verify if the opening is enough and further allowing for the epidural dissection (phantom electrode). Thereafter, the electrode is gently placed with careful attention to any significant bleeding at the epidural space, and a correct positioning is verified under radiographic imaging (Figs. 2 and 3).

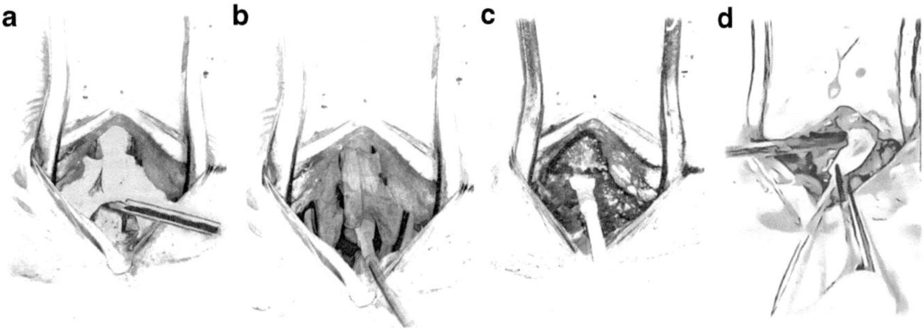

Fig. 2 Paddle lead insertion technique at the thoracolumbar region. (**a**) Small laminectomy or hemilaminectomy is performed, and the ligamentum flavum is opened; (**b** and **c**) Phantom lead is inserted in the epidural space, and (**d**) the paddle lead is inserted under radiographic and electrophysiologic supervision

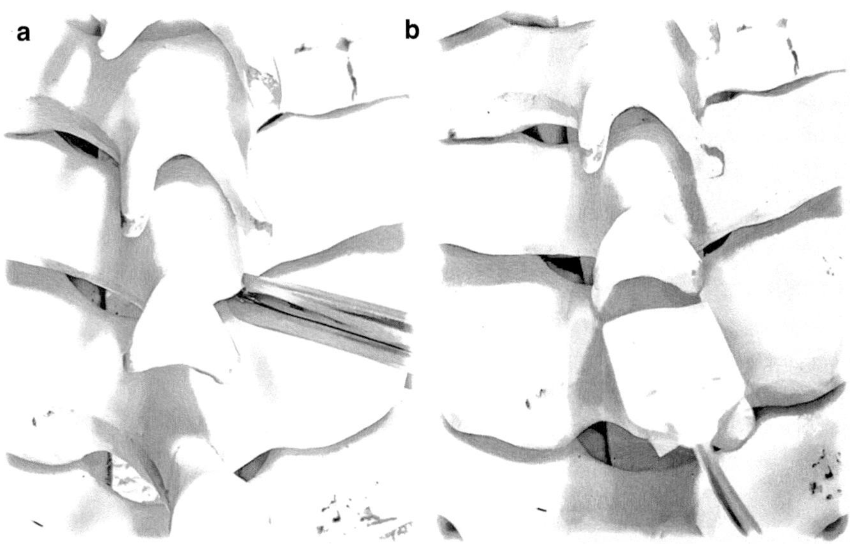

Fig. 3 Paddle lead insertion technique in cervicothoracic region. (**a**) Small laminectomy or hemilaminectomy is performed, and the ligamentum flavum is opened; (**b**) phantom lead is inserted followed by the insertion of the paddle lead

An efficient fixation of the electrodes is done with anchoring pieces provided by the electrode companies. They should be done to steady anatomical structures, such as aponeurosis.

An extension wire is connected to the electrodes and is tunneled through the subcutaneous tissue to the exit site that should be at least 20 cm away from the surgical incision. Special care is taken to keep all the electrodes in a sterile fashion inside the patient so that only the extension is taken to a counter opening.

Impedance tests are done to verify for any disconnection or breakage and an extra radiographic image is done. At last, a careful wound closure is done, and the extension wire is anchored.

Rigoard et al. described an optic transligamentar minimally invasive surgery apparatus intended to induce a smaller muscle retraction and to promote a better visualization of the anatomical structures [51, 52].

Implant of Pulse Generator

After a trial period of 4–14 days, the patient is evaluated for the pain improvement result. Most authors establish a minimum of at least 50% pain relief to consider a permanent implant. In our opinion, when the patient has a suboptimal palliation of pain or when there is doubt if the system is beneficial, the surgical incision is reopened, and the paddle electrode is withdrawn.

Before taking out the paddle lead (in case of an insufficient improvement) or before connecting the lead to the pulse generator, the external portion of the extension wire is cut in order to remove all material that may be colonized and potentially infected.

If the patient has a significant pain relief, the patient is advised to implant a definitive pulse generator. Common implantation of this pulse generator is in the subcutaneous tissue in the abdomen, in the lateral portion of the lumbar region, or in the gluteal tissue. The final site should be discussed previously with the patient considering their expectations and preferences, including previous surgical scars. If the patient has no preference, we mostly recommend the gluteal region. Before entering the surgical room, a nurse is sent to check with the patient the correct placement, including the creation of a scar that may be easily hidden under the clothes.

The most common paddle leads available at the market nowadays are long enough to connect directly with the pulse generator, so a subcutaneous tunneling is done between the incision of the lead and the pulse generator site. The wires are connected to the generator and screwed.

When there is a thick subcutaneous tissue in the generator site, we recommend that the excess fat tissue should be removed, so that the patient can have an easier connection with the external platform for either the battery charging as well as for further increments or decrements in the amplitude and adjustments.

The pulse generator should be sutured in the aponeurotic tissue, avoiding further displacement, and finally, the layers are closed carefully.

The patient should have a radiographic evaluation one day after the surgery for long-term follow-up (Figs. 4, 5, and 6).

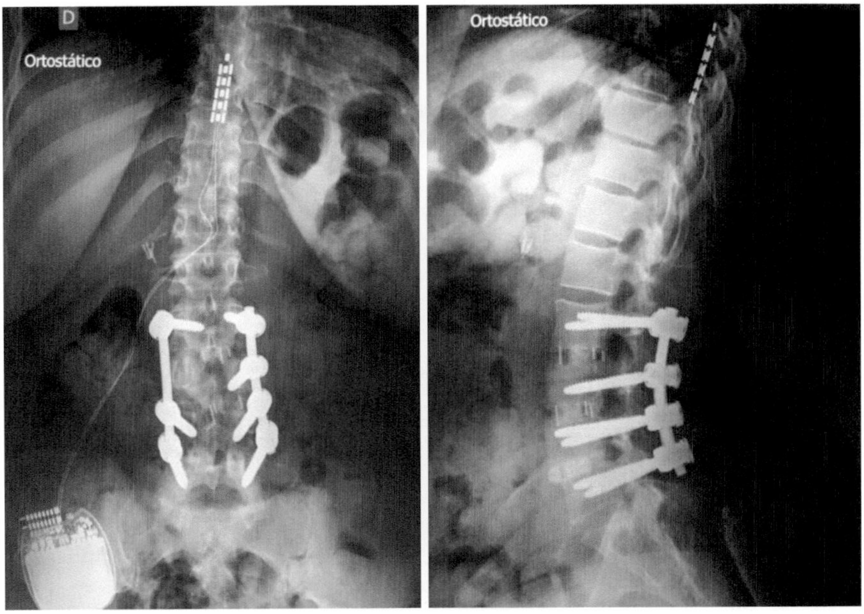

Fig. 4 Paddle lead spinal cord stimulation for the treatment of lumbar and lower limbs' pain. The lead is usually inserted mostly from the T8 to T12 epidural space

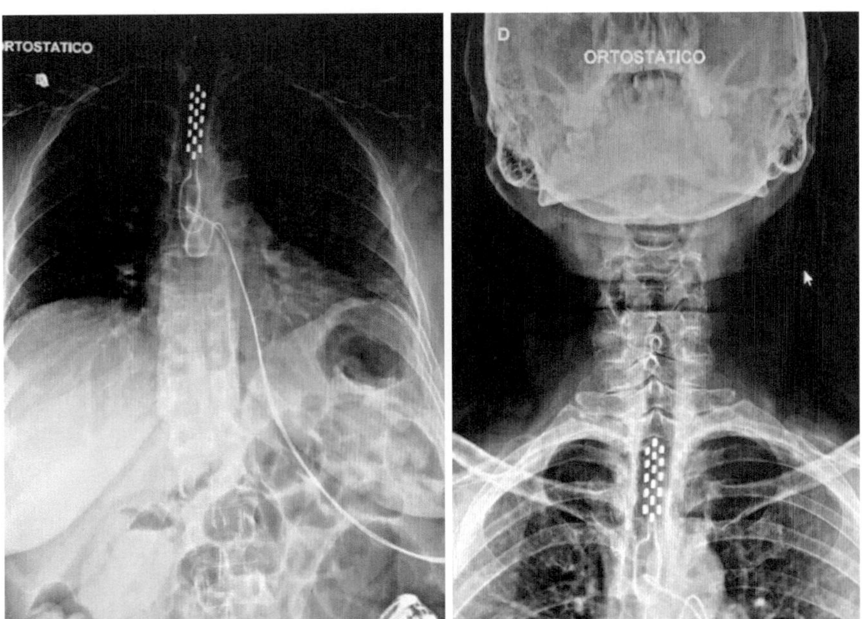

Fig. 5 Paddle lead for spinal cord stimulation for upper thoracic pain

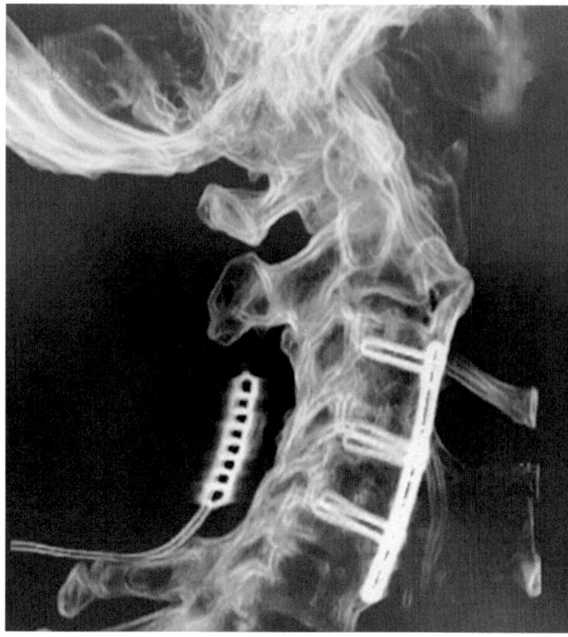

Fig. 6 Tomographic view of a paddle lead inserted in a patient with the previous laminectomy in the cervical region (traumatic spinal pain)

Spinal Cord Stimulation in Upper Thoracic and Cervical Regions

In most services, the most common site of SCS implants is located in the lower thoracic spinal cord, aiming for the treatment of pain in the lumbar and gluteal region as well as in the lower limbs.

However, other spinal cord regions are suitable for this implantation as well. They include the upper thoracic spine (less common indication) for the treatment of pain in the upper thoracic region and cervical or cervicomedullary junction.

Deer et al. published a review board-approved, prospective, multicenter analysis of patients that were submitted to cervical implants of SCS in 16 centers, either in the United States or in an additional 3 international centers [53]. A total of 38 patients were then analyzed, where 28 (73.7%) were implanted with percutaneous leads, while 10 (26.3%) received paddle leads. They were evaluated after 3, 6, and 12 months. The mean percentage of pain relief described by the patients was 54.2% at 3-month, 60.2% at 6-month, and 66.8% at 12-month follow-up. Similarly, the analysis of the Patient Disability Index showed a significant improvement (decreasing from 49.6 at baseline to 34.5, 33.4, and 28.4, respectively at 3, 6, and 12 months later). The quality of life was reported as improved or greatly improved in 80.7% of patients at 3-month evaluation, with minor changes (80.9 and 62.6%) at 6- and 12-month evaluations. A total of 92.4% of the patients considered themselves as very satisfied or satisfied at 3 months (with rates of 85.7 at 6 months and 87.6% at 12 months). They concluded that the results of cervical SCS in pain control, disability, and quality of life were comparable with those with thoracic implantation.

In this study, involving many centers, the tip of the electrode was placed in C2 in half of the patients while an additional 39.4% had the tip at the C3 or C4 space [53]. Similar studies show that in most cases, the tip of the electrode is placed at C2 space [54].

Other articles reviewed the results of cervical SCS, including case series, retrospective studies, and prospective non-randomized studies. The most common indications were complex regional pain syndrome, brachial plexus lesion, failed neck surgery syndrome, cervical radicular pain, ischemic pain, and peripheral nerve lesion [36, 54–59].

One prospective study analyzed the results of cervical SCS in patients with systemic scleroderma and Raynaud's syndrome [60], with electrodes being placed between C4 and C7. The authors found a significant improvement, with Raynaud's episodes decreasing in 93% of patients, as well as a reduction in edema in 86% of patients and improvement in the ulceration in 100% of cases.

While in most cases, the paddle lead is directed upward, with the insertion coming from the lower cervical or upper thoracic lesion, some authors propose the insertion in the C1-C2 space where the space around the spinal cord is bigger, where they were supposed to promote a smaller rate of complications [57].

A retrospective review of cases from a single neurosurgeon [61] analyzed the results of 100 patients that had paddle leads at the cervical or cervicomedullary regions after a successful trial. Twenty-five of them had a cervicomedullary implant to painful conditions such as trigeminal deafferentation pain, trigeminal neuropathic pain, postherpetic neuralgia, and occipital neuralgia. The main goal was to stimulate the nucleus caudalis. The surgical technique included a small C1 hemilaminectomy in the side of the pain plus a small occipital craniectomy (when the pain achieved the upper facial region). According to this study, the vast majority of patients with trigeminal neuropathic pain (including postherpetic) had a significant benefit. In contrast, occipital neuralgia had a lower rate of success.

Complications

Despite the safety and effectiveness of SCS, both the patient and the pain physician should be aware of the possibility of complications. An extra caution and vigilance should always be taken. These complications vary from mild to the most feared spinal cord injury.

A systematic review of the literature showed that life-threatening complications were rare, while other adverse events had an incidence of 34% of cases who had a stimulator [62]. They were due to superficial infection (4.5%), infection in deeper structures (0.1%), pain in the region of the neurostimulator (5.8%), other biological complications (2.5%), and equipment failure (10.2%). A stimulator revision needing additional surgery occurred in 23.1% of patients, and stimulator removal was needed in 11% of cases.

The most common complication in percutaneous SCS is lead migration, but the rate is much lower when using paddle leads [31]. If there is a slight migration, small changes in the generator programming are usually enough. But if this is not possible, an extra surgery may be needed. For this reason, a careful anchoring should be an essential part of the surgical procedure. At the end of the anchoring procedure, a gentle pull in the electrode is done to certify that the electrode is immobile. The surgeon should be careful to anchor the electrode in a steady structure, often the aponeurosis.

Hardware malfunction or breakage is not uncommon when dealing with patients with SCS. Newer technology is warranted to avoid this complication that, in most cases, patients are treated with the exchange of the affected material. It includes electrode or extension wire fracture, disconnections, and pulse generator failures.

Pain in the pulse generator site is seen in some patients and may be due to causes such as fluid or blood accumulation, positioning into sensible areas of the body, or poor fixation of the generator. Sometimes, the patient spins constantly the generator under the skin, sometimes causing the electrode or the extension wire to break.

Infection is a feared complication as well. A multisite retrospective review showed a rate of 2.45% of infection after SCS [63]. Revision surgeries had a higher incidence of infections but without statistical significance. Implants performed at academic centers had a higher incidence of infections when compared with nonacademic hospitals.

The rate of infection did not show significant differences when performed by physicians of different specialties or when comparing percutaneous versus paddle leads. Diabetes, tobacco use, or obesity did not show to be a significant risk factor for infection. The use of postoperative antibiotics as well as the application of an occlusive dressing decreased the incidence of infections.

Levy et al. published a review of the incidence and frequency of neurologic complications after paddle lead implantation. The number was based on the literature and FDA analysis in addition to the three paddle lead manufacturer's reports and data. They found an incidence of less than 0.6% overall spinal cord injury, including motor dysfunction caused by epidural hematomas (0.19%), motor dysfunction without epidural hematoma (0.13%), sensory dysfunction (0.1%), and autonomic dysfunction (0.013%). The vast majority of cases had a complete or partial recovery [64].

Petraglia et al. reviewed 8326 patients that underwent percutaneous or paddle lead SCS (5458 vs 2868 patients, respectively). Unlike the previous study mainly based on manufacturer's data, their information was based on the Thomson Reuters' MartketScan database, which contains records from employers, health plans, and government and public organizations of over 158 million patients in the United States. They also studied the incidence of spinal cord injury and spinal hematoma not only in paddle leads but also with percutaneous leads. The overall incidence of spinal cord injury was 2.13% (percutaneous: 2.35% versus paddle: 1.71%). The main weakness in their review is that they could not evaluate the severity or the duration of the neurologic deficits [65].

The Future of Spinal Cord Stimulation

SCS is a growing technology. New and future advances may help to increase the rate of success, as well as finding solutions to improve the comfort of both the patient and the physician.

Newer paddle leads have been developed, producing thinner plates, with more available contacts, at distances that have been shown to produce better coverage and with materials that are more flexible and durable. At the same time, rechargeable pulse generators with increasing delivery of energy and with multiple capacities have been created. New waveforms and configurations such as burst, high frequency, high density, and differential target multiplexed (DTM) are some examples of how neurophysiological studies and engineering may help patients throughout the world.

At the same time, there is a great solicitude that the whole apparatus (leads, cables, and generators) should be compatible with magnetic resonance imaging (MRI). It is clear that there is an increasing need for the use of this diagnostic modality in modern medicine. Analysis of SCS patients has shown that approximately 82–84% of these patients are expected to need at least one MRI in the next 5 years [66].

The list of recommendations for the future development of neurostimulation (Neuromodulation Appropriateness Consensus Committee by International Neuromodulation Society) has focused on some priorities for the development of new devices. They include concerns such as (a) improved safety, (b) miniaturization, (c) cost utility, (d) better cosmetic results, (e) impact on intended targets, while sparing unintended targets, (f) increasing longevity of devices, and (g) increasing safety for the neural tissue. Furthermore, the study of new neural targets, modification of current delivery and waveforms, newer and safer materials, as well as the role of technologies such as wireless, image-guided implantation, and closed-loop technology should bring better results and security [12].

Conclusions

Spinal cord stimulation is a safe and effective technique for the treatment of chronic refractory pain. The use of paddle leads has been related to a better outcome when compared to percutaneous leads. However, the rate of complications in the short term is higher in the paddle group, despite that, in the long term, they have a lower rate of complications and surgeries, such as in lead migration.

The surgeon should be aware of some technical issues for a better outcome.

References

1. Eriksen J, Jensen MK, Sjøgren P, Ekholm O, Rasmussen NK. Epidemiology of chronic non-malignant pain in Denmark. Pain. 2003;106(3):221–8. https://doi.org/10.1016/s0304-3959(03)00225-2.
2. Melzack R, Wall PD. Pain mechanisms: a new theory. Science. 1965;150(3699):971–9. https://doi.org/10.1126/science.150.3699.971.
3. Cavuoto J. The birth of an industry. In: Krames E, Peckham PH, Rezai A, editors. Neuromodulation. Academic Press; 2009. https://doi.org/10.1016/B978-0-12-374248-3.00006-9.
4. Shealy CN, Mortimer JT, Reswick JB. Electrical inhibition of pain by stimulation of the dorsal columns: preliminary clinical report. Anesth Analg. 1967;46(4):489–91.
5. Gildenberg PL. History of electrical neuromodulation for chronic pain. Pain Med. 2006;7(suppl_1):S7–S13. https://doi.org/10.1111/j.1526-4637.2006.00118.x.
6. Burchiel KJ, Raslan AM. Contemporary concepts of pain surgery. J Neurosurg. 2019;130(4):1039–49. https://doi.org/10.3171/2019.1.JNS181620.
7. Miller JP, Eldabe S, Buchser E, Johanek LM, Guan Y, Linderoth B. Parameters of spinal cord stimulation and their role in electrical charge delivery: a review. Neuromodulation. 2016;19(4):373–84. https://doi.org/10.1111/ner.12438.
8. Ji RR, Berta T, Nedergaard M. Glia and pain: is chronic pain a gliopathy? Pain. 2013;154 Suppl 1(0 1):S10–28. https://doi.org/10.1016/j.pain.2013.06.022.
9. Sato KL, Johanek LM, Sanada LS, Sluka KA. Spinal cord stimulation reduces mechanical hyperalgesia and glial cell activation in animals with neuropathic pain. Anesth Analg. 2014;118(2):464–72. https://doi.org/10.1213/ANE.0000000000000047.
10. Caylor J, Reddy R, Yin S, Cui C, Huang M, Huang C, Ramesh R, Baker DG, Simmons A, Souza D, Narouze S, Vallejo R, Lerman I. Spinal cord stimulation in chronic pain: evidence and theory for mechanisms of action. Bioelectron Med. 2019;5:12. https://doi.org/10.1186/s42234-019-0023-1.
11. Dones I, Levi V. Spinal cord stimulation for neuropathic pain: current trends and future applications. Brain Sci. 2018;8(8):138. https://doi.org/10.3390/brainsci8080138.
12. de Vos CC, Meier K, Zaalberg PB, Nijhuis HJ, Duyvendak W, Vesper J, et al. The appropriate use of neurostimulation: new and evolving neurostimulation therapies and applicable treatment for chronic pain and selected disease states. Neuromodulation. 2014;17(6):599–615. https://doi.org/10.1111/ner.12204.
13. Kapural L, Peterson E, Provenzano DA, Staats P. Clinical evidence for spinal cord stimulation for failed back surgery syndrome (FBSS): systematic review. Spine (Phila Pa 1976). 2017;42(Suppl 14):S61–6. https://doi.org/10.1097/BRS.0000000000002213.
14. Thomson S. Failed back surgery syndrome - definition, epidemiology and demographics. Br J Pain. 2013;7(1):56–9. https://doi.org/10.1177/2049463713479096.
15. North RB, Kidd DH, Farrokhi F, Piantadosi SA. Spinal cord stimulation versus repeated lumbosacral spine surgery for chronic pain: a randomized, controlled trial. Neurosurgery. 2005;56(1):98–106. https://doi.org/10.1227/01.neu.0000144839.65524.e0.
16. North RB, Ewend MG, Lawton MT, Kidd DH, Piantadosi S. Failed back surgery syndrome: 5-year follow-up after spinal cord stimulator implantation. Neurosurgery. 1991;28(5):692–9.
17. Kumar K, Taylor RS, Jacques L, Eldabe S, Meglio M, Molet J, et al. Spinal cord stimulation versus conventional medical management for neuropathic pain: a multicentre randomised controlled trial in patients with failed back surgery syndrome. Pain. 2007;132(1–2):179–88. https://doi.org/10.1016/j.pain.2007.07.028.
18. Schultz DM, Webster L, Kosek P, Dar U, Tan Y, Sun M. Sensor-driven position-adaptive spinal cord stimulation for chronic pain. Pain Physician. 2012;15(1):1–12.
19. Perruchoud C, Eldabe S, Batterham AM, Madzinga G, Brookes M, Durrer A, et al. Analgesic efficacy of high-frequency spinal cord stimulation: a randomized double-blind placebo-controlled study. Neuromodulation. 2013;16(4):363–9. https://doi.org/10.1111/ner.12027.

20. Schu S, Slotty PJ, Bara G, von Knop M, Edgar D, Vesper J. A prospective, randomised, double-blind, placebo-controlled study to examine the effectiveness of burst spinal cord stimulation patterns for the treatment of failed back surgery syndrome. Neuromodulation. 2014;17(5):443–50. https://doi.org/10.1111/ner.12197.
21. Kapural L, Yu C, Doust MW, Gliner BE, Vallejo R, Sitzman BT, et al. Novel 10-kHz high-frequency therapy (HF10 therapy) is superior to traditional low-frequency spinal cord stimulation for the treatment of chronic back and leg pain: the SENZA-RCT randomized controlled trial. Anesthesiology. 2015;123(4):851–60. https://doi.org/10.1097/ALN.0000000000000774.
22. Mekhail N, Visnjevac O, Azer G, Mehanny DS, Agrawal P, Foorsov V. Spinal cord stimulation 50 years later: clinical outcomes of spinal cord stimulation based on randomized clinical trials-a systematic review. Reg Anesth Pain Med. 2018;43(4):391–406. https://doi.org/10.1097/AAP.0000000000000744.
23. Pergolizzi JV, LeQuang JA, Nalamachu S, et al. The Budapest criteria for complex regional pain syndrome: the diagnostic challenge. Anaesthesiol Clin Sci Res. 2018;2(1):1–10.
24. Kemler MA, Barendse GA, van Kleef M, de Vet HC, Rijks CP, Furnée CA, et al. Spinal cord stimulation in patients with chronic reflex sympathetic dystrophy. N Engl J Med. 2000;343(9):618–24. https://doi.org/10.1056/NEJM200008313430904.
25. Deer TR, Levy RM, Kramer J, Poree L, Amirdelfan K, Grigsby E, et al. Dorsal root ganglion stimulation yielded higher treatment success rate for complex regional pain syndrome and causalgia at 3 and 12 months: a randomized comparative trial. Pain. 2017;158(4):669–81. https://doi.org/10.1097/j.pain.0000000000000814.
26. de Vos CC, Meier K, Zaalberg PB, Nijhuis HJ, Duyvendak W, Vesper J, et al. Spinal cord stimulation in patients with painful diabetic neuropathy: a multicentre randomized clinical trial. Pain. 2014;155(11):2426–31. https://doi.org/10.1016/j.pain.2014.08.031.
27. Pluijmsl WA, Slangenl R, Joostenl EA, Kesselsl AG, Merkiesl ISJ, Schaperl NC, et al. Electrical spinal cord stimulation in painful diabetic polyneuropathy, a systematic review on treatment efficacy and safety. Eur J Pain. 2011;15(8):783–8. https://doi.org/10.1016/j.ejpain.2011.01.010.
28. Dua A, Lee CJ. Epidemiology of peripheral arterial disease and critical limb ischemia. Tech Vasc Interv Radiol. 2016;19(2):91–5. https://doi.org/10.1053/j.tvir.2016.04.001.
29. Kinfe TM, Pintea B, Vatter H. Is spinal cord stimulation useful and safe for the treatment of chronic pain of ischemic origin? A review. Clin J Pain. 2016 Jan;32(1):7–13. https://doi.org/10.1097/ajp.0000000000000229.
30. Dobias M, Michalek P, Neuzil P, Stritesky M, Johnston P. Interventional treatment of pain in refractory angina. A review. Biomed Pap Med Fac Univ Palacky Olomouc Czech Repub. 2014;158(4):518–27. https://doi.org/10.5507/bp.2014.028.
31. Bendersky D, Yampolsky C. Is spinal cord stimulation safe? A review of its complications. World Neurosurg. 2014;82(6):1359–68. https://doi.org/10.1016/j.wneu.2013.06.012.
32. Kapural L, Nagem H, Tlucek H, Sessler DI. Spinal cord stimulation for chronic visceral abdominal pain. Pain Med. 2010;11(3):347–55. https://doi.org/10.1111/j.1526-4637.2009.00785.x.
33. Aiyer R, Barkin RL, Bhatia A, Gungor S. A systematic review on the treatment of phantom limb pain with spinal cord stimulation. Pain Manag. 2017;7(1):59–69. https://doi.org/10.2217/pmt-2016-0041.
34. Peng L, Min S, Zejun Z, Wei K, Bennett MI. Spinal cord stimulation for cancer-related pain in adults. Cochrane Database Syst Rev. 2015;2015(6):CD009389. https://doi.org/10.1002/14651858.CD009389.pub3.
35. Fama CA, Chen N, Prusik J, Kumar V, Wilock M, Roth S, et al. The use of preoperative psychological evaluations to predict spinal cord stimulation success: our experience and a review of the literature. Neuromodulation. 2016;19(4):429–36. https://doi.org/10.1111/ner.12434.
36. Doleys DM. Psychological factors in spinal cord stimulation therapy: brief review and discussion. Neurosurg Focus. 2006;21(6):E1. Published 2006 Dec 15. https://doi.org/10.3171/foc.2006.21.6.4.

37. Davis CE 3rd, Kyle BN, Thorp J, Wu Q, Firnhaber J. Comparison of pain, functioning, coping, and psychological distress in patients with chronic low back pain evaluated for spinal cord stimulator implant or behavioral pain management. Pain Med. 2015;16(4):753–60. https://doi.org/10.1111/pme.12526.
38. Sparkes E, Raphael JH, Duarte RV, LeMarchand K, Jackson C, Ashford RL. A systematic literature review of psychological characteristics as determinants of outcome for spinal cord stimulation therapy. Pain. 2010;150(2):284–9. https://doi.org/10.1016/j.pain.2010.05.001.
39. Taylor RS, Desai MJ, Rigoard P, Taylor RJ. Predictors of pain relief following spinal cord stimulation in chronic back and leg pain and failed back surgery syndrome: a systematic review and meta-regression analysis. Pain Pract. 2014;14:489–505. https://doi.org/10.1111/papr.12095.
40. Mekhail N, Mehanny D, Armanyous S, Saweris Y, Costandi S. The impact of obesity on the effectiveness of spinal cord stimulation in chronic spine-related pain patients. Spine J. 2019 Mar;19(3):476–86. https://doi.org/10.1016/j.spinee.2018.08.006.
41. North RB, McNamee JP, Wu L, Piantadosi S. Artificial neural networks: application to electrical stimulation of the human nervous system. Neurosurg Focus. 1997;2(1):e1. https://doi.org/10.3171/foc.1997.2.1.1.
42. Babu R, Hazzard MA, Huang KT, Ugiliweneza B, Patil CG, Boakye M, et al. Outcomes of percutaneous and paddle lead implantation for spinal cord stimulation: a comparative analysis of complications, reoperation rates, and health-care costs. Neuromodulation. 2013;16(5):418–27. https://doi.org/10.1111/ner.12065.
43. Villavicencio AT, Leveque JC, Rubin L, Bulsara K, Gorecki JP. Laminectomy versus percutaneous electrode placement for spinal cord stimulation. Neurosurgery. 2000;46(2):399–406. https://doi.org/10.1097/00006123-200002000-00025.
44. Duarte RV, Thomson S. Trial versus no trial of spinal cord stimulation for chronic neuropathic pain: cost analysis in United Kingdom National Health Service. Neuromodulation. 2019;22:208–14. https://doi.org/10.1111/ner.12898.
45. Hussaini SMQ, Murphy KR, Han JL, Elsamadicy AA, Yang S, Premji A, et al. Specialty-based variations in spinal cord stimulation success rates for treatment of chronic pain. Neuromodulation. 2017;20(4):340–7. https://doi.org/10.1111/ner.12582.
46. Pahapill PA. Surgical paddle-lead placement for screening trials of spinal cord stimulation. Neuromodulation. 2014;17(4):346–8. https://doi.org/10.1111/ner.12084.
47. Lee JJ, Simpson RK, Dalm B. Permanent paddle-lead trial for spinal cord stimulation. Cureus. 2018;10(5):e2645. Published 2018 May 18. https://doi.org/10.7759/cureus.2645.
48. García March G, Bordes V, Roldán P, Real L, González Darder JM. Estimulación medular crónica y síndrome de cirugía de espalda fallida. Resultados clínicos con la utilización de electrodos planos quirúrgicos [Spinal cord stimulation and failed back surgery syndrome. Clinical results with laminectomy electrodes]. Neurocirugia (Astur). 2015;26(2):78–83. https://doi.org/10.1016/j.neucir.2014.09.009.
49. Guo YP, Wong PM, Li Y, Or PP. Is double-gloving really protective? A comparison between the glove perforation rate among perioperative nurses with single and double gloves during surgery. Am J Surg. 2012;204(2):210–5. https://doi.org/10.1016/j.amjsurg.2011.08.017.
50. Walsh KM, Machado AG, Krishnaney AA. Spinal cord stimulation: a review of the safety literature and proposal for perioperative evaluation and management. Spine J. 2015;15(8):1864–9. https://doi.org/10.1016/j.spinee.2015.04.043.
51. Rigoard P, Luong AT, Delmotte A, Raaholt M, Roulaud M, Monlezun O, et al. Multicolumn spinal cord stimulation lead implantation using an optic transligamentar minimally invasive technique. Neurosurgery. 2013;73(3):550–3. https://doi.org/10.1227/neu.0000000000000008.
52. Monlezun O, Voirin J, Roulaud M, Ingrand P, Veyrieras C, Brandet C, et al. "MAST" prospective study: value of minimal access spine technologies technique for multicolumn spinal cord stimulation surgical lead implantation in the context of a French multicentre randomized controlled trial (ESTIMET study). Neurochirurgie. 2015;61(Suppl 1):S125–30. https://doi.org/10.1016/j.neuchi.2014.06.004.

53. Deer TR, Skaribas IM, Haider N, Salmon J, Kim C, Nelson C, et al. Effectiveness of cervical spinal cord stimulation for the management of chronic pain. Neuromodulation. 2014;17(3):265–71. https://doi.org/10.1111/ner.12119.
54. Hunter CW, Carlson J, Yang A, Deer T. Spinal cord stimulation for the treatment of failed neck surgery syndrome: outcome of a prospective case series. Neuromodulation. 2018;21(5):495–503. https://doi.org/10.1111/ner.12769.
55. Simpson BA, Bassett G, Davies K, Herbert C, Pierri M. Cervical spinal cord stimulation for pain: a report on 41 patients. Neuromodulation. 2003;6(1):20–6. https://doi.org/10.1046/j.1525-1403.2003.03003.x.
56. Forouzanfar T, Kemler MA, Weber WE, Kessels AG, van Kleef M. Spinal cord stimulation in complex regional pain syndrome: cervical and lumbar devices are comparably effective. Br J Anaesth. 2004;92(3):348–53. https://doi.org/10.1093/bja/aeh072.
57. Whitworth LA, Feler CA. C1-c2 sublaminar insertion of paddle leads for the management of chronic painful conditions of the upper extremity. Neuromodulation. 2003;6(3):153–7. https://doi.org/10.1046/j.1525-1403.2003.03022.x.
58. Wolter T, Kieselbach K. Cervical spinal cord stimulation: an analysis of 23 patients with long-term follow-up. Pain Physician. 2012;15(3):203–12.
59. Wolter T, Winkelmüller M. Continuous versus intermittent spinal cord stimulation: an analysis of factors influencing clinical efficacy. Neuromodulation. 2012;15(1):13–20. https://doi.org/10.1111/j.1525-1403.2011.00410.x.
60. Francaviglia N, Silvestro C, Maiello M, Bragazzi R, Bernucci C. Spinal cord stimulation for the treatment of progressive systemic sclerosis and Raynaud's syndrome. Br J Neurosurg. 1994;8(5):567–71. https://doi.org/10.3109/02688699409002949.
61. Chivukula S, Tempel ZJ, Weiner GM, Gande AV, Chen C-J, Ding D, et al. Cervical and cervicomedullary spinal cord stimulation for chronic pain: efficacy and outcomes. Clin Neurol Neurosurg. 2014;127:33–41. https://doi.org/10.1016/j.clineuro.2014.09.023.
62. Turner JA, Loeser JD, Deyo RA, Sanders SB. Spinal cord stimulation for patients with failed back surgery syndrome or complex regional pain syndrome: a systematic review of effectiveness and complications. Pain. 2004;108(1–2):137–47. https://doi.org/10.1016/j.pain.2003.12.016.
63. Hoelzer BC, Bendel MA, Deer TR, Eldrige JS, Walega DR, Wang Z, et al. Spinal cord stimulator implant infection rates and risk factors: a multicenter retrospective study. Neuromodulation. 2017;20(6):558–62. https://doi.org/10.1111/ner.12609.
64. Levy R, Henderson J, Slavin K, Simpson BA, Barolat G, Shipley J, et al. Incidence and avoidance of neurologic complications with paddle type spinal cord stimulation leads. Neuromodulation. 2011;14(5):412–22. https://doi.org/10.1111/j.1525-1403.2011.00395.x.
65. Petraglia FW III, Farber SH, Gramer R, Verla T, Wang F, Thomas S, et al. The incidence of spinal cord injury in implantation of percutaneous and paddle electrodes for spinal cord stimulation. Neuromodulation. 2016;19(1):85–90. https://doi.org/10.1111/ner.12370.
66. Desai MJ, Hargens LM, Breitenfeldt MD, Doth AH, Ryan MP, Gunnarsson C, et al. The rate of magnetic resonance imaging in patients with spinal cord stimulation. Spine (Phila Pa 1976). 2015;40(9):E531–7. https://doi.org/10.1097/BRS.0000000000000805.

The Penta Implant as I Do it

Joshua Feler and Claudio A. Feler

Status of SCS

While SCS and neuromodulation have seen far-reaching changes since their conceptual inception and initial clinical efforts, it is our belief that certain clinical syndromes are more likely to respond to SCS than others; in spite of the evolution of devices, both electrodes and current generators, as well as numerous newer programming modes, some pathologies remain resistant to therapy.

The evolution of SCS technologies has been animated by both the need to provide for patient care and to accumulate profits. In pursuit of establishing and preserving market share, some companies have limited their devices to identifiably unique and limited stimulation and implantation parameters; these may evolve through time with shifts in implanter preference but perhaps at a slower rate than is warranted by available data establishing best practices. Our thought is that patients and their pathologies vary, and having the ability to treat all comers within a treatable group is sensible and provides the best care for most patients. A single lead that supports a diverse rather than limited set of anatomical and stimulation profiles is most consistent with this perspective.

J. Feler
Neurosurgery Resident, Brown University, Providence, RI, USA

C. A. Feler (✉)
Carbondale, CO, USA

T. d. S. Freitas et al. (eds.), *Neuromodulation Techniques for Pain Treatment*,
https://doi.org/10.1007/978-3-030-84778-4_4

Why Penta

The Penta lead was designed to obtain paresthetic overlap across multiple, distinct, and varied areas of anatomy from a single lead implant. It was designed to allow both a multitude of cathodal and anodal positions with tight spacing and small contacts (Fig. 1) such that paresthesia might be moved around the patient's anatomy by using multiple program sets employing a combination of cathodal activation and anodal blocking. The lead has a domed shape to better fit the relatively peaked roof of the dorsal spinal canal. Figure 2 shows the electrode number scheme. Notably, there are 20 contacts, with the lateral columns arranged in paired sets such that the final count is 16 separate contacts. The surfaces are microtextured to increase the

Description		Penta, 3 mm
Electrodes are shown facing down (anteriorly)		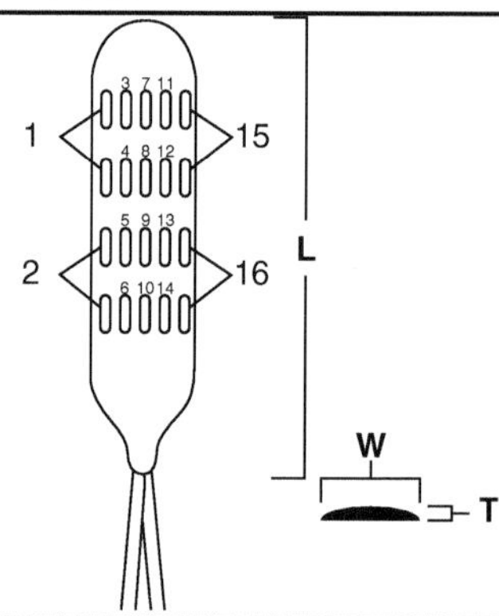
Lead length and model	60 cm	3228
Lead diameter		1.4 mm
Electrodes		
Number		16
Configuration		5 columns of 4
Length		4 mm
width		1 mm
Longitudinal spacing		3 mm
Lateral spacing		1 mm
Array length		25 mm
Array width		9 mm
Paddles		
Length (L, includes taper)		46 mm
width (W)		11 mm
Thickness (T)		2 mm
Lead resistance (for all lengths)		< 10ohms
Differentiation band signifies		Electrodes 1-8

Fig. 1 Engineering specifications for Penta electrode

Table 1 Prognosis for pain relief dependent on pain location and features

	Constant/steady	Mechanical	Responsive to sympathetic block	Unresponsive to sympathetic block
Leg pain	Excellent response expected	Poor response expected	Good response expected	Uncertain response, reasonable to trial
Back pain	Good response expected	Poor response expected	Not relevant	Not relevant
Arm pain	Excellent response expected	Poor response expected	Good response expected	Uncertain response, reasonable to trial
Neck pain	Poor response expected	Poor response expected	Not relevant	Not relevant

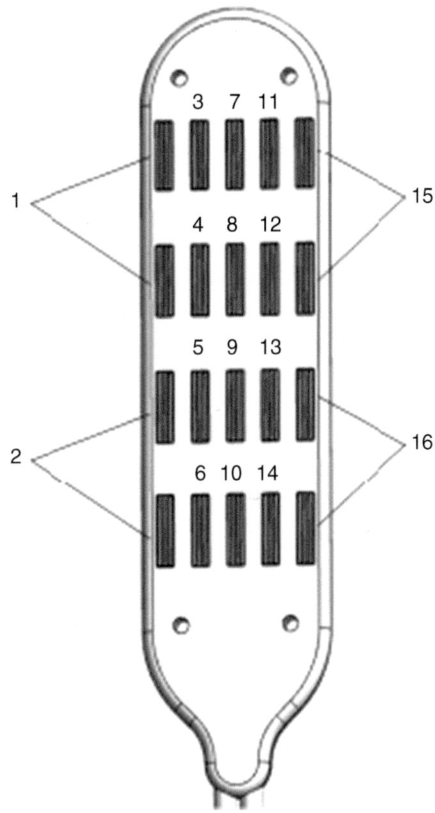

Fig. 2 Channel designations for Penta electrode

contact surface area, limiting current density. Although the generator could have been used to limit power output and thereby current density, if the lead were attached by an implanter to another manufacturer's generator, then unsafe current densities would be possible. This was thought to be unsafe; hence, the microtexturing option was adopted to provide safety in unexpected use cases by clinicians.

The lead has flexible function once implanted. Because of the array and lead dimensions, it provides redundancy such that multiple programs may yield similar effective paresthesia overlap. If a patient prefers a non-paresthesia-producing program, Penta provides this capability while leaving open the possibility of implementing a conventional program when needed. Initial results were presented at NANS in 2009. (Ref. [1])

Indicated Patients

While I recognize that patient selection is not simple, I do my best to select patients for SCS procedures that have significant neuropathic pain. Patients with either CRPS-1 or CRPS-2 are optimally considered, particularly those that describe more than 50% constant, steady pain or have more than 50% pain reducible by repeated sympathetic injections. The greater percentage of appendicular pain vs axial pain, the greater the opportunity for a good outcome. On occasion, patients with CRPS-1 are selected that do not have this proportion of appendicular symptoms, but in my experience, outcomes are inferior in this group. Leg and arm pain is more treatable than back or neck pain. I have found that neck pain is very difficult to treat even with good stimulation overlap. Success in the low back target is dependent on the patient's complaint being constant rather than mechanical.

We understand that many implanters select patients more liberally than we do; nonetheless, our practice is to exclude from trial implantation those patients who report pains that are described in mechanical terms when these complaints exceed 50% of the total pain complaint. With this strategy, I recognize that I likely exclude some patients who would experience some clinical benefit, in pursuit of obtaining better than expected outcomes in those that I do an implant. We do not trial patients to "see if they respond," believing that the trial of stimulation is not a reliable means of assessing a patient's response to permanent implantation.

Our strategy is to select patients carefully based on their clinical characteristics and then to do a percutaneous trial assessing their experience with stimulation: whether or not they like stimulation, how much positional stimulation is obtained, whether or not they prefer non-paresthetic producing programs or conventional paresthesia producing programs, whether or not they note any functional improvement, and what their experience with pain relief is. It is important to manage expectations by educating patients as to which elements of their pain may be treatable and to which I do not expect to respond. Anecdotally, I would note that patients who experience no pain relief with a well-placed, properly functioning stimulator will not have any benefit with a permanent implant. Patients who report intermediate pain relief will likely respond similarly to permanent stimulation. Finally, patients who report "complete" pain relief have the most difficulty predicting long-term outcomes based on the trial of stimulation because these patients may be experiencing a short-term placebo effect that will ultimately fade.

Prior to any intervention with any lead, MRI or myelography should be obtained to assess the intraspinal anatomy in the area through which the lead will pass. This step is fundamental to avoid injury to neural elements during the procedure.

Identification of unexpected areas of degenerative stenosis or disc prolapse is essential.

Preoperative Evaluation

All patients undergo clinical and psychometric evaluation. In my practice, an MMPI-2 has been the standard, along with a formal evaluation with a psychologist. Utilizing the MMPI-2, I exclude patients from consideration if their conversion V (hysteria, hypochondriasis, and depression scores) is exaggeratedly deep. It has been my experience that psychologists are more effective at identifying psychiatric disorders and drug-seeking behaviors that may impact outcomes. I have had the surprising experience of implanting a patient with a dissociative identity disorder. Fortunately, all five of the patient's personalities both liked and got benefit from their stimulation. I feel strongly that a patient should have formal psychological evaluation and clearance prior to the trial of SCS whenever possible to avoid the discovery of contraindications after a "successful" trial. When a patient who has not had formal psychological evaluation is referred for a permanent implant after a successful trial, they are sent for formal evaluation. Many fail to pass the scrutiny of a psychologist. My practice is to not implant these patients. In summary, the entire evaluation team should confer on each patient. Patients who are deemed appropriate for permanent implantation then undergo a trial of stimulation.

Medically, those patients with a history of bleeding diathesis, severe cardiac disease (unless the implant is for off-label use for angina), history of infections with procedures, uncontrolled diabetes, etc. are given consideration, but these patients must be handled with extraordinary care to avoid complications. These typically will require subspecialty consultation to assess their true risk in undergoing a procedure.

Patients are well educated prior to trial or permanent so that they have a full appreciation of what to expect. This education is best provided by both the clinician and the stimulation company's representative.

Operative Method

Implantation of laminectomy electrodes should only be done by physicians properly trained for these procedures and the management of the procedural complications that may occur. This would include neurosurgeons and orthopedic spine surgeons.

Anesthetic methods vary, including local anesthesia with sedation, epidural anesthesia, subarachnoid anesthesia, and general anesthesia. My preference is for general anesthesia with a short-acting paralytic agent during induction. This approach allows for both motor stimulation and EMG monitoring. Some implanters prefer other methods and tout them as safer and more precise; however, in my hands, that has not been the case. Using a general anesthetic, the patient is still, and the procedure is comfortable. If the implanting surgeon has also performed the trial, there is greater awareness and control over lead positioning. Intraoperative stimulation confirms laterality. EMG monitoring also contributes to good positioning.

Once the anesthesia has been established, the patient is placed in a prone position for a thoracic implant. The radiolucent Wilson frame is used to offload the abdomen. This positioning reduces intraspinal venous pressure and improves lordosis to facilitate the approach through the dorsal spinal roof, easing lead advancement.

The surgical approach is determined based on the need for a centrally placed lead or a primarily unilaterally placed lead. While it is possible to place a central lead from a unilateral approach via hemilaminotomy, it is far easier to place a central lead through a midline dissection. The downside to a midline dissection is the removal of the dorsal tension band which may later produce localized mechanical pain (Figs. 3 and 4).

Imaging is used to localize the target and the translaminar entry point, which, for back and leg targets, is T10–11, ultimately placing the lead such that the top of the Penta is near the disk space of T9 and no lower than the mid-pedicle of T9.

Preoperative antibiotics are infused at a time appropriate for the antibiotic selected. This selection depends on local hospital and community bacteriograms and potential known patient hypersensitivities. Antibiotics are continued postoperatively for 24 hours in a permanent implant. This may require an overnight stay.

The incision is planned such that one-third of the incision is cephalad to the planned bony removal and two-thirds of the incision is caudal to that point. This allows the lead to be placed from a caudal direction, lowering the approach angle of the lead to the dura, diminishing the potential impact of the lead onto the spinal cord. Once the skin incision has been made, dissection is carried to the dorsal fascia

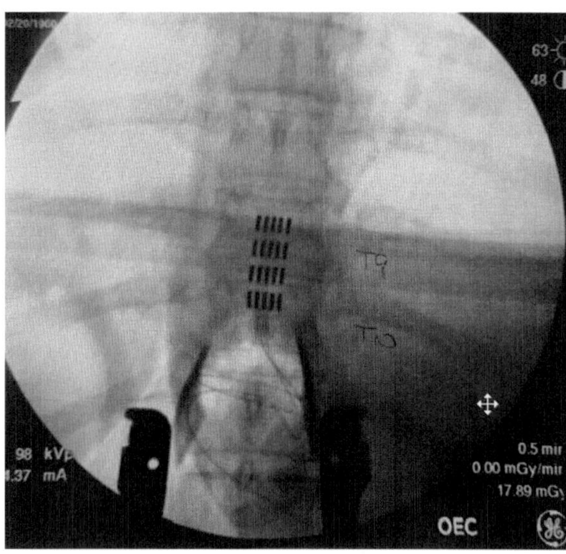

Fig. 3 Penta electrode implanted through a midline dissection at T9–10

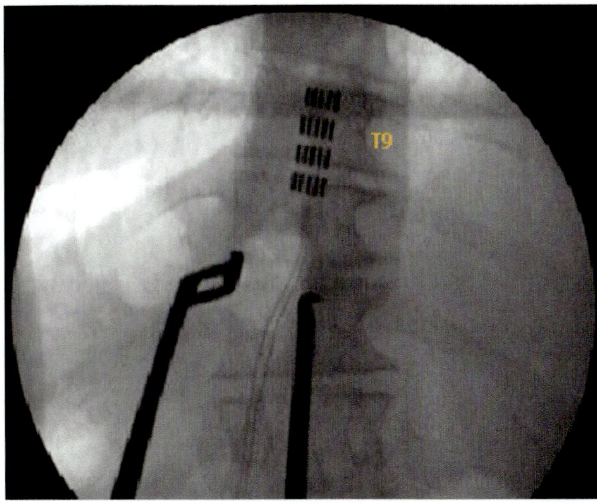

Fig. 4 Penta electrode implanted through a unilateral approach. Respects the midline

with pen cautery, maintaining hemostasis. Retractors are placed to hold the skin and subcutaneous tissue, and if a unilateral approach has been selected, fascia is divided unilaterally, the paraspinous musculature is dissected away for spinous process and laminae, and a unilateral retractor is placed. If a midline dissection is planned, then the supraspinous and interspinous ligaments are divided, following which a portion of both the T10 and T11 spinous processes are resected, with more bone being removed from the T11 process to facilitate a low angle of approach to the spine with the Penta lead.

While magnification is not required for this operation, we use the operating microscope for magnification as well as excellent lighting to visualize the bony elements and, more importantly, the dura when it presents. A high-speed drill is used to remove lamina down to the ligamentum flavum. Once the ligamentum flavum is exposed, a 1 or 2 mm Kerrison Punch with a cervical footplate is used to remove any ligament and remaining bone to create an access corridor through which to deliver the lead. The corridor should be 2–3 millimeters wider and taller than the lead so that there is no friction between the lead and bone/ligament. This allows good tactile feedback from the epidural space. Any sensation of obstructions will be felt and not pushed through. If there is resistance while passing the lead, then an appropriate epidural dissector may be used to dissect further, following which the lead may be placed. As a matter of habit, I do not like to introduce lead blanks prior to placing the lead. Usually, the lead can be placed safely on the first pass, eliminating a step that could create complications to the spinal cord. It is imperative, however, that the lead be placed gently. X-rays should be checked, and intraoperative stimulation is then used to confirm lead placement.

If at all possible, avoid doing complete laminectomies over the lead's final position. Removing the roof of the spinal canal increases the distance from the lead's body to the spinal cord, markedly reducing the efficiency of stimulation. This negatively impacts the ability to cover the needed topography of pain with stimulation and reduces generator efficiencies.

Once the lead's position is felt to be acceptable, the lead is secured to the residual T 11 spinous process with 2–0 Vicryl.

The carrier tubes are then tunneled to a separate generator incision and attached to the generator. Irrigation is copious, following which hemostasis is assessed, particularly from within the spinal canal. If there is any intraspinal bleeding noted, Flowseal™ may be used, followed by additional irrigation, repeating until clear. Consideration for a drain is also reasonable, if brought out through a separate stab wound. After confirming hemostasis, the dorsal lumbar fascia is closed with absorbable suture, and strain relief coils are placed over the fascia as well as deep into the generator. Again the wounds are irrigated and then closed in layers with absorbable sutures and staples for the skin. Other skin closures may be used; however, staples are the least likely to produce wound complications, and they require removal, which mandates an office visit at approximately a week for a wound check.

Initial programming is accomplished immediately postop or no later than the morning after surgery. Patients are followed closely for wound checks and optimization of their programs.

Caveats

1. Place the lead in a position that will provide proper paresthetic overlap even if you initially intend to treat it with a paresthesialess program.
2. Locate the skin incision such that two-thirds of it is caudal to the intended site of bony entry into the spinal canal; this allows for a low angle of approach to the epidural space.
3. Remove sufficient bone and ligament to allow frictionless passage of the lead into the epidural space, allowing good tactile feedback from the epidural space.
4. Avoid doing complete laminectomies at the location of the lead.
5. Obtain excellent hemostasis. Consider using a drain.
6. Leave generous strain relief coils at both incisions.

In patients having a Penta placed for high cervical indications, the positioning is prone with the head restrained in a pin and tong headrest. Chest rolls are placed. This approach has been well described previously (Ref. [2]). The Penta's design provides for coverage of both upper extremities and sometimes the lower extremities from this position. Importantly, the approach is retrograde from above the ring of C1 projecting under the rings of C1 and C2 (Fig. 5). This location is much safer than the mid-cervical canal due to the large epidural space at this location. The lead is anchored to the residual atlanto-occipital membrane with 4–0 suture via the lead body suture hole. An additional lead anchor is not used because this might cause tension between the lead body and the anchor point at the carrier tubes, later leading to a distraction failure secondary to the patient's neck potion.
Summary Comments

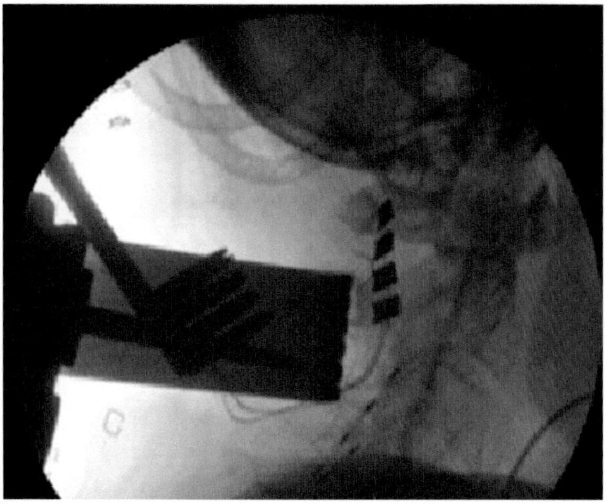

Fig. 5 High cervical implant of a Penta electrode

Proper patient and device selection is essential to obtaining a good result for the patient. Similarly, these devices are highly nuanced and must be implanted in the correct location with skill.

Penta is a lead designed to evoke stimulation either narrowly or broadly via a platform that, because of its relatively small size, is easily implanted. This chapter provides adequate direction for one skilled in the art of spinal surgery to properly place this device.

References

1. North American Neuromodulation Society Annual Meeting. Selective dermatome activation using a novel five-column spinal cord stimulation paddle Lead: a case series Claudio Feler, MD, Semmes-Murphey Neurologic & Spine Institute, Memphis, TN; Jason Garber, MD, Western regional Center for Brain and Spine Surgery. NV: Las Vegas; 2009.
2. Whitworth Louis A, Feler Claudio A. C1-C2 sublaminar insertion of paddle leads for the management of chronic painful conditions of the upper extremity. Neuromodulation. 2003:6.

Deep Brain Stimulation for Pain: Indications and Technique

Clement Hamani

Introduction

Deep brain stimulation is a therapy that involves the delivery of electrical current to the brain parenchyma through implanted electrodes. These are usually placed in specific brain targets with the aid of stereotactic techniques and connected to a pulse generator via extension cables. Parameters that may vary with the use of DBS are the stimulation frequency, pulse width, current amplitude, the use of monopolar or bipolar stimulation, as well as the electrode contacts selected as cathodes or anodes.

The use of electrical stimulation for the treatment of pain has almost 70 years and was one of the first applications of this technique in functional neurosurgery [1–3]. Nevertheless, it was only in the 1970s and 1980s that the use of brain stimulation for pain became more widespread with surgeons in multiple centers worldwide delivering this therapy to the thalamus and internal capsule, as well as the periaqueductal (PAG)/periventricular gray matter (PVG) [4–26]. More recently, stimulation of the anterior cingulum (ACC) has been advocated [27–30]. Despite its relatively widespread use, there has recently been a progressive decline in the number of chronic pain patients treated and centers offering DBS for chronic pain. This is due to several factors, including the development of medications and alternative treatments for nociceptive pain, the poor results of two double-blinded multicenter trials sponsored by a DBS system manufacturer [31–33], and the lack of approval for the use of DBS to treat chronic neuropathic pain in many countries.

C. Hamani (✉)
Sunnybrook Research Institute, Toronto, ON, Canada

Harquail Centre for Neuromodulation, Sunnybrook Health Sciences Centre, Toronto, ON, Canada

Division of Neurosurgery, Sunnybrook Health Sciences Centre, University of Toronto, Toronto, ON, Canada
e-mail: clement.hamani@sunnybrook.ca

T. d. S. Freitas et al. (eds.), *Neuromodulation Techniques for Pain Treatment*,
https://doi.org/10.1007/978-3-030-84778-4_5

In this chapter, we review selection criteria, technical aspects, clinical results, and complications of DBS for the treatment of pain.

Indications and Surgical Aspects

The first step to understand which procedure and brain target to select is the definition of the type of chronic pain (neuropathic or nociceptive), the region of the body compromised, and the clinical condition associated with the development of pain. Despite the lack of comparative studies, it seems that stimulation of the sensory thalamus (e.g. nucleus ventralis caudalis; Vc) has been more commonly indicated for neuropathic pain, whereas historically PAG/PVG stimulation has been offered to nociceptive pain [34–38]. The latter, however, has also been used to treat neuropathic pain, particularly when allodynia is present. Further, many centers implant electrodes in both Vc and PAG/PVG. Anterior cingulum DBS has been more commonly offered in investigational studies to patients with chronic pain intractable to medication who may have failed DBS in the PAG/PVG and/or sensory thalamus, presenting with whole-body or hemibody pain [27]. Other targets investigated in the past and not routinely used to date include the internal capsule [11, 39], septal region [40, 41], and medial thalamus [42–45].

As described above, a slight difference exists between common etiological diagnoses in patients with neuropathic pain treated with DBS. While thalamic stimulation has been more frequently used to treat poststroke pain, spinal cord injury, multiple sclerosis, and phantom limb pain, PAG/PVG has also been used for the treatment of nociceptive pain, including failed back syndrome (FBS) [26].

Surgical candidates are patients who have severe and refractory pain and tried and failed all reasonable medical treatments and physiotherapy. As trying multiple medical therapies is a long process, it usually takes years prior to referral for surgery. An important aspect is that patients need to be screened for psychological or psychosocial overlay and secondary gain. Patients with conditions that contraindicate brain surgery (e.g. coagulopathy) are often not suitable DBS candidates.

From a technical perspective, most centers target the sensory thalamus based on magnetic resonance imaging and indirect coordinates based on the anterior-posterior (AC-PC) commissural plane and midcommissural point (MCP) [26]. The somatosensory thalamic target is the ventralis caudalis nucleus contralateral to the side of the worse pain. Commonly used coordinates are 2–3 mm anterior to PC at the level of the AC-PC plane. Due to the somatotopical representation of the body in the thalamus, the mediolateral coordinate in relation to the midline varies from 12–13 mm lateral for facial pain, to 14–15 mm lateral for upper extremity pain, to 16–17 mm lateral for lower extremity pain. In contrast to the somatosensory thalamus, PAG/PVG may be largely targeted based on direct neuroimaging visualization, as this structure lies near the boundaries of the III ventricle and cerebral aqueduct. Standard coordinates for placement of the electrodes in the region of the PVG are

2–5 mm anterior to PC, 2 mm lateral to the medial wall of the third ventricle, at the level of the AC-PC plane [32, 33, 39, 46].

In addition to neuroimaging, several centers corroborate the precise target for electrode placement using electrophysiology, including microelectrode recordings and micro/macro stimulation. In the sensory thalamus (Vc) [20, 47–50], stimulation with lower current amplitudes leads to perceived paresthesias in projected fields. These are also used to define the placement of actual DBS electrodes. Once in place, stimulation is delivered through electrode contacts to assess whether paresthesias are perceived in the correspondent body region where pain is perceived. During PVG stimulation, patients sometimes report a warm sensation that may be even pleasurable [32, 39, 51]. Ventrally placed electrodes in the region of the PAG may sometimes lead to stimulation-induced sensations of anxiety and fear [32, 39, 51].

Protocols for the postoperative management of chronic pain patients receiving DBS vary according to center. While some externalize the lead for further testing, others implant and connect the pulse generator with the leads in the same surgical procedure. The first allows what is called "test stimulation trial". This consists of the stimulation delivery through externalized wires while patients are still in the hospital. During the test trial, different stimulation settings are delivered to the patient in a tentative to characterize the ones associated with the greatest amount of analgesia and the coverage of the area of pain. In most centers, a trial is considered to be successful if a >50% reduction in pain is achieved with stimulation. Under these circumstances, electrodes are connected to the pulse generator and the DBS system initially programmed according to settings considered to be optimal. If the test trial is negative, the electrode and the extension cable are removed. On average, it is estimated that 60% of trialed patients have a positive response and end up being implanted with an IPG [26].

Postoperative Aspects and Results

During programming sessions, an important aspect is to deliver stimulation to painful regions at settings that induce paresthesias considered to be pleasant [19, 32, 39, 51]. Commonly used parameters for thalamic stimulation are frequencies around 100 Hz, 60–210 microseconds of pulse width, and 2–5 V [19, 24, 26, 32, 33, 39, 51]. In the PVG, one searches for stimulation-induced warmth sensations. Commonly used settings are 10–25 Hz, 60–210 microseconds, and 1-5 V [13, 33, 46, 51, 52].

The long-term outcome of DBS for the treatment of chronic neuropathic pain is quite variable, with most studies showing a response in 20–70% of the patients [7, 10, 14, 17–19, 21, 23, 24, 32–39, 46, 51, 53–57]. Part of the variability seems to be due to the fact that there are multiple conditions treated with DBS at different targets, the parallel use of analgesic medications, the inclusion of all patients vs. only those who present a positive stimulation trial, and the length of follow-up. In general, neuropathic pain patients seem to fare worse than those with nociceptive pain and studies that only include patients who did well in the test stimulation trial tend to show a better response [26]. Another aspect believed to influence the outcome is the diagnosis associated with chronic neuropathic pain. Those forecasting a better analgesic response include complex regional pain syndrome (CRPS), phantom limb, and peripheral neuropathies, compared to postherpetic neuralgia, brachial plexus avulsion, or thalamic pain [33, 35–38, 58–61]. In some studies, a long-term outcome following DBS was shown to be worse than at short term [26]. Reasons to explain the loss of benefit recorded over time are unclear but may involve plasticity of neuronal circuits and tolerance, predominantly described after PAG/PVG stimulation [39, 62]. Independent on the reason, the variability in study results, the sometimes reported loss of benefit over time, combined with the poor outcome reported in two open-labeled multicenter studies sponsored by one of the manufacturers of the stimulators (Medtronic) [63], substantially reduced the interest in the field.

In a recent series of studies, the ACC was investigated as a potential DBS target in patients with chronic pain [27–30]. Following a test stimulation trial, most patients ended up implanted with pulse generators. At 6 months and 1 year postoperatively, numerical rating pain scores improved by 60% and 43%, respectively [27]. In addition to pain relief, ACC DBS was associated with improvements in affective components of pain [27, 28]. A major complication of anterior cingulum DBS seems to be the development of afterdischarges and seizures [27, 64]. Though these can be somewhat controlled following changes in cycling patterns and the ramping of stimulation delivery, these side effects are fairly concerning [27, 64].

Another target recently proposed to modulate affective components of pain was the ventral striatum/anterior limb of the internal capsule (VS/ALIC) [65]. In a recent report, patients with poststroke pain were implanted with VS/ALIC electrodes and randomized to blindly receive active or sham DBS [65]. Though no significant differences were found between active or sham stimulation on the Pain Disability Index (primary outcome variable), significant differences were found on outcome measures related to the affective sphere of pain [65].

Finally, it is worth mentioning that DBS is also being investigated for cluster headaches. Substantial reductions in the frequency and duration of cluster episodes have been reported in open-label studies [66–71], with no significant differences being recorded in trials conducting blinded assessments of active versus sham stimulation [72].

Hardware- and surgical-related adverse effects of DBS for pain are somewhat similar to those recorded in other conditions [35–38, 73]. The most common ones are intracranial hemorrhages (1–2% risk), lead migration, breakage of the wires and leads that need to be repositioned (approximately 5%), and infections (3–5%) [74].

Conclusions

Despite the promising results of open-label studies, more recent series and two double-blinded multicenter trials sponsored by one of the manufacturers of the device have shown worst outcomes compared to the older literature [31–33]. That said, patients who respond to DBS often present striking results. As DBS is often considered to be one of the last resort alternatives for the clinical management of refractory chronic pain patients, further research is definitely required. With recent progress on imaging modalities, new electrode designs, electrophysiological testing, and the better appreciation of clinical phenotypes, the development of biomarkers capable of predicting treatment response is of great urgency. This, combined with technological advancements, may revitalize the field.

References

1. Heath RG. Studies in schizophrenia: a multidisciplinary approach to mind-brain relationships. Cambridge, MA: Harvard University Press; 1954.
2. Heath RG, Mickle WA. Evaluation of seven years' experience with depth electrode studies in human patients. In: Ramey ER, O'Doherty DS, editors. Electrical studies on the unanesthetized human brain. New York: Paul B. Hoeber, Inc.; 1960. p. 214–47.
3. Pool JL, Clark WK, Hudson P, Lombardo M. Steroid hormonal response to stimulation of electrodes implanted in the subfrontal parts of the brain. In: Fields WS, Guillemin R, Carton CA, editors. Hypothalamic-hypophysial interrelationships, a symposium. Sprigfield: Charles C. Thomas; 1956. p. 114–24.
4. Mazars G, Merienne L, Cioloca C. [Treatment of certain types of pain with implantable thalamic stimulators]. Neurochirurgie. 1974;20(2):117–24.
5. Mazars G, Merienne L, Ciolocca C. [Intermittent analgesic thalamic stimulation. Preliminary note]. Rev Neurol (Paris). 1973;128(4):273–9.
6. Mazars G, Rogé R, Mazars Y. Résultats de la stimulation du faisceau spinothalamique et leur incidence sur la physiopathologie de la douleur. Rev Neurol (Paris). 1960;103(2):136–8.
7. Mazars GJ. Intermittent stimulation of nucleus ventralis posterolateralis for intractable pain. Surg Neurol. 1975;4(1):93–5.
8. White JC, Sweet WH. Pain and the neurosurgeon: a 40-year experience. Springfield: Charles C. Thomas; 1969.
9. Hosobuchi Y, Adams JE, Rutkin B. Chronic thalamic stimulation for the control of facial anesthesia dolorosa. Arch Neurol. 1973;29(3):158–61.
10. Hosobuchi Y, Adams JE, Rutkin B. Chronic thalamic and internal capsule stimulation for the control of central pain. Surg Neurol. 1975;4(1):91–2.
11. Adams JE, Hosobuchi Y, Fields HL. Stimulation of internal capsule for relief of chronic pain. J Neurosurg. 1974;41(6):740–4.
12. Fields HL, Adams JE. Pain after cortical injury relieved by electrical stimulation of the internal capsule. Brain. 1974;97(1):169–78.
13. Richardson DE, Akil H. Long term results of periventricular gray self-stimulation. Neurosurgery. 1977;1(2):199–202.
14. Richardson DE, Akil H. Pain reduction by electrical brain stimulation in man. Part 2: chronic self-administration in the periventricular gray matter. J Neurosurg. 1977;47(2):184–94.
15. Richardson DE, Akil H. Pain reduction by electrical brain stimulation in man. Part 1: acute administration in periaqueductal and periventricular sites. J Neurosurg. 1977;47(2):178–83.
16. Hosobuchi Y, Adams JE, Linchitz R. Pain relief by electrical stimulation of the central gray matter in humans and its reversal by naloxone. Science. 1977;197(4299):183–6.
17. Dieckmann G, Witzmann A. Initial and long-term results of deep brain stimulation for chronic intractable pain. Appl Neurophysiol. 1982;45(1–2):167–72.
18. Gybels J, Kupers R. Central and peripheral electrical stimulation of the nervous system in the treatment of chronic pain. Acta Neurochir Suppl (Wien). 1987;38:64–75.

19. Hosobuchi Y. Subcortical electrical stimulation for control of intractable pain in humans. Report of 122 cases (1970-1984). J Neurosurg. 1986;64(4):543–53.
20. Lenz FA, Tasker RR, Dostrovsky JO, Kwan HC, Gorecki J, Hirayama T, et al. Abnormal single-unit activity recorded in the somatosensory thalamus of a quadriplegic patient with central pain. Pain. 1987;31(2):225–36.
21. Plotkin R. Results in 60 cases of deep brain stimulation for chronic intractable pain. Appl Neurophysiol. 1982;45(1–2):173–8.
22. Siegfried J, Lazorthes Y, Sedan R. Indications and ethical considerations of deep brain stimulation. Acta Neurochir Suppl (Wien). 1980;30:269–74.
23. Tasker RR, Vilela FO. Deep brain stimulation for neuropathic pain. Stereotact Funct Neurosurg. 1995;65(1–4):122–4.
24. Turnbull IM, Shulman R, Woodhurst WB. Thalamic stimulation for neuropathic pain. J Neurosurg. 1980;52(4):486–93.
25. Young RF, Kroening R, Fulton W, Feldman RA, Chambi I. Electrical stimulation of the brain in treatment of chronic pain. Experience over 5 years. J Neurosurg. 1985;62(3):389–96.
26. Hamani C, Fontaine D, Lozano AM. DBS for persistent non-cancer pain. In: Lozano AM, Gildenberg PL, Tasker RR, editors. Textbook of stereotactic and functional neurosurgery. Berlin/Heidelberg: Springer; 2009. p. 2227–38.
27. Boccard SGJ, Prangnell SJ, Pycroft L, Cheeran B, Moir L, Pereira EAC, et al. Long-term results of deep brain stimulation of the anterior cingulate cortex for neuropathic pain. World Neurosurg. 2017;106:625–37.
28. Boccard SG, Fitzgerald JJ, Pereira EA, Moir L, Van Hartevelt TJ, Kringelbach ML, et al. Targeting the affective component of chronic pain: a case series of deep brain stimulation of the anterior cingulate cortex. Neurosurgery. 2014;74(6):628–35; discussion 35–7.
29. Boccard SG, Pereira EA, Moir L, Van Hartevelt TJ, Kringelbach ML, FitzGerald JJ, et al. Deep brain stimulation of the anterior cingulate cortex: targeting the affective component of chronic pain. Neuroreport. 2014;25(2):83–8.
30. Spooner J, Yu H, Kao C, Sillay K, Konrad P. Neuromodulation of the cingulum for neuropathic pain after spinal cord injury. Case report. J Neurosurg. 2007;107(1):169–72.
31. Coffey RJ, Lozano AM. Neurostimulation for chronic noncancer pain: an evaluation of the clinical evidence and recommendations for future trial designs. J Neurosurg. 2006;105(2):175–89.
32. Hamani C, Schwalb JM, Rezai AR, Dostrovsky JO, Davis KD, Lozano AM. Deep brain stimulation for chronic neuropathic pain: long-term outcome and the incidence of insertional effect. Pain. 2006;125(1–2):188–96.
33. Rasche D, Rinaldi PC, Young RF, Tronnier VM. Deep brain stimulation for the treatment of various chronic pain syndromes. Neurosurg Focus. 2006;21(6):E8.
34. Bittar RG, Kar-Purkayastha I, Owen SL, Bear RE, Green A, Wang S, et al. Deep brain stimulation for pain relief: a meta-analysis. J Clin Neurosci. 2005;12(5):515–9.
35. Levy RM. Deep brain stimulation for the treatment of intractable pain. Neurosurg Clin N Am. 2003;14(3):389–99, vi.
36. Levy RM, Lamb S, Adams JE. Treatment of chronic pain by deep brain stimulation: long term follow-up and review of the literature. Neurosurgery. 1987;21(6):885–93.
37. Rezai AR, Lozano AM. Deep brain stimulation for chronic pain. In: Burchiel KJ, editor. Surgical management of pain. New York: Thieme Medical Publishers, Inc; 2002. p. 565–74.
38. Wallace BA, Ashkan K, Benabid AL. Deep brain stimulation for the treatment of chronic, intractable pain. Neurosurg Clin N Am. 2004;15(3):343–57, vii.
39. Kumar K, Wyant GM, Nath R. Deep brain stimulation for control of intractable pain in humans, present and future: a ten-year follow-up. Neurosurgery. 1990;26(5):774–81; discussion 81–2.
40. Schvarcz JR. Chronic stimulation of the septal area for the relief of intractable pain. Appl Neurophysiol. 1985;48(1–6):191–4.
41. Schvarcz JR. Long-term results of stimulation of the septal area for relief of neurogenic pain. Acta Neurochir Suppl (Wien). 1993;58:154–5.

42. Andy OJ. Parafascicular-center median nuclei stimulation for intractable pain and dyskinesia (painful-dyskinesia). Appl Neurophysiol. 1980;43(3–5):133–44.
43. Andy OJ. Thalamic stimulation for chronic pain. Appl Neurophysiol. 1983;46(1–4):116–23.
44. Schvarcz JR. Chronic self-stimulation of the medial posterior inferior thalamus for the alleviation of deafferentation pain. Acta Neurochir Suppl (Wien). 1980;30:295–301.
45. Thoden U, Doerr M, Dieckmann G, Krainick JU. Medial thalamic permanent electrodes for pain control in man: an electrophysiological and clinical study. Electroencephalogr Clin Neurophysiol. 1979;47(5):582–91.
46. Owen SL, Green AL, Stein JF, Aziz TZ. Deep brain stimulation for the alleviation of post-stroke neuropathic pain. Pain. 2006;120(1–2):202–6.
47. Davis KD, Kiss ZH, Tasker RR, Dostrovsky JO. Thalamic stimulation-evoked sensations in chronic pain patients and in nonpain (movement disorder) patients. J Neurophysiol. 1996;75(3):1026–37.
48. Lenz FA, Dostrovsky JO, Tasker RR, Yamashiro K, Kwan HC, Murphy JT. Single-unit analysis of the human ventral thalamic nuclear group: somatosensory responses. J Neurophysiol. 1988;59(2):299–316.
49. Lenz FA, Kwan HC, Martin R, Tasker R, Richardson RT, Dostrovsky JO. Characteristics of somatotopic organization and spontaneous neuronal activity in the region of the thalamic principal sensory nucleus in patients with spinal cord transection. J Neurophysiol. 1994;72(4):1570–87.
50. Tasker RR. Microelectrode findings in the thalamus in chronic pain and other conditions. Stereotact Funct Neurosurg. 2001;77(1–4):166–8.
51. Kumar K, Toth C, Nath RK. Deep brain stimulation for intractable pain: a 15-year experience. Neurosurgery. 1997;40(4):736–46; discussion 46–7.
52. Young RF, Chambi VI. Pain relief by electrical stimulation of the periaqueductal and periventricular gray matter. Evidence for a non-opioid mechanism. J Neurosurg. 1987;66(3):364–71.
53. Nandi D, Aziz TZ. Deep brain stimulation in the management of neuropathic pain and multiple sclerosis tremor. J Clin Neurophysiol. 2004;21(1):31–9.
54. Owen SL, Green AL, Nandi DD, Bittar RG, Wang S, Aziz TZ. Deep brain stimulation for neuropathic pain. Acta Neurochir Suppl. 2007;97(Pt 2):111–6.
55. Siegfried J. Monopolar electrical stimulation of nucleus ventroposteromedialis thalami for postherpetic facial pain. Appl Neurophysiol. 1982;45(1–2):179–84.
56. Bittar RG, Burn SC, Bain PG, Owen SL, Joint C, Shlugman D, et al. Deep brain stimulation for movement disorders and pain. J Clin Neurosci. 2005;12(4):457–63.
57. Nandi D, Smith H, Owen S, Joint C, Stein J, Aziz T. Peri-ventricular grey stimulation versus motor cortex stimulation for post stroke neuropathic pain. J Clin Neurosci. 2002;9(5):557–61.
58. Whitworth LA, Fernandez J, Feler CA. Deep brain stimulation for chronic pain. Semin Neurosurg. 2004;15(2–3):183–93.
59. Boccard SG, Pereira EA, Moir L, Aziz TZ, Green AL. Long-term outcomes of deep brain stimulation for neuropathic pain. Neurosurgery. 2013;72(2):221–30; discussion 31.
60. Frizon LA, Yamamoto EA, Nagel SJ, Simonson MT, Hogue O, Machado AG. Deep brain stimulation for pain in the modern era: a systematic review. Neurosurgery. 2020;86(2):191–202.
61. Pereira EA, Boccard SG, Linhares P, Chamadoira C, Rosas MJ, Abreu P, et al. Thalamic deep brain stimulation for neuropathic pain after amputation or brachial plexus avulsion. Neurosurg Focus. 2013;35(3):E7.
62. Tsubokawa T, Yamamoto T, Katayama Y, Hirayama T, Sibuya H. Thalamic relay nucleus stimulation for relief of intractable pain. Clinical results and beta-endorphin immunoreactivity in the cerebrospinal fluid. Pain. 1984;18(2):115–26.
63. Coffey RJ. Deep brain stimulation for chronic pain: results of two multicenter trials and a structured review. Pain Med. 2001;2(3):183–92.
64. Huang Y, Cheeran B, Green AL, Denison TJ, Aziz TZ. Applying a sensing-enabled system for ensuring safe anterior cingulate deep brain stimulation for pain. Brain Sci. 2019;9(7):150.

65. Lempka SF, Malone DA Jr, Hu B, Baker KB, Wyant A, Ozinga JG, et al. Randomized clinical trial of deep brain stimulation for poststroke pain. Ann Neurol. 2017;81(5):653–63.
66. Seijo F, Saiz A, Lozano B, Santamarta E, Alvarez-Vega M, Seijo E, et al. Neuromodulation of the posterolateral hypothalamus for the treatment of chronic refractory cluster headache: experience in five patients with a modified anatomical target. Cephalalgia. 2011;31(16):1634–41.
67. Leone M, Franzini A, Broggi G, Bussone G. Hypothalamic stimulation for intractable cluster headache: long-term experience. Neurology. 2006;67(1):150–2.
68. Leone M, Franzini A, Broggi G, May A, Bussone G. Long-term follow-up of bilateral hypothalamic stimulation for intractable cluster headache. Brain. 2004;127(Pt 10):2259–64.
69. Leone M, Franzini A, Bussone G. Stereotactic stimulation of posterior hypothalamic gray matter in a patient with intractable cluster headache. N Engl J Med. 2001;345(19):1428–9.
70. Franzini A, Messina G, Cordella R, Marras C, Broggi G. Deep brain stimulation of the posteromedial hypothalamus: indications, long-term results, and neurophysiological considerations. Neurosurg Focus. 2010;29(2):E13.
71. Bartsch T, Pinsker MO, Rasche D, Kinfe T, Hertel F, Diener HC, et al. Hypothalamic deep brain stimulation for cluster headache: experience from a new multicase series. Cephalalgia. 2008;28(3):285–95.
72. Fontaine D, Lazorthes Y, Mertens P, Blond S, Geraud G, Fabre N, et al. Safety and efficacy of deep brain stimulation in refractory cluster headache: a randomized placebo-controlled double-blind trial followed by a 1-year open extension. J Headache Pain. 2010;11(1):23–31.
73. Hamani C, Ewerton FI, Bonilha SM, Ballester G, Mello LE, Lozano AM. Bilateral anterior thalamic nucleus lesions and high-frequency stimulation are protective against pilocarpine-induced seizures and status epilepticus. Neurosurgery. 2004;54(1):191–5; discussion 5–7.
74. Hamani C, Lozano AM. Hardware-related complications of deep brain stimulation: a review of the published literature. Stereotact Funct Neurosurg. 2006;84(5–6):248–51.

Introduction to Dorsal Root Ganglion Stimulation an Overview of the Field

Keith-Austin Scarfo, Pavli S. Demian, Natalie Strand, Corey Hunter, and Timothy R. Deer

Introduction

The application of neuromodulation started in the late 1960s with the advent of dorsal column stimulation for surgical treatment of chronic pain as first described by Shealy in 1967. While traditional SCS has provided efficacious and cost-effective treatment for patients with chronic pain, there have been challenges with regard to focal pain or CRPS, particularly in the feet [1–4]. Evidence shows that SCS fairs no better than physical therapy over time with CRPS [5], largely due to the inability to consistently capture the focal areas like the foot or the creation of unwanted paresthesias in unaffected areas. It was not until recently that the dorsal root ganglion, itself, was discovered to be directly implicated in the creation and perpetuation of neuropathic pain [6].

Numerous attempts have been made with limited success to utilize techniques and hardware from dorsal column stimulation to directly target the DRG. These attempts have ultimately resulted in failure due to anatomical and hardware

K.-A. Scarfo (✉)
Department of Neurosurgery, Warren Alpert Medical School of Brown University, Providence, RI, USA

Rhode Island Hospital, Norman Prince Spine Insititue, Providence, RI, USA
e-mail: kscarfo@lifespan.org

P. S. Demian
The Pain Management Center, Hamilton Township, NJ, USA

N. Strand
Mayo Clinic Arizona, Phoenix, AZ, USA

C. Hunter
Ainsworth Institute of Pain Management, New York, NY, USA

T. R. Deer
The Spine and Nerve Center of The Virginias, Charleston, WV, USA

T. d. S. Freitas et al. (eds.), *Neuromodulation Techniques for Pain Treatment*,
https://doi.org/10.1007/978-3-030-84778-4_6

considerations ranging from lead placement in the neuroforamen to the delivery of significant overstimulation of the DRG. Neuromodulation, with its multiple uses, continued to have a significant shortcoming to include the relative lack of reliability in delivering stimulation and subsequent pain relief in focal neuropathic pain, nerve injury, and neuropathy [1–6].

As far back as the mid-twentieth century, the dorsal root ganglion was thought to be predominantly a support structure with an accessory role in sensory transmission and thus was targeted for chronic pain [7]. However, it was not until the early 1990s when direct stimulation of the DRG for the treatment of chronic pain was first studied in an animal model. Almost 20 years would transpire before animal research was translated into a human feasibility study for DRG stimulation by Deer et al. in 2009 (Fig. 1). Ultimately, the decision was made to target the dorsal root ganglion over the dorsal column for the purpose of regulating the passage of action potentials via the T-junction of the neuronal cell bodies contained within the ganglion as well as providing focal stimulation to specific regions of the body. In 2011, a larger international study further demonstrated the safety and efficacy of DRG stimulation [8, 9].

In 2012, a prospective, single-arm, pilot study demonstrated the potential for use of dorsal root ganglion stimulation to treat chronic pain targeting difficult-to-reach

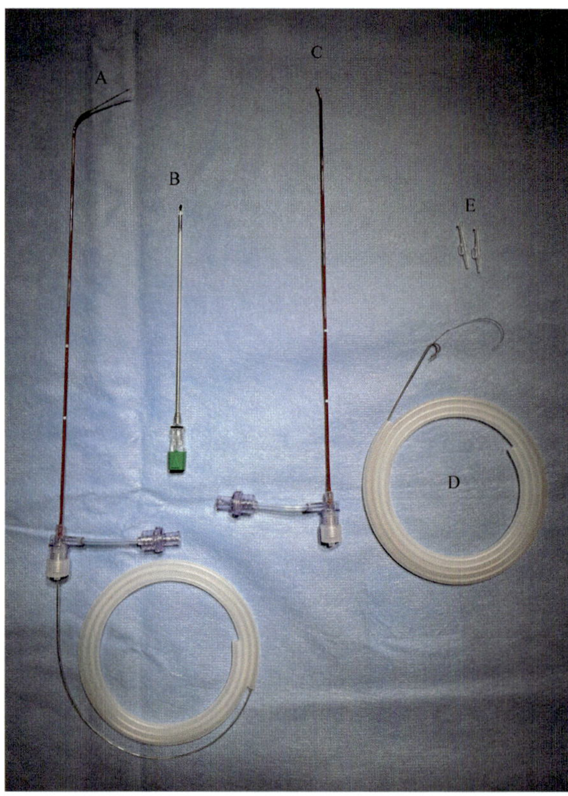

Fig. 1 (**a**) Delivery sheath with big curve and lead inserted. (**b**) Delivery needle. (**c**) Delivery sheath small curve. (**d**) Guidewire and lead stylet. (**e**) Lead anchors

anatomic regions such as the foot. As the potential for DRG stimulation was realized, indications grew to include pelvic pain, complex regional pain syndrome, post-thoracotomy pain, phantom limb pain, post-hernia pain, postsurgical pain, and painful peripheral diabetic neuropathy. These added indications have broadened the awareness of multiple specialties that previously were not involved in the management of chronic pain and provided an option for patients who previously had none. After careful review of safety and efficacy data, Food and Drug Administration granted premarket approval to Axium Neurostimulator Systems in 2016 [10–18].

Real-World Evidence

The use of DRG for the treatment of neuropathic pain syndromes has been shown to be efficacious and is supported by peer-reviewed evidence. Given the variety of neuropathic pain syndromes, the decision to treat with DRG stimulation should be evaluated based on the currently available evidence for each specific neuropathic process [19].

Complex regional pain syndrome has been one of the most highly studied and well-established indications for DRG stimulation given the ACCURATE study which demonstrated superiority to SCS stimulation for subjects with diagnosed CRPS over 12 months [12]. A prospective case series by Van Buyten et al. in which 8 out of 11 subjects with unilateral or bilateral lower extremity CRPS were implanted with DRG stimulation devices. At one-month follow-up, average self-reported pain was reduced by 62% as compared to baseline. Some subjects had improvement in edema and trophic changes associated with CRPS [20].

DRG stimulation has been shown to be helpful in the treatment of painful diabetic peripheral neuropathy (PDPN) as demonstrated in two retrospective case studies. Schu et al. implanted seven patients following a successful trial with cervical and lumbar leads to target patients PDPN and followed patients through 25 months demonstrating sustained 50% improvement in subjects' pain [16]. A second series trialed ten male patients with diabetes and a diagnosis of DPDN in the lower limbs. Seven of the ten patients proceeded to implantation with at least 50% improvement in pain after the trial. At 6-month follow-up, there was an average of 58.4% VAS improvement. Nondiabetic peripheral neuropathies (idiopathic, HIV-related, chemotherapy-induced) are also associated with severe pain, and the effect of DRG stimulation has been less frequently studied. A retrospective analysis of DRG stimulation did evaluate eight patients with mixed neuropathic diagnoses. After 6 weeks, 4 out of the 5 patients with poly-sensory neuropathy, 1 patient with chronic radiculopathy, and 2/2 PDPN patients had greater than 50% response in VAS improvement. The mean overall improvement in pain at 6 weeks was a 79.5% reduction in VAS as compared to baseline [21, 22].

Chronic postsurgical pain (CPSP; excluding CRPS I&II) after surgical intervention including joint replacement, abdominal surgery, thoracotomy, and mastectomy is common [13, 23, 24]. Espinet conducted a retrospective single-center case series in which 16 patients were implanted with DRG systems following a successful trial (>50% pain relief). Most of the diagnoses were either abdominal pain or knee pain with lead placement from T1 through S4 DRGs (Fig. 2). At 6 months post implant, there was shown an average of 77.2% VAS improvement compared to baseline [25]. A similar noncontrolled study of CPSP by Liam et al. implanted DRG stimulation systems in 29 of 36 patients with CPSP [26]. At 3 and 6 months, overall and segmental pain relief were 64.0% ($N = 16$) and 76.4% ($N = 24$) respectively [15, 24]. Breel et al. reported on 30 subjects with chronic postsurgical neuropathic pain with pain located in the trunk/groin/abdomen among other body locations. Of the 30 patients, 26 proceeded to implantation. At 6 months of treatment, patients had an average of 45% pain reduction, and 83% of patients reported pain relief in their normal pain areas. Fifty percent of the patients were at subthreshold stimulation [27]. A retrospective review was performed by Schu et al. on neuropathic groin pain (Fig. 3). Twenty-five of 29 patients were implanted with the DRG system after a successful trial at target DRGs between T12 and L4. At approximately 28 weeks, the average VAS pain reduction was 71.4%, and 19 of 23 patients experienced a >50% reduction in their pain. Of note, a sub-analysis of the post-herniorrhaphy cohort also showed significant improvement [15]. A case series demonstrated L1/S2 lead placement as a potentially effective long-term treatment modality for chronic pelvic pain [11].

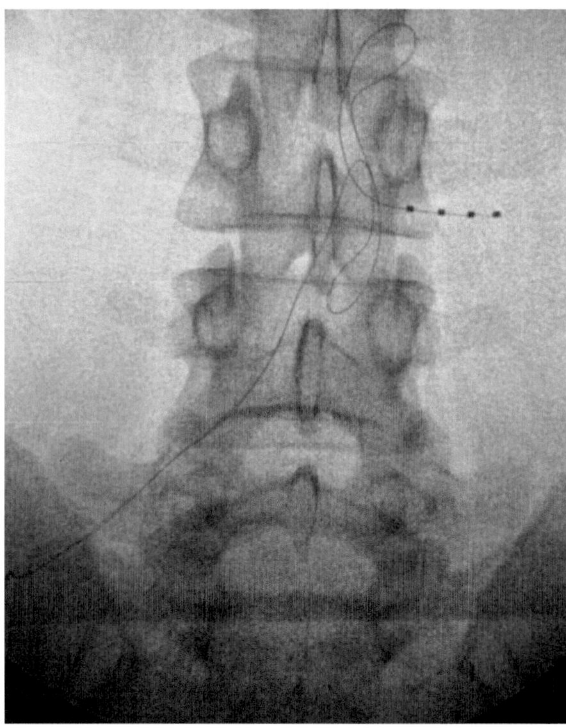

Fig. 2 Lead placement in the anterior-posterior view. The right L3 DRG is targeted for the treatment of knee pain

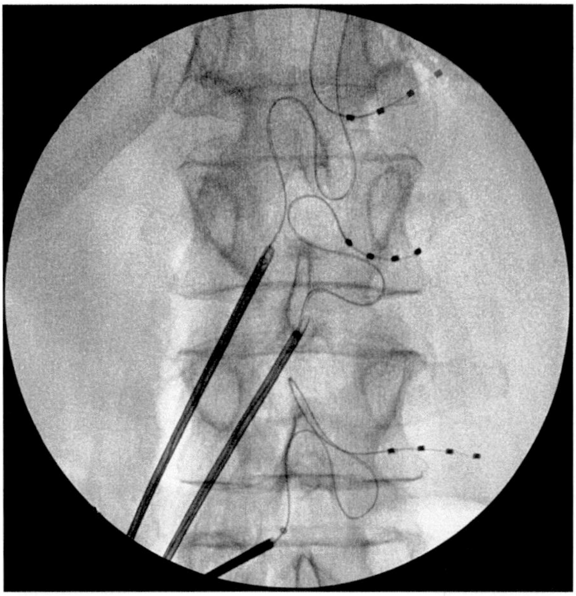

Fig. 3 Lead placement in the anterior-posterior view. The right T12, L1, and L2 DRGs are targeted for the treatment of hip and groin pain. Note the different approaches for epidural needle placement to accommodate varying lead delivery techniques

DRG has also shown significant promise in the treatment of post-herpetic neuralgia [PHN] given the focal nature of this neuropathic pain syndrome [28, 29]. There continues to be discussion regarding lead placement, at the level of injury verses above and below, due to the DRG being damaged in PHN [19].

Phantom limb pain [PLP] is another condition with focal neuropathic pain perceived in an amputated limb. Eldabe et al. performed an eight-patient retrospective study with average baseline pain of 85.5 mm. At follow-up (mean 14.4 months), pain was rated 43.5 mm with improvement in subjective ratings of quality of life and functional improvement. Some patients reduced or eliminated pain medications [14]. Hunter et al. published similar findings on the utility of DRG for the treatment of post amputee pain in a four-patient study using radiofrequency ablation to "map" which dorsal root ganglion should be targeted during the trial and subsequent implant.

Clinical Efficacy

The feasibility of targeting the dorsal root ganglion was established in a prospective, multicenter, single-arm, pilot study which enrolled 10 subjects with chronic intractable neuropathic pain of the trunk and/or limbs. Patients were implanted with an average of 2.9 leads attached to an external generator. At baseline, the overall mean VAS score was 73 ± 10 mm. The average pain reduction between baseline and final visit 4 weeks later was 70 ± 32%. The average decrease in back pain was 84 ± 22%. The average decrease in leg and foot pain was 80 ± 26% and 70 ± 30%, respectively.

There were no changes in stimulation output due to changes in body position and leads were removed and subjects exited the study after the last follow-up [3].

The long-term viability of neurostimulation of the DRG was furthered in a study by Liem et al. Thirty-two subjects were implanted with DRG stimulation and followed for 6 months with 2 weeklong "washout" periods (posttrial and 4 weeks post implant). At all assessments, more than half of the subjects reported pain relief of 50% or better. At 6 months post implant, average overall pain ratings were 58% lower than baseline [$p < 0.001$], and the proportions of subjects experiencing 50% or more reduction in pain specific to back, leg, and foot regions were 57%, 70%, and 89%, respectively. When stimulation was discontinued for a short time, pain returned to baseline levels [4].

The ACCURATE trial is a prospective, randomized, controlled, multicenter study to evaluate the safety and efficacy of the DRG stimulation compare to traditional spinal cord stimulation in subjects with chronic complex regional pain. After a successful trial period (50% pain relief), a total of 115 subjects were implanted with the device [DRG-61, 54-SCS]. Subjects were followed up for 12 months with 3-, 6-, 9-month intervals post implant. Superiority was also established with DRG as compared to traditional SCS with DRG subjects experiencing significantly less postural variation in perceived paresthesia as compared to SCS. Other endpoints included SF-36, POMS, BPI, subject satisfaction, stimulation specificity, and percentage change in VAS which demonstrated non-inferiority with DRG and superiority with SF-36 and BPI [12].

Further studies demonstrated additional indications for DRG stimulation. A retrospective review showed that lead placement between T12 and L4 demonstrated an improvement in groin pain, including post-herniorrhaphy pain over 6 months [15]. A case series demonstrated L1/S2 lead placement as a potentially effective long-term treatment modality for chronic pelvic pain [7]. DRG was also found to be effective in low back pain due to FBSS that did not respond to SCS through 12 months [30].

Safety of Dorsal Root Ganglion Stimulation

There have been multiple publications addressing the safety of dorsal root ganglion stimulation. Most notable are the ACCURATE study and the retrospective review published by Sivanesan which utilize data from the MAUDE database. In a follow-up to the ACCURATE study, a post-market safety analysis of DRG was also carried out by Deer et al. utilizing a large consecutive cohort of patients obtained from the manufacture.

ACCURATE was a prospective, multicenter trial which enrolled 152 patients and randomized 76 of them to DRG therapy and the remaining 76 patients to dorsal column stimulation [SCS]. Adverse events were collected and categorized as an unfavorable and/or unintended sign, symptom, or disease temporarily associated with the use of the implanted device. The authors stratified adverse events as serious if they were immediately life-threatening and resulting in persistent, permanent disability as well as necessitating invasive intervention to prevent permanent impairment or death, resulting in the need for a 24-hour hospital stay or longer. The safety analysis reported 8 severe adverse events of 76 patients in the DRG arm or 10.5% as compared to SCS with 11 of 76 patients or 14.5%. There was no statistical difference comparing severe adverse events between these DRG and SCS ($P = 0.62$). Throughout the study period, there were no unanticipated SAE or stimulation-induced neurological deficits and no deaths of study subjects. There were 52 procedure-related events reported by 35 patients in the DRG arm or 46.1% as compared to 29 procedure-related events reported by 20 patients in the SCS arm or 26.3%. The adverse event data showed a statistical difference between the DRG and SCS arms of the study ($P = 0.018$). The authors hypothesize that the additional procedure time (average 107.2 vs 75.7 minutes) and the number of leads (3 or 4 vs 1 or 2) required for the placement of DRG as compared to SCS most likely contributed to this difference. For both DRG and SCS, the most common procedure-related adverse event reported was pain at the procedure site. Device-related adverse events showed no statistical difference ($P = 0.22$) when DRG is compared head-to-head with SCS [12, 31].

In 2019, a post-market safety analysis of DRG stimulation was published in a follow-up to the ACCURATE study. This post-market surveillance utilized records for both DRG stimulation and SCS obtained from the manufacturer, Abbott Neuromodulation (Chicago, IL, USA), dating between April of 2016 and March of 2018 compiled the safety and compliance associated with DRG therapy as compared to spinal cord stimulation (SCS). Device manufactures are required to maintain compliant event data providing Deer et al. with accurate and complete reporting for a cohort study. The manufacturer's data revealed a large consecutive cohort of patient adverse event data for >500 DRG and >2000 spinal cord stimulator implants for analysis. The adverse event rate for DRG and SCS were 3.2% and 3.1%, respectively. The most common adverse event reported for both DRG and SCS was infection at a comparable rate of 1.08% and 1.12%, respectively, followed by device-related pain at a rate of 0.30% for SCS and 0.54% for DRG.

In 2019, Sivanesan et al. published a retrospective safety analysis that utilized data from the FDA-supported MAUDE (Manufacturer and User Facility Device Experience) database. The study examined publicly reported safety events for DRG stimulation including both trials and implants. The authors' queried data entries termed "dorsal root ganglion stimulator for pain relief" between May 2016 and December 2017 and categorized complications based on the event description. A total of 979 unique events were identified, and analysis was used to stratify events based on the severity of the adverse outcome. Combining the data of both trials and permanent implants, 47% of the reported events were categorized as device-related complications. Device-related complications may include migration, erosion, lead damage or failure, hardware malfunction, and difficult insertion or removal. Procedural complications accounted for 24% with the remainder of episodes included patient complaints, 12.4%; serious adverse events, 2.4%; and the remaining 4.6% categorized as other. The most common device-related complications included migration or lead damage which was reported at 272 and 99, respectively. Unfortunately, the total number of procedures performed during the 20-month period is unknown, and therefore the incidence of complications cannot be calculated based on this data set. Of note, the prevalence of adverse events associated with DRG was similar to those reported with SCS.

DRG stimulation has an excellent safety profile with an adverse event rate equal to or better than SCS. This has been demonstrated not only in a tightly controlled setting, the ACCURATE study, but also through the analysis of real-world data over the first 2 years post FDA approval and the analysis from the FDA's MAUDE database. While no study is without its individual limitations, their combined data reveals a safety profile on par with SCS [32–34].

MRI Safety

At the time of this chapter being written, DRG is considered MR conditional. The Proclaim™ DRG IPG component should be implanted in the upper buttock, low back, flank, or abdomen, and the lead tip must be placed in the epidural space between T10 and S2. Approved areas for scanning include the head, lower extremities (excluding the hip), and the upper extremities (excluding the shoulder). Scan requirements include the use of a 1.5 Tesla cylindrical bore magnet with horizontal field orientation. Patients should be positioned supine with arms at their sides. Total active scan time cannot exceed 30 minutes per session. If additional scans are necessary, they may be performed after 30 minutes of waiting [35].

Regulatory Requirement

Currently, the Food and Drug Administration requires implanting physicians in the United States should be experienced in the diagnosis and treatment of chronic pain syndromes and have undergone surgical and device implantation training for DRG neurostimulation systems. Abbott neuromodulation has developed a comprehensive training program for physicians who desire to utilize this therapy [36].

Conclusion

Dorsal root ganglion stimulation has been extensively studied for the treatment of complex regional pain syndrome and focal painful conditions. The device provides significant pain relief with an excellent safety profile and an adverse event rate equal to or better when compared to SCS.

References

1. Shealy CN, Mortimer JT, Rewick JB. Electrical inhibition of pain by stimulation of the dorsal columns: preliminary clinical report. Anesth Analg. 1967;4:489–91.
2. Bevan S, Yeats J. Protons activate a cation conductance in a sub-population of rat dorsal root ganglion neurons. J Physiol. 1991;43:145–61.
3. Deer TR, Grigsby E, Weiner RL, et al. A prospective study of dorsal root ganglion stimulation for the relief of chronic pain. Neuromodulation. 2013;16:67–71.
4. Liem L, Russo M, Huygen FJPM, et al. A multicenter, prospective trial to assess the safety and performance of the spinal modulation dorsal root ganglion neurostimulator system in the treatment of chronic pain. Neuromodulation. 2013;16(5):471–82.
5. Kemler MA, de Vet HC, Barendse GA, van den Wildenberg FA, van Kleef M. Effect of spinal cord stimulation for chronic complex regional pain syndrome type I: five-year final follow-up of patients in a randomized controlled trial. J Neurosurg. 2008;108:292.
6. Krames ES. The dorsal root ganglion in chronic pain and as a target for neuromodulation: a review. Neuromodulation. 2015;18:24–32.
7. Soresi A. Control of "intractable pain" by spinal ganglia block. Am J Surg. 1949;77(1):72–8.
8. Shanthanna H, Chan P, McChesney J, Thabane L, Paul J. Pulsed radiofrequency treatment of the lumbar dorsal root ganglion in patients with chronic lumbar radicular pain: a randomized, placebo-controlled pilot study. J Pain Res. 2014;7:47–55. Published 2014 Jan 10. https://doi.org/10.2147/JPR.S55749.
9. van Boxem K, van Eerd M, Brinkhuizen T, Patijn J, van Kleef M, van Zundert J. Radiofrequency and pulsed radiofrequency treatment of chronic pain syndromes: the available evidence [published correction appears in Pain Pract. 2010 Mar-Apr;10[2]:164. Brinkhuize, Tjinta [corrected to Brinkhuizen, Tjinta]]. Pain Pract. 2008;8(5):385–93. https://doi.org/10.1111/j.1533-2500.2008.00227.x.
10. Deer TR, Grigsby E, Weiner RL, Wilcosky B, Kramer JM. A prospective study of dorsal root ganglion stimulation for the relief of chronic pain. Neuromodulation. 2013;16:67–71.
11. Hunter CW, Yang A. Dorsal root ganglion stimulation for chronic pelvic pain: a case series and technical report on a novel lead configuration. Neuromodulation. 2019;22(1):87–95. https://doi.org/10.1111/ner.12801.
12. Deer TR, Levy RM, Kramer J, et al. Dorsal root ganglion stimulation yielded higher treatment success rate for complex regional pain syndrome and causalgia at 3 and 12 months: a randomized comparative trial. Pain. 2017;158(4):669–81. https://doi.org/10.1097/j.pain.0000000000000814.
13. Bayman EO, Brennan TJ. Incidence and severity of chronic pain at 3 and 6 months after thoracotomy: meta-analysis. J Pain. 2014;15:887–97.
14. Eldabe S, Burger K, Moser H, et al. Dorsal root ganglion [DRG] stimulation in the treatment of phantom limb pain [PLP]. Neuromodulation. 2015;18:610–7.
15. Schu S, Gulve A, Eldabe S, et al. Spinal cord stimulation of the dorsal root ganglion for groin pain-a retrospective review. Pain Pract. 2015;15:293–9.
16. Schu S, Mutagi H, Kapur S, et al. Sustained pain relief in painful diabetic neuropathy [PDN] achieved through targeted spinal cord stimulation [SCS]: a retrospective case series. Neuromodulation. 2015;18:e91.
17. Hunter CW, Yang A, Davis T. Selective radiofrequency stimulation of the dorsal root ganglion (DRG) as a method for predicting targets for neuromodulation in patients with post amputation pain: a case series. Neuromodulation. 2017;20(7):708–18.
18. Antony A, Schultheis C, Jolly N, et al. Neuromodulation of the dorsal root ganglion for chronic postsurgical pain. Pain Med. 2019;20(1):S41–6.
19. Deer TR, et al. The neuromodulation appropriateness consensus committee on best practices for dorsal root ganglion stimulation. Neuromodulation. 2019;22:1–35.

20. Van Buyten JP, Smet I, Liem L, Russo M, Huygen F. Stimulation of dorsal root ganglia for the management of complex regional pain syndrome: a prospective case series. Pain Pract. 2015;15:208–16.
21. Eldabe S, Espinet A, Kang P, et al. Dorsal root ganglia stimulation for painful diabetic peripheral neuropathy: a preliminary report. Neuromodulation. 2017;20:e51.
22. Falowski S, Pope J, Cusack W. Early US experience with stimulation of the dorsal root ganglia for the treatment of peripheral neuropathy in the lower extremities: a multicenter retrospective case series. Abstract from: International Neuromodulation Society - 13th World Congress; 2017; Edinburgh, Scotland, UK.
23. Kehlet H, Jensen TS, Woolf CJ. Persistent postsurgical pain: risk factors and prevention. Lancet. 2006;367:1618–25.
24. Wang L, Guyatt GH, Kennedy SA, et al. Predictors of persistent pain after breast cancer surgery: a systematic review and meta-analysis of observational studies. CMAJ. 2016;188:E352–61.
25. Espinet AJ. Stimulation of dorsal root ganglion [DRG] for chronic post-surgical pain [CPSP]: a retrospective single centre case series from Australia using targeted spinal cord stimulation [SCS]. Neuromodulation. 2015;18:e93.
26. Liem L, Nijhuis H, Huygen FJPM, et al. Treatment of chronic post-surgical pain [CPSP] using spinal cord stimulation [SCS] of the dorsal root ganglion [DRG] neurostimulation: results from two prospective studies. Pain Pract. 2014;14:3–4.
27. Breel J, Zuidema X, Schapendonk J, Lo B, Wille FF. Treatment of chronic post-surgical pain with dorsal root ganglion [DRG] stimulation [10701]. Neuromodulation. 2016;19:e15.
28. Vesper J, Schu S, Slotty P, et al. Cervical and high-thoracic dorsal root ganglion stimulation [DRG] in chronic pain [10317]. Neuromodulation. 2016;19:388.
29. Sullivan R, Teddy P. Stimulation of dorsal root ganglion [DRG] for chronic intractable pain: a retrospective single Centre case series from Australia using targeted spinal cord stimulation [SCS]. Neuromodulation. 2015;18:e95.
30. Huygen F, Liem L, Cusack W, Kramer J. Stimulation of the L2–L3 dorsal root ganglia induces effective pain relief in the low back. Pain Pract. 2018;18(2):205–13. https://doi.org/10.1111/papr.12591.
31. Deer T, Pope J, Hunter C, Falowski S, Kapural L, Kramer J, Levy R. Safety analysis of dorsal root ganglion stimulation in the treatment of chronic pain. Neuromodulation: Technology at the Neural Interface; 2019. https://doi.org/10.1111/ner.12941.
32. Sivanesan E, Bicket MC, Cohen SP. Retrospective analysis of complications associated with dorsal root ganglion stimulation for pain relief in the FDA MAUDE database. Reg Anesth Pain Med. 2019;44(1):100–6. https://doi.org/10.1136/rapm-2018-000007.
33. Mironer YE, Brown C, Satterhwaite JR, et al. A new technique of "midline anchoring" in spinal cord stimulation dramatically reduces lead migration. Neuromodulation. 2004;7:32–7.
34. Hagedorn JM, Demian PS, Scarfo KA, Engle AM, Deer TR. Proclaim™ DRG Neurostimulator System for the management of chronic, intractable pain [published online ahead of print, 2020 May 19]. Pain Manag. 2020;10.2217/pmt-2020-0010. https://doi.org/10.2217/pmt-2020-0010.
35. Abbott MRI procedure information, Clinician's manual.
36. Abbott Proclaim™ DRG Implantable Pulse Generator Model 3664, Clinician's Manual.

Percutaneous/Paddle Techniques: Values and Pearls

José Luiz de Campos

Introduction

Researches show that spinal cord neurostimulation has better quality when implanting at least 2 (two) columns of leads in the epidural space [1–5]. This necessarily implies the use of 2 (two) percutaneous cylindrical leads (Fig. 1) or a paddle lead with more than one column. It is believed that a minimum of 2 (two) columns of leads result in a greater number of combinations and a greater number of possibilities for adjustments, promoting better results in analgesia as well as device programming [2–5]. In such manner, it is possible to act in larger areas of the posterior horn of the spinal cord [6–8].

The most commonly found paddle leads have between 2 (two) to 5 (five) columns. Currently, paddle leads with only 1 (one) column of 4 or 8 electrodes (S-Series) (Fig. 1) [4, 7–9] are also available on the market and are mostly used for percutaneous passage. Statistically, however, the implantation of percutaneous leads worldwide occurs in greater numbers than that of paddle leads, mainly due to its low invasiveness [9].

Multicolumn paddle leads normally require more invasive surgical procedures such as laminectomy or laminotomy. In the case of surgical implants, there will be total or partial removal of the bone structure superior to the epidural space. This structure works as a protective layer for the spinal cord and also plays a role in stability. In addition to this, the risk of epidural hematomas and neurological injuries is greatly increased [10]. In most cases, these procedures require the patient to undergo general anesthesia which makes it more invasive, time-consuming, and costly.

J. L. de Campos (✉)
Anaesthesiology and Pain Management Hospital Vera Cruz and Clinica Adora em, Campinas, SP, Brazil

Physician Responsible for the Teaching and Training Center for Specialization in Pain, CET/SBA, Hospital Vera Cruz, Campinas, SP, Brazil

T. d. S. Freitas et al. (eds.), *Neuromodulation Techniques for Pain Treatment*, https://doi.org/10.1007/978-3-030-84778-4_7

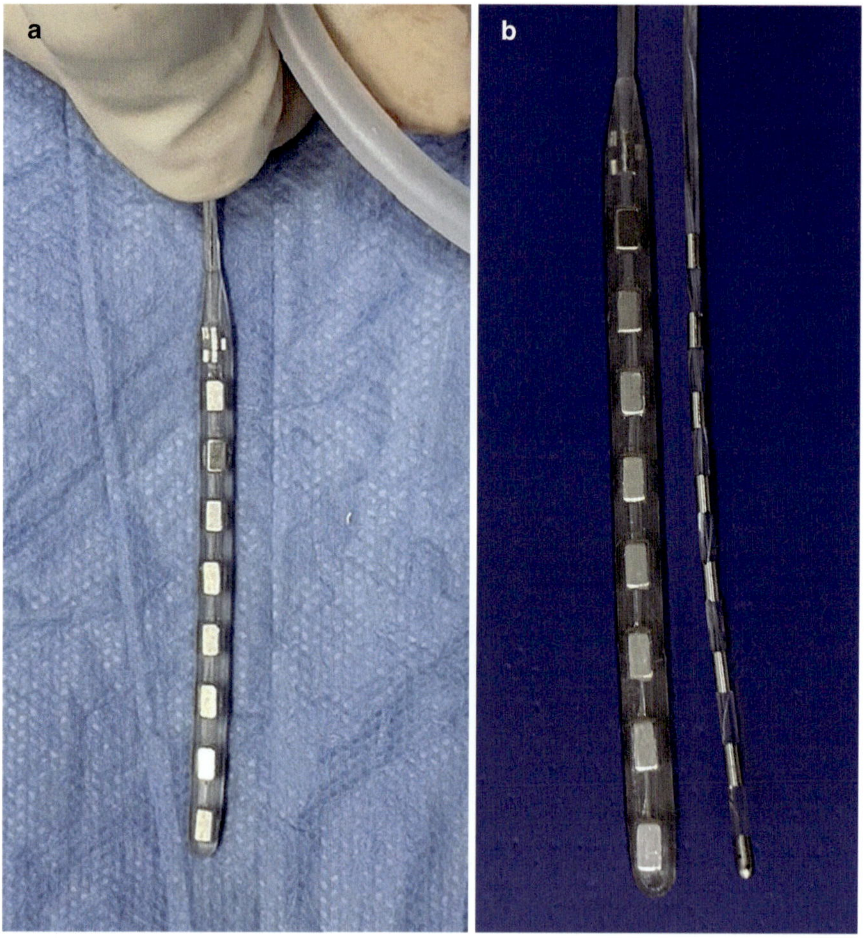

Fig. 1 Figures (**a**, **b**) Percutaneous Cylindrical Leads or Paddle Leads (S- Series Type). Figure (**a**): Paddle Lead (S-8). Figure (**b**): Padle Lead (S-8) and Octrode Cylindrical Lead

Also, in order to use at least 2 (two) percutaneous cylindrical leads, 2 (two) punctures must be performed in the epidural space. Each puncture requires the use of 1 (one) 14-Ga Tuohy needle through which the leads are introduced. The puncture and passage of the leads, especially in these cases, are followed by 2 (two) incisions made around each needle to promote the anchoring of each lead in the paravertebral region. This happens because it is unlikely that 2 (two) punctures will be performed next to each other, thus making only 1 (one) incision in the skin and soft tissues [11].

Delivery devices with larger gauges have been developed for some time now, allowing simultaneous introduction of at least 2 (two) percutaneous leads into the epidural space. Therefore, only 1 (one) puncture is performed, and consequently, only 1 (one) incision is needed to anchor them [9].

The 7-gauge metal needle [1] was a device used in the past, but it was often necessary to use a hammer to overcome the resistance of the interlaminar cleft as well

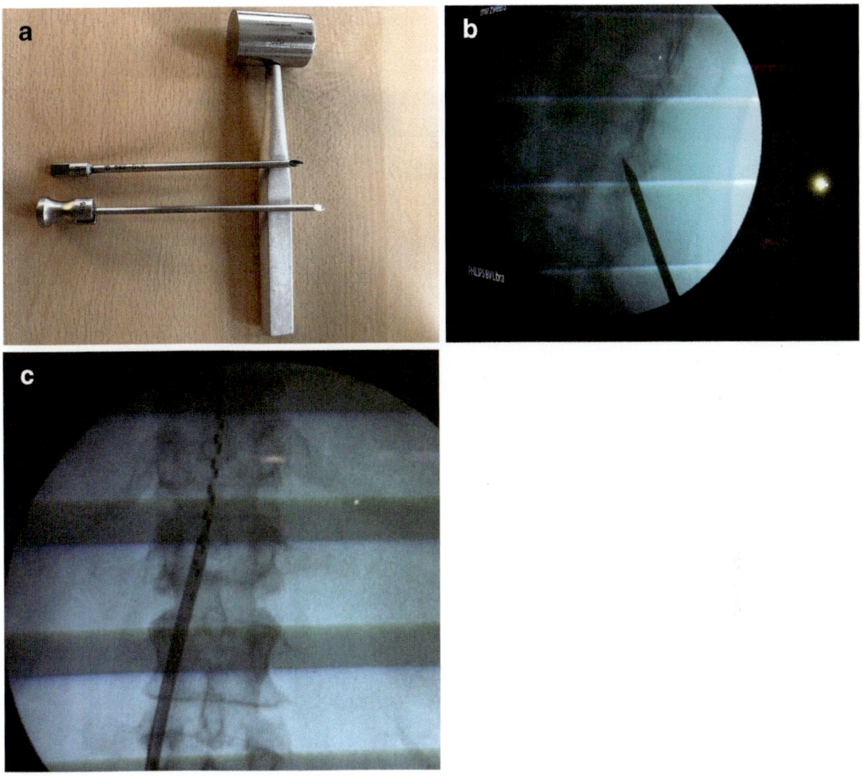

Fig. 2 Paddle Lead (S-8) and Octrode Cylindrical Lead. (Figures **a**, **b**, **c**) Figure (**a**): Hammer, The 7-gauge and 5 gauge metal needle. Figure (**b**): Entry into Epidural Space. Lateral View. Figure (**c**): Placing 2 electrodes simultaneously. (1): this device was used in the past to enable the passage of more than one lead

as that of the ligamentum flavum (Fig. 2). This metallic needle allowed the passage of 2 (two) or 3 (three) percutaneous leads as well as the passage of 1 (one) or 2 (two) paddle leads with a column of 8 electrodes each (S-Series) through a single puncture. However, during the use of this device at the time of the epidural puncture, there was a greater likelihood of an inadvertent puncture of the dura mater, and fear regarding the incidence of major damage to the nervous system in the spinal canal was instilled. Therefore, due to these risks, this system was abandoned.

Since 2009 in Europe and 2011 in the United States of America, a new lead delivery system called Epiducer (Abbott) has been used [1, 8, 12]. It is a minimally invasive lead delivery device that enables the implantation of a wide array of possible lead configurations: multiple cylindrical leads, S-Series leads, or even combined [11, 13] leads. This device uses the Seldinger technique, at which a metallic guidewire is inserted and the needles of different and progressively larger gauges are exchanged. Such needles serve to gradually dilate the epidural space just as the technique performed for vascular puncture accesses, promoting greater safety to the procedure.

Materials

The Epiducer system has the following components (Fig. 3):

A. 14-gauge non-cutting Tuohy needle: made of 304 stainless steel which is a special steel alloy. The 14-Ga Tuohy needle is traditionally used for punctures of

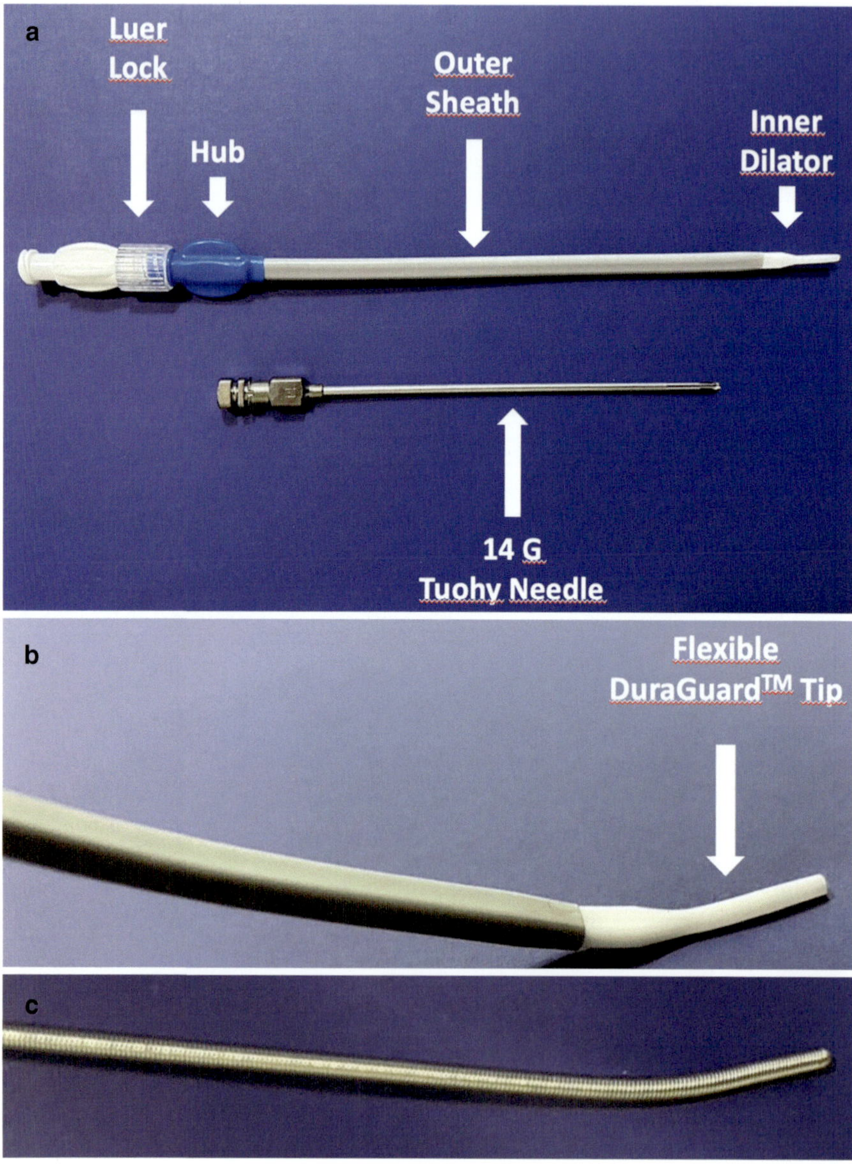

Fig. 3 (Figures **a**, **b**, **c**) The Epiducer system components. Figure (**a**): The Epiducer and Tuohy needles. Figure (**b**): The flexible DuraGuard tip of the inner dilator. Figure (**c**): The guidewire of Epiducer system

the epidural space and comes in two different lengths to allow its use in patients of different sizes.

B. Malleable guidewire: made of 304 stainless steel (special steel alloy) with an internal metallic stylet that has a curved tip and penetrates the epidural space. This guidewire allows the exchange between the 14-Ga Tuohy needle and the Epiducer needle using the Seldinger technique.
C. Epiducer needle: it has 2 (two) radiopaque components – a rigid external system with a sheath made of high-density polyethylene with barium sulfate and an internal dilator made of low-density polyethylene with barium sulfate with a malleable and conical tip. The rigid outer sheath will be the final guide for the passage of the leads. The malleable component with the conical tip works as an epidural space dilator.

   It is important to ensure that the Luer Lock of the internal malleable system is fully locked clockwise before using the whole set. Otherwise, when applying force to progress the system, the progression of the external rigid system may occur, inadvertently causing neural or dura mater injury. The Epiducer system comes in 2 (two) different lengths, 13 cm (5 inches) and 19 cm (7.5 inches), to suit the patient's biotype variations
D. Cylindrical percutaneous leads: accepted in MRI exams, they can be quadripolar or octapolar. They have a rigid metallic wire with a straight tip and a steerable metallic wire with a curved tip.
E. Percutaneous plate leads (S-Series): not accepted in MRI exams, they can also be quadripolar or octapolar. The dimensions of octapolar type S leads are as follows: blade length of 67 mm (allows coverage of 2 vertebral segments), width of 4 mm, thickness of 1.8 mm, length of contact 4 mm, and contact width of 2.5 mm. It is possible to observe in Fig. 4, the differences between a percutaneous lead and an S-Series lead, the 14-Ga Tuohy needle, and the Epiducer at its distal ends. They have straight and curved metallic guidewires.

Technique and Methods

The same is true for other spinal neural stimulation techniques where the procedure is performed with the patient in the prone position [1, 8, 13–15].

Standard anesthetic monitoring is used for local interventions. Anesthetic sedation associated with local anesthesia or deep sedation, such as general anesthesia, can be used with the patient preferably not curarized [14–15].

Fluoroscopy, using a C-arc, is configured to determine the desired input level as well as to monitor the progression of the various stages during implantation [1, 8, 11, 13].

After ensuring aseptic procedures and setting up the surgical field, local anesthesia is applied (Xylocaine 2% with adrenaline 1:200,000).

The introduction of the Epiducer system should preferably be in the L1/L2 interlaminar space or below it [1, 8, 11, 13–14]. This recommendation aims to reduce the

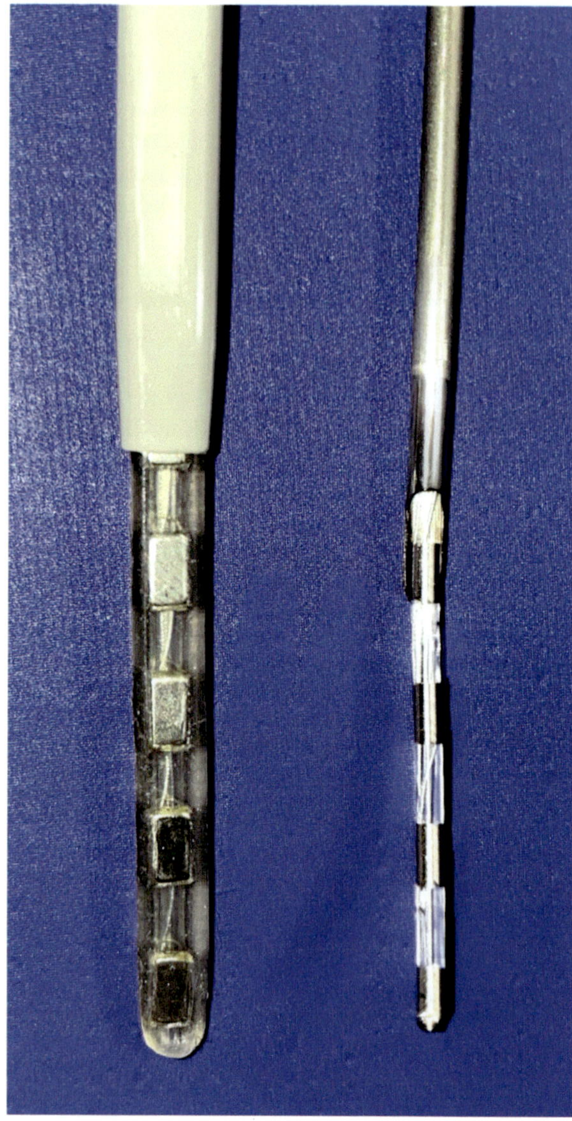

Fig. 4 The different diameters of the cylindrical percutaneous lead and S-Series lead both coming out of the needle tips (Tuohy and Epiducer, respectively)

risk of spinal cord injury. Based on clinical and anatomical evidence, the implant can occur above L1. However, if this decision is made, the procedure should only be performed after a thorough analysis of the risks and benefits to the patient.

Initially, a small puncture can be made under the dermal layers with a scalpel blade number 11, facilitating the introduction of the non-cutting 14-Ga Tuohy needle. The chosen entry point should be approximately 2 (two) vertebral levels below the desired epidural entry point. The approach is performed with a small paramedian angle, preferably of less than 30° as well as a midline approach between the 14-Ga Tuohy needle and the skin at a maximum of 30° [1, 8] (Fig. 5). The 14-Ga

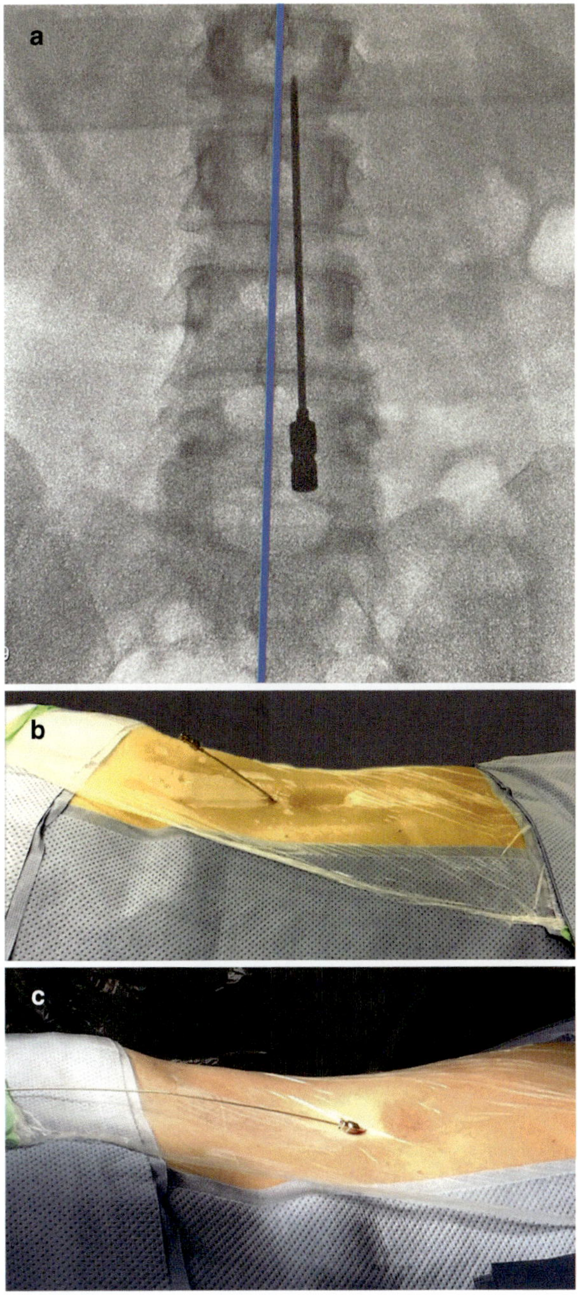

Fig. 5 (Figures **a**, **b**, **c**) The Tuohy needle approach with skin and midline (less than 30°) Figure (**a**): AP View Approach., Figure (**b**): Puncture Angle., and Figure (**c**): Inserting GuideWire

Tuohy needle is introduced under fluoroscopic guidance (AP view) through the deeper layers of the soft tissue and toward the interlaminar opening. The loss of resistance technique (LOR) can be used to confirm the correct puncture of the epidural space under fluoroscopic lateral view (L view).

Once the correct puncture of the epidural space is confirmed, the metallic, malleable, and steerable guidewire is inserted. It should be placed in the posterior epidural space which corresponds to the epidural sensitive area (Fig. 6) (L view). During the insertion of the leads, the same path must be followed since this is the target site for adequate neurostimulation.

In patients in which the guidewire finds resistance to pass through the epidural space, Epiducer should not be used, and alternative strategies should be employed. Some options include the placement of a conventional percutaneous lead or a radical change of technique such as the laminectomy approach.

At this moment, the scalpel incision should be increased in order to allow the passage of the Epiducer system.

The replacement or exchange of the needles begins by using the Seldinger technique. The 14-Ga Tuohy needle is removed, and the guidewire remains in the epidural space. It is important to remember the imperative need to fully twist the Luer Lock (Fig. 3) clockwise, allowing the Epiducer internal system to be properly locked to the external system before its introduction. The shape of the inner sheath of the Epiducer is tapered and has the purpose of gradually dilating the soft tissues and the epidural space (L view). Secondly, the radiopaque and flexible tip of this internal component, called DuraGuard, serves to protect the dura mater during insertion. Its conical shape closely follows the guidewire from its entry into the

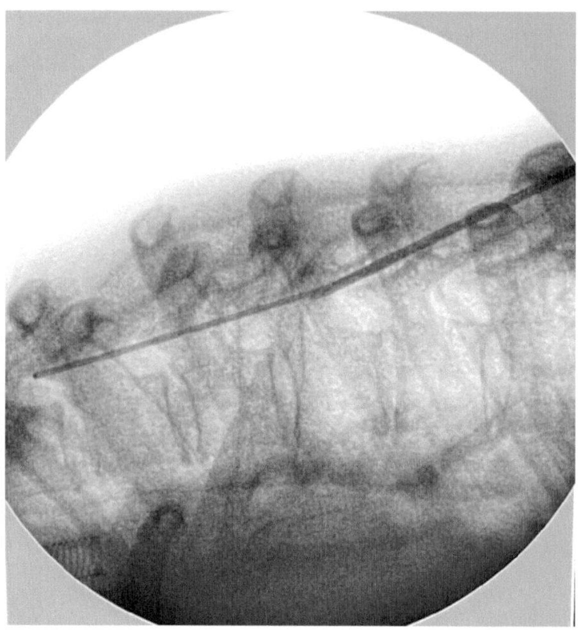

Fig. 6 Steerable guidewire is inserted. It should be placed in the posterior epidural space

epidural space to a more advanced site where, even after its removal, it will allow the outer sheath of the Epiducer to remain anchored within the epidural space. This conical tip provides visual confirmation through fluoroscopy as well as the proper position of the system (Fig. 7). The blue hub of the Epiducer has lateral flaps that indicate that the system is advancing in alignment with the patient's nervous system while it is being introduced (Fig. 8).

The internal dilator is detached from the outer sheath by turning the Luer Lock counterclockwise and then removed along with the guidewire, leaving only the outer sheath anchored to the epidural space (Fig. 9).

It is important to draw attention to the fact that the entire procedure, using the Seldinger technique to replace the 14-Ga Tuohy needle with the Epiducer, must be performed without applying too much force on the system. This action can lead to

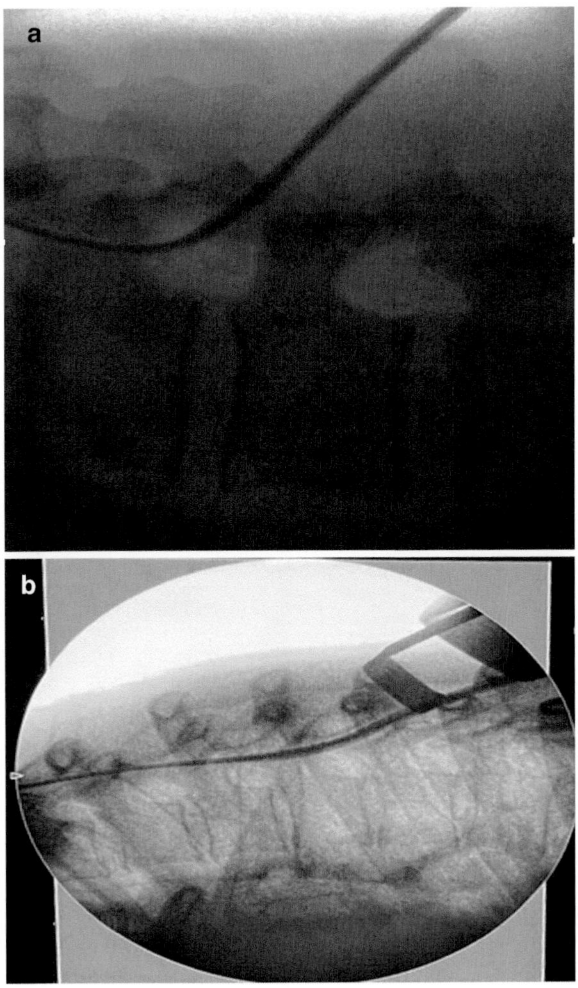

Fig. 7 (**a**, **b**) Epiducer's conical tip confirmation via fluoroscopy in epidural space. (**a**) Epiducer introduction. Lateral view – lumbar puncture. (**b**) Epiducer introduction. Lateral view – thoracic puncture

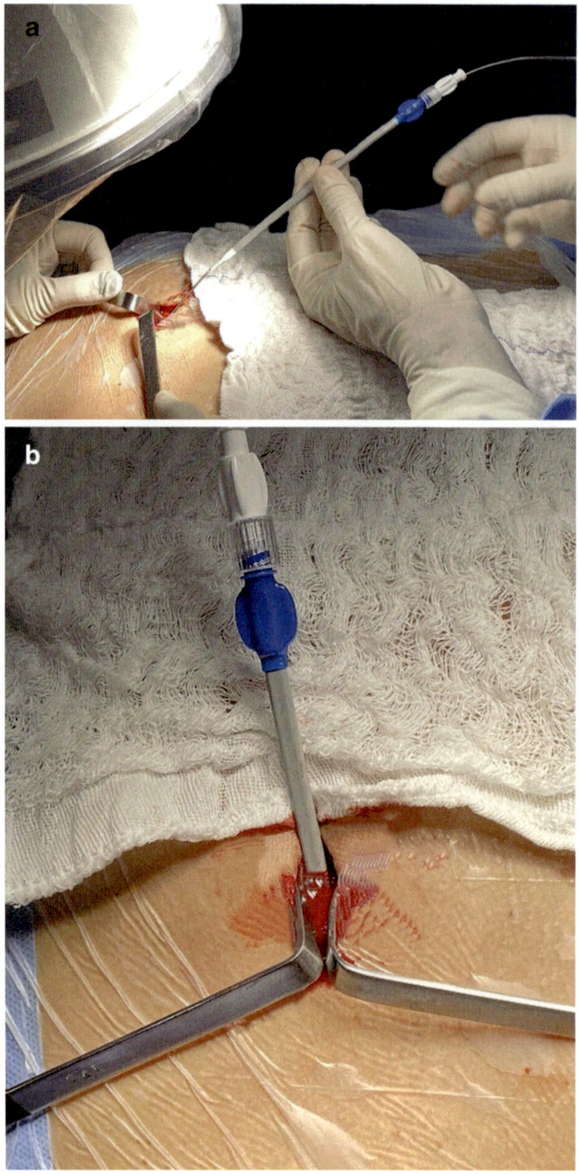

Fig. 8 (**a** and **b**) Epiducer must advance in alignment with midline, and the blue hub must advance in plane parallel to the patient's spine. (**a**) Epiducer must advance in alignment with midline. (**b**) The blue hub must advance in plane parallel to the patient's spine

folds and/or deformities in it, as it is a plastic alloy component. As previously mentioned, if the Epiducer system cannot be inserted properly due to any anatomical condition of the patient's interlaminar or epidural space, the Epiducer system must be replaced by a new one to avoid damage. Also, still due to difficulties that might arise, it is advisable to replace the technique with either a cylindrical lead implant through the 14-Ga Tuohy needle itself or even a laminectomy.

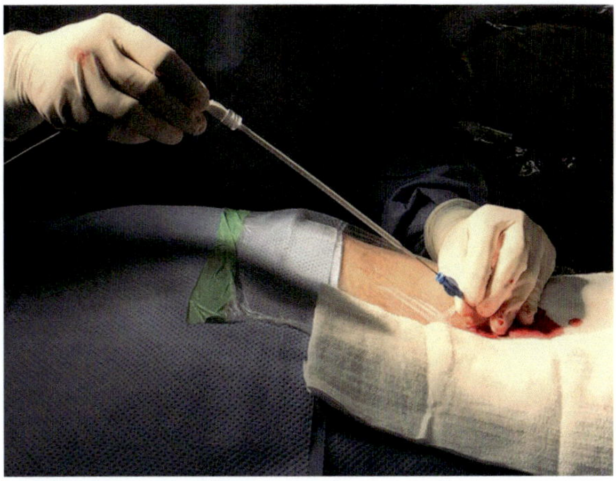

Fig. 9 The internal dilator is detached from the outer sheath by turning the Luer Lock counterclockwise and then removed along with the guidewire

At this moment, when the outer sheath is correctly positioned in the epidural space, the leads are introduced [1, 8, 11, 13–16]. This device allows several leads to be introduced in the same angle, facilitating the alignments as well as the unique access into the epidural space for the placement of multiple leads, reducing the time of the procedure and also enabling the introduction of an S-Series lead without the need for laminectomy.

All leads, whether cylindrical or type S paddle, can be introduced through the Epiducer with the use of a curved-tip guidewire. The leads must be kept in the most central and posterior regions of the epidural space, preventing their progression to the lateral and anterior regions (AP and L view) (Fig. 10). The stimuli applied to the lateral regions can be uncomfortable for patients because they cause root stimuli. The anterior region is motor and is, therefore, not pertinent to the analgesia therapy [10].

The S-Series leads must always be inserted with the electrodes facing downward, toward the medullary cone (conus medullaris) (Fig. 11). The S-Series leads also have a radiopaque marker that enables to verify that the leads are facing toward the dorsal cord. (Fig. 12) [8, 12, 13]. After confirming the correct location of the leads, through intraoperative stimulation, homeostasis is revised in the incision area, and the surgical focus is explored while the Epiducer gray external sheath protects the leads (Fig. 13). Next, in the aponeurosis of the paravertebral musculature, a preferably nonelastic multifilament wire is passed in order to anchor the leads. The sheath is withdrawn, using once again the technique in which the lead is kept in place while the system is retracted, placing the lead in the ideal location. The lead is anchored to the fascia after the removal of the steerable mandrel. The advantage of the Epiducer is that it allows several lead options to be implanted through an entry point: 1 (one) S-Series lead, with 1 (one) or 2 (two) percutaneous leads or up to 3 (three) percutaneous leads. The advantage is that the epidural space only needs to be approached once, reducing the risk of puncture of the dura mater with the sharper 14-Ga Tuohy needle (Fig.13).

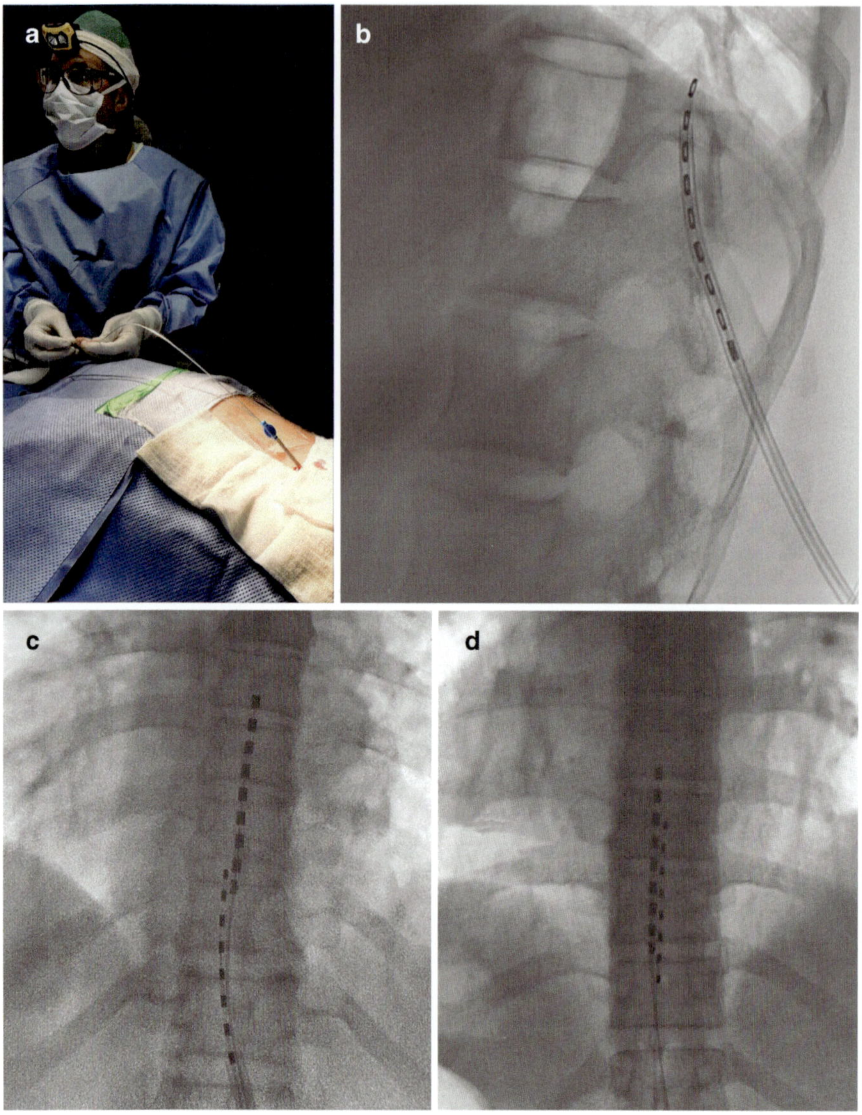

Fig. 10 (**a**) Lead navigation. (**b**) Paddle lead advance showing the electric poles facing the medullary canal. (**c**) Cylindrical electrode passage after passing the paddle lead. (**d**) Leads final position. Paddle and cylindrical leads. (**e**) Leads final position. 2 Paddle leads final position

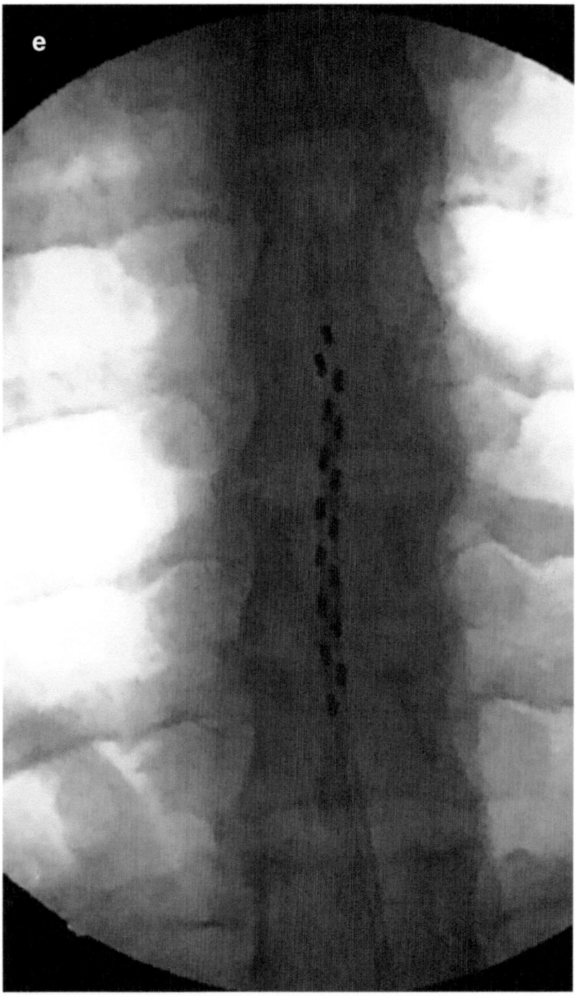

Fig. 10 (continued)

When programming the placement of 2 (two) S-Series leads (Fig. 14), an adaptation to the technique must be made. The width of the type S lead does not allow another type S lead to pass along inside the outer sheath of the Epiducer. There is a peculiar way of doing it to minimize the risks or the need to introduce another contralateral 14-Ga Tuohy needle. With the Epiducer still in place, the guidewire is reinserted into the epidural space. Then, the outer sheath is removed, and the guidewire and the first S-Series lead are implanted in place. The entire Epiducer system is assembled again by locking the Luer Lock of the internal dilator to the outer sheath and advancing specifically over the guidewire [8, 13, 17–18]. From this point on, the procedure is similar to that described previously, with the implantation of a new S-Series lead parallel to the first. Usually, the second approach is facilitated due to the previous dilation of the tissues.

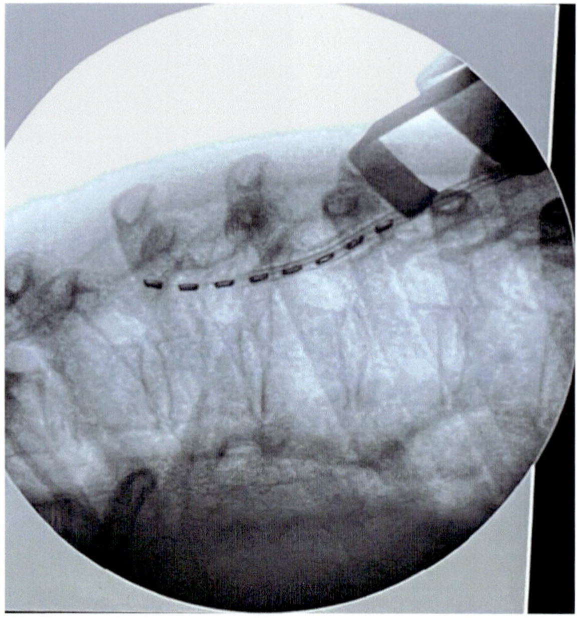

Fig. 11 The S-Series leads must always be inserted with the electrodes facing downward, toward the medullary cone (conus medullaris)

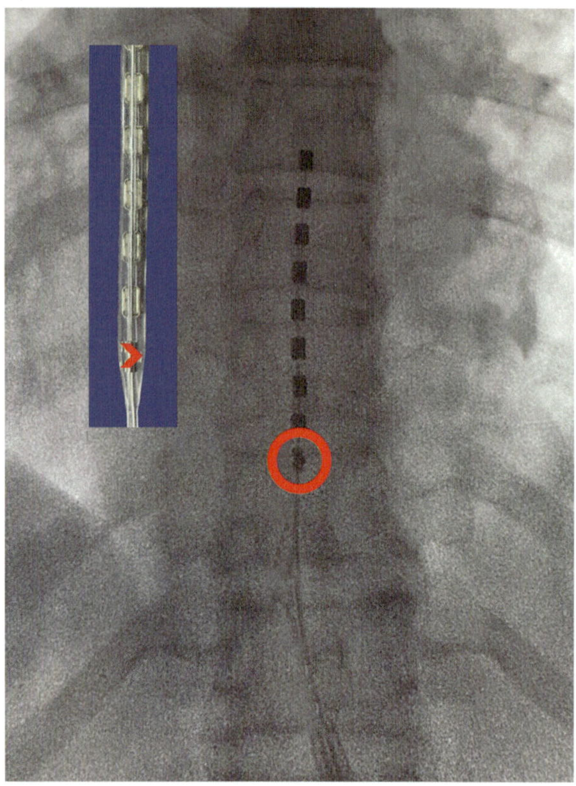

Fig. 12 The radiopaque marker of S-series leads to confirm that the leads are facing toward the spinal cord

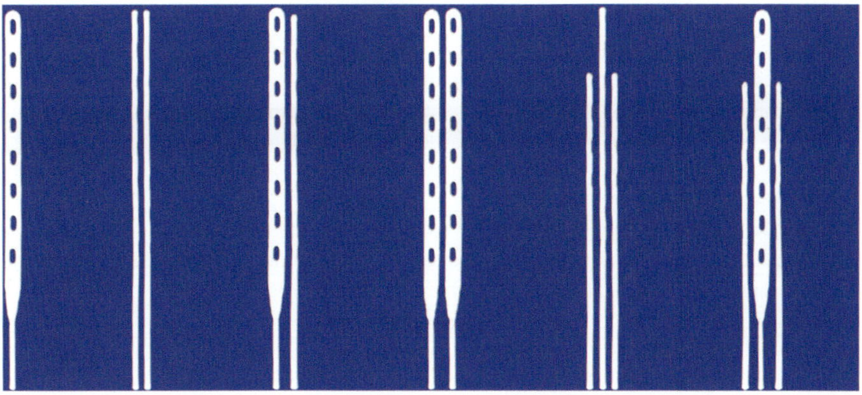

Fig. 13 Schematic drawing showing some possible lead configurations during implantation using the Epiducer system

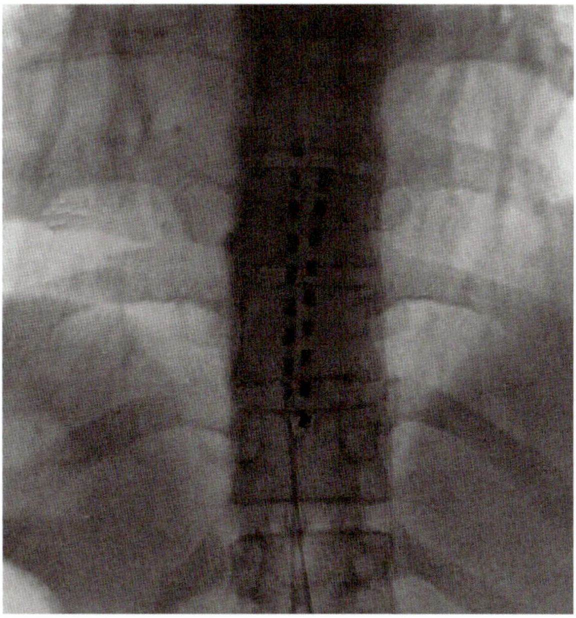

Fig. 14 Two S-Series leads implanted

Closing of the skin is accomplished by first closing the subcutaneous layers. The procedure tips and pearls are shown in Table 1.

Final Considerations

Epiducer has proven to be safe during the implantation technique and has maintained the same success and complication rates found in other implantation techniques for spinal cord neurostimulation [1, 8, 14, 18–20]. The literature shows

Table 1 Tips and Pearls

1.	Patient selection – Patients who presented lumbar and thoracic spine within the anatomical limits of normality (MRI and CT studies of the spinal canal)
2.	Entry angle (AP view) – Uses the lumbar paramedian approach with an angle of less than 30° degrees with the skin and with the central axial line of the spine
3.	Fluoroscopic lateral view – To enter the epidural space, pass the guidewire and introduce the Epiducer using the guidewire
4.	Lock the Luer lock before introducing the Epiducer
5.	Change the Epiducer if there is any damage to the system during the attempted introduction
6.	Inject saline into the epidural space to enable the entry of the lead(s)
7.	Only insert the S-series lead with the electrodes facing down
8.	When using two or more S-series leads, the guidewire must be reintroduced and the Epiducer removed. Then, the Epiducer is reintroduced through the lateral view (fluoroscopy) specifically over the guidewire, and one S-series lead is introduced at a time. It is also possible to use two Epiducer systems
9.	Attention to anchoring is vital for the successful prognosis of the technique

doctors' satisfaction and the same rates of effectiveness, and good results are confirmed.

In the same way, complications and/or adverse effects have shown a statistically similar occurrence when compared to other percutaneous techniques. All reported adverse events correspond to risks already known and inherent to the SCS procedure and/or surgery in general and were not specifically related to the percutaneous implantation of spinal leads using the Epiducer lead application system. The most common adverse events are migration and infection [1, 8, 16, 21]. There are no reports of serious neurological damage related to the use of this system.

The review of some articles suggests that the implantation of leads using the Epiducer lead delivery system is as safe as the standard lead placement technique [1, 8, 22–28]. The adverse events identified in the literature review were captured during the course of the studies with much longer follow-ups than implant studies with the Epiducer. Longer evaluations of the performance of the S-Series and cylindrical leads with this system are necessary in order to establish real long-term performance.

Currently, no serious adverse events have been reported. These included dural punctures, spinal fluid leaks, permanent paralysis, epidural hematomas, or others that required hospitalization.

There are reports of implants lasting 9 minutes per lead [1, 8, 22–28] using the technique described with an insertion angle that varies between 30° degrees to 40° degrees with a paramedian approach of 73.6% of patients undergoing this procedure.

Therefore, literature reviews demonstrate the feasibility and safety of using the Epiducer lead delivery system for percutaneous implantation of S-Series and cylindrical leads [1, 6, 8]. When compared to surgical techniques, there are benefits to this technique such as lower invasiveness, less pain complaints regarding the procedure in the postoperative period, and reports of faster return of patients to their usual activities.

References

1. Logé D, De Coster O, Washburn S. Technological innovation in spinal cord stimulation: use of a newly developed delivery device for introduction of spinal cord stimulation leads. Neuromodulation. 2012;15(4):392–401.
2. Mironer E, Bernstein CA, Mason R, et al. A prospective clinical evaluation of a rechargeable implantable pulse generator (IPG) in combination with a tripolar lead array: final analysis of sustainability of spinal cord stimulation therapy for chronic lower back pain. Poster presented at: 2011 bi-annual meeting of the international Neuromodulation society. London, England; May 25, 2011.
3. Barolat G, Oakley JC, Law JD, North RB, Ketcik B, Sharan A. Epidural spinal cord stimulation with a multiple electrode paddle lead is effective in treating intractable low back pain. Neuromodulation. 2001;4:59–66.
4. North RB, Kidd DH, Petrucci L, Dorsi MJ. Spinal cord stimulation electrode design: a prospective, randomized, controlled trial comparing percutaneous with laminectomy electrodes: part II—clinical outcomes. Neurosurgery. 2005;57:990–6. discussion 990–996.
5. Villavicencio AT, Leveque JC, Rubin L, Bulsara K, Gorecki JP. Laminectomy versus percutaneous electrode placement for spinal cord stimulation. Neurosurgery. 2000;46:399–405. discussion 405–406.
6. Verrills P, Sinclair C, Barnard A. A review of spinal cord stimulation systems for chronic pain. J Pain Res. 2016;9:481–92.
7. Martinez GJ, Lautenschlager KA, Aden JK, Maani CV, Lopez EM, McCallin JP. Effects of multimodal analgesia on recovery from percutaneous spinal cord stimulator implantation [published online ahead of print, 2019 Dec 18]. Neuromodulation.
8. Deer T, Bowman R, Schocket SM, et al. The prospective evaluation of safety and success of a new method of introducing percutaneous paddle leads and complex arrays with an epidural access system. Neuromodulation. 2012;15:21–9.
9. De Coster O, Forget P, Moens M, Matic M, Choustoulakis L, Poelaert J. A new minimally invasive technique for lead revision of perc-paddle leads. Acta Neurochir. 2018;160(4):831–3.
10. Mekhail N, Visnjevac O, Azer G, Mehanny DS, Agrawal P, Foorsov V. Spinal cord stimulation 50 years later: clinical outcomes of spinal cord stimulation based on randomized clinical trials-a systematic review. Reg Anesth Pain Med. 2018;43(4):391–406.
11. Deer TR, Mekhail N, Provenzano D, et al. The appropriate use of neurostimulation: avoidance and treatment of complications of neurostimulation therapies for the treatment of chronic pain. Neuromodulation appropriateness consensus committee. Neuromodulation. 2014;17(6):571–98.
12. Raso LJ, Deer TR, Schocket SM, et al. Use of a newly developed delivery device for percutaneous introduction of multiple lead configurations for spinal cord stimulation. Neuromodulation. 2014;17(5):465–71.
13. Logé D, De Coster O, Pollet W, Vancamp T. A novel percutaneous technique to implant plate-type electrodes. Minim Invasive Neurosurg. 2011;54(5–6):219–22.
14. Sastry S, Berger K. Troubleshooting and problem solving: the nuances of the Epiducer. Neuromodulation. 2014;17:93–5.
15. Carolis G. Spinal cord stimulation with a Slimline paddle Lead Introductioned under local anaesthesia: a new technique for the treatment of failed Back surgery syndrome. Reg Anesth Pain Med. 2012;37(7):225.
16. Lan W, Ahmad A, Poply K. A prospective single Centre pilot study to investigate the duration of time and radiation exposure following Epiducer delivery system in patients undergoing anatomical placement of percutaneous-paddle Lead for spinal cord stimulation with intractable lumbar spinal neuropathic. PainNeuromodulation. 2017;20:630.
17. Oh BH, Kim HT, Yim KH, Park YS. Percutaneously inserted unilateral Lead migration salvaged with a paddle electrode. Pain Pract. 2020;20(5):2–6.

18. Forget P, Billet B, Hanssens K, Raza A, Coster O. Dual cervical and thoracic/lumbar Lead placements in spinal cord stimulation using an Epiducer. Neuromodulation. 2019;22:E63.
19. De Coster O, Forget P, Moens M, Matic M, Choustoulakis L, Poelaert J. A new minimally invasive technique for lead revision of perc-paddle leads. Acta Neurochir. 2018;160(4):831–3.
20. Colini Baldeschi G, De Carolis G. The Italian experience with octopolar perc-paddle leads. Neuromodulation. 2014;17(4):349–53.
21. Bara G, Schu S, Vesper J. Infection rates of percutaneously implanted leads for SCS after a trial phase: 6 years of follow-up. Neuromodulation. 2016;19:E39.
22. Petraglia FW 3rd, Farber SH, Gramer R, et al. The incidence of spinal cord injury in implantation of percutaneous and paddle electrodes for spinal cord stimulation. Neuromodulation. 2016;19(1):85–90.
23. Barolat G, Oakley JC, Law JD, North RB, Ketcik B, Sharan A. Epidural spinal cord stimulation with a multiple electrode paddle lead is effective in treating intractable low back pain. Neuromodulation. 2001;4:59–66.
24. DuyvendakW. Spinalcordstimulationwithadualquadripolarsurgicalleadplaced in general anesthesia is effective in treating intractable low back and leg pain. Neuromodulation. 2007;10:113–9.
25. Rosenow JM, Stanton-Hicks M, Rezai AR, Henderson JM. Failuremodesofspinalcord stimulation hardware. J Neurosurg Spine. 2006;5:183–90.
26. Loge D, De Coster O. Use of a newly developed delivery device for percutaneous introduction of SCS leads. Poster presented at: 2011 bi-annual meeting of the international Neuromodulation society. London, England; May 25, 2011.
27. Kemler MA, de Vet HC, Barendse GA, van den Wildenberg FA, van Kleef M. Effect of spinal cord stimulation for chronic complex regional pain syndrome type I: five-year final follow-up of patients in a randomized controlled trial. J Neurosurg. 2008;108:292–8.
28. Weigel R, Capelle HH, Flor H, Krauss JK. Event-related cortical processing in neuropathic pain under long-term spinal cord stimulation. Pain Physician. 2015;18:185–94.

Peripheral Nerve Field Stimulation (PNfS)

Dawood Sayed, Daniel Lee Neuman, and Stanley Golovac

Introduction

Neuromodulation generally involves the selective application of a programmable pulse waveform through a series of electrodes within a lead to stimulate afferent nerve fibers and, subsequently, reduce the perception of pain. This treatment is most indicated in cases of severe localized pain, intractable to analgesics and other conventional therapies. The use of electrical stimulation for the treatment of pain dates back to the late 1800s when Julius Althaus applied alternating current electrotherapy to peripheral nerves for pain relief [1]. However, it was not until the publications by Melzack and Wall as well as Shealy and colleagues did neuromodulation in the form of spinal cord stimulation (SCS) become a noted alternative to traditional pain management [2, 3].

Historically, SCS has primarily been used for widespread leg, buttock, and to some extent back pain, particularly following failed back surgery. In some cases, SCS becomes ineffective over time with some contributing factors postulated to stem from original lead placement, lead migration, and changes in pain patterns [4,

D. Sayed (✉)
The American Society of Pain and Neuroscience, Pain Medicine, Interventional Pain, The Marc Asher Comprehensive Spine Center, The Center of Neuromodulation, Kansas City, Kansas, USA

D. L. Neuman
Resident Physician, Department of Anesthesiology, The University of Kansas Health System, Kansas City, Kansas, USA

S. Golovac
Space Coast Pain Institute, Merritt Island, FL, USA

Florida Pain, Melbourne, FL, USA

Golovac Consulting, Coral Gables, FL, USA

Surgery Partners, Merritt Island, FL, USA

Physician Partners of America, Tampa, FL, USA

T. d. S. Freitas et al. (eds.), *Neuromodulation Techniques for Pain Treatment*,
https://doi.org/10.1007/978-3-030-84778-4_8

5]. Traditionally, SCS has not adequately covered and helped to diminish axial back pain [6]. In addition, it has failed to address pain in key regions such as the face and trunk, leading to experimentation with the placement of subcutaneous leads within these "peripheral" areas [7].

The following chapter will focus on and discuss peripheral nerve field stimulation (PNfS), in particular its proposed mechanism, advantages, the process of candidate selection, as well as trialing and implantation.

Proposed Mechanism

Similar to SCS and peripheral nerve stimulation (PNS), the mechanism of PNfS is believed to be based on the gate control theory, which suggests that pain perception by the brain is generated by spinal cord signals transmitted by Aβ fibers (non-nociceptive stimuli) and C fibers (responsible for carrying painful, or nociceptive, stimuli). It was further postulated that the activation of the Aβ fibers "closes" the gate through dorsal horn interneurons, inhibiting subsequent nociceptive transmission of C fibers. By activating nociceptive fibers, the gate then "opens" via excitation of projection neurons that results in impedance of inhibitory interneurons [2, 8–10]. The gate control theory of pain provides the foundation for understanding how activation of large myelinated nerve fibers inhibits the transmission of pain impulses from the peripheral nervous system to high centers [9–13].

Mathematical modeling allowed for the determination of optimal implantation depth (10 to 15 mm below the skin surface), which resulted in the greatest degree of activation of Aβ fibers and minimal Aδ fibers, reaffirming that PNfS acts through the Aβ fiber [14–17]. PNfS may also modulate descending pathways of the upper central nervous system by stimulating the subcutaneous electrode, leading to localized analgesia. This is separate from the effects on segmental spinal cord regulation. Furthermore, it has been demonstrated that local electrical stimulation can reduce inflammation of the cutaneous nerve fibers, depolarizing the cell membrane and reducing circulating catecholamine sensitivity [17, 18].

The potential mechanisms for PNfS also include influencing local receptor and tissue excitability in the painful area, affecting local blood circulation [9], the conduction of the spinal and thalamic pathways, the function of sympathetic efferents, and by regulation of neurotransmitter levels [19]. Although no true consensus has been made regarding the mechanisms of PNfS, most believe that endogenous enkephalins are impacted, leading to changes in the nociceptive threshold in the target area [14]. Further human studies are needed to corroborate potential mechanisms.

Modality Advantages

In PNfS, leads are subcutaneously placed to stimulate the region of affected nerves, cutaneous afferents, or the dermatomal distribution of the nerves, which converge back to the spinal cord. Original insight into treating craniofacial pain with neurostimulation was first observed by Wall and Sweet in the 1960s. They implanted an electrode into their own infraorbital foramina, resulting in a decrease in pain perception during the period of stimulation [20].

As time evolved, many new applications and sites have been discovered and used to treat ongoing chronic neuropathic pain, including craniofacial [12, 21–24] (Fig. 1), thoracic and intercostal [25, 26] (Fig. 2), low back [18, 27–33], abdominal [34, 35], inguinal and genital [36–38], pelvic [39], and more distal peripheral nerves [40, 41]. PNfS may be utilized alongside traditional SCS for back and leg pain [30, 31]; however, the benefit of stimulating an area locally allows for the stimulation field to remain concentrated and precisely over the intended painful area. This also supports easy operation with less trauma.

In addition:

- PNfS is easily reversible and has low morbidity and few side effects.
- Implantation of the system is minimally invasive; leads can be inserted percutaneously, which avoids the more invasive nature of surgical dissection required with PNS.
- Percutaneous insertion of electrodes allows for an appropriate assessment of the patient's response while trialing in the precise location of pain.
- Analgesia associated with PNfS may contribute to the reduction or elimination of opioids.
- Developments in programmable systems and patient-controlled devices allow patients to alter stimulation to mirror pain severity.
- Electrodes continually improve in design and longevity [42, 43].

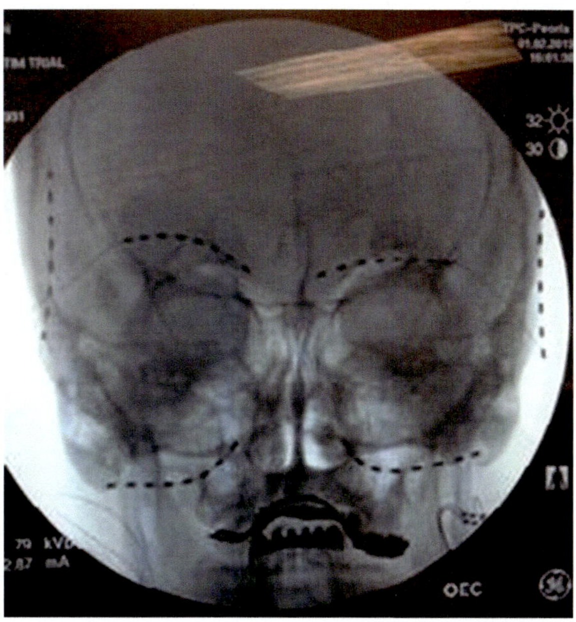

Fig. 1 Craniofacial octrode lead placement. (With permission from Stanley Golovac, MD)

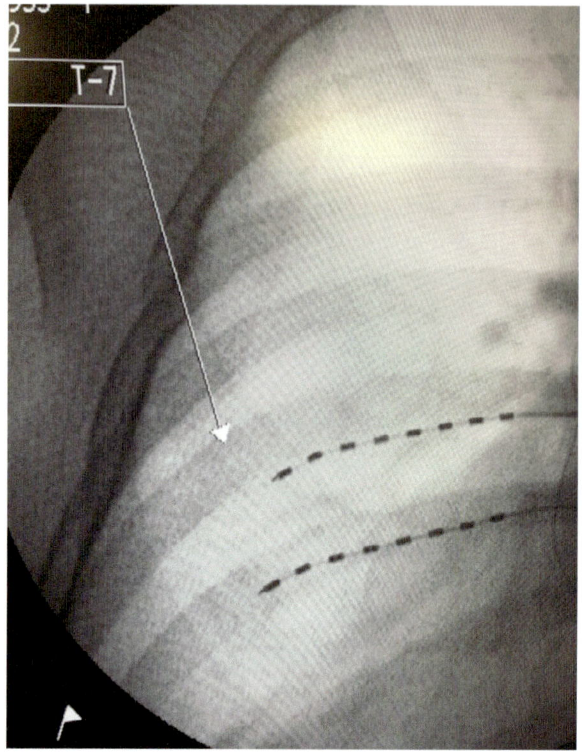

Fig. 2 Chest wall/intercostal nerve octrode lead placement. (With permission from Dawood Sayed, MD)

Candidate Selection

Failure of traditional or conservative management of neuropathic or mixed nociceptive/neuropathic pain is typically a prerequisite to PNfS candidacy, but the physician must also consider the innervation of the specific area of complaint and know that electrical current may influence the affected area. An inaccessible innervation or too large of a field may necessitate the implantation more proximally. The decision to implant a permanent peripheral lead is similar to that of spinal cord stimulation, and must answer the following questions:

- Does the patient experience significant pain reduction by visual analog score?
- Is the stimulation tolerable, i.e., pleasant and comfortable?
- Is function improved during the temporary period of stimulation [28, 42, 44, 45]? (Table 1)

Neuropsychological Testing

The presence of a psychopathological disorder is a crucial consideration when evaluating the appropriateness of any therapy but is especially important in candidates for implant. This evaluation is necessary because neuromodulatory therapy does not

Table 1 Inclusion and exclusion criteria for PNfS testing [33, 42, 45]

Inclusion criteria	Exclusion criteria
Neuropathic and nociceptive pain	Inability to obtain consent
Lack of response or contraindication to guideline-based conventional or conservative therapies	Infection in the target area for implantation or severe immunocompromise
PNfS alone or concomitant with epidural leads for the treatment of axial back pain related to FBSS	Allergy to injectate
Diagnostic testing of the spine unrevealing for alternative indication for operation	Coagulopathy
	Lack of patient compliance or presence of untreated psychopathological condition
	Cognitive impairment with stimulator management
	Lack of improvement in the trial phase

remove the cause of the painful experience but it instead modulates the afferent nociceptive input. Therefore, the presence of disorders of somatization, affect, conversion, personality, or substance should be ruled out [33, 42, 45–47].

PNfS Trial

The temporary trial placement is essential in determining whether the patient experiences pain relief over the target and first must be preceded by identifying the areas and associated intensities of pain. Many physicians utilize marking to outline the nerve or nerves responsible for sensation to the painful area. A marking pen also acts as a visual aid between patient and physician to reinforce the understanding that the correct area is being targeted [33, 42, 45]. Skipping this seemingly elementary step may be a likely contributor to modality failure [42].

The decision-making process then occurs once the area is clearly demarcated. Considerations include dense or overlapping paresthesia and its potential benefits, deployment ease, stability of the permanent system, patient safety, and the ability to create a montage of paresthesia using a single implantable pulse generator (IPG). Traditionally, painful areas that are smaller and more superficial may benefit from a single PNfS lead. Conversely, larger areas may be more suitable for one or more leads with the idea that cross-talking (i.e., current transmittance from one lead to a more distant lead) may increase the area of paresthesia [48]. PNfS lead placement may seem facile, but unsuspected difficulties may exist. Naturally, pain outside the confines of paresthesia will never diminish [42]. By using the length of the array as an advantage, lines of current transect the area of pain. It is also important to note that multiple electrodes do not always confer greater effectiveness. PNfS targets the terminal sensory nerve fibers that exist within the deep dermis; therefore, depth becomes an impactful consideration [15, 16]. A needle coursing through the dermis is painful, and so will be the lead and electrode array that follows. Similarly, a lead placed too deep may inadvertently recruit muscle fiber, which also leads to discomfort. Hence, the lead is optimally positioned at the junction between dermis and fat [33, 42, 45].

After sterile preparation, local anesthetic is delivered subcutaneously in a wheal fashion to prime skin for incision and subsequent needle entry. With constant palpation, the needle remains parallel to the dermis and should be easily advanced with minimal resistance; horizontal depression of the needle produces minimal inflection when traversing the correct layer. The lead body is marginally detectable once deployed. Some newer devices may even allow for real-time testing by using a nerve stimulator prior to lead placement [42].

Sedation is the preferred choice of anesthetic for this reason in order to avoid using excessive amounts of local anesthetic, which may lead to a falsely negative outcome while testing [42, 45]. Testing at the time of the trial procedure does not guarantee that the area will demonstrate pain improvement but will help to assure that the "zone" of pain is the intended area to target. Even in the appropriate layer, paresthesia may be uncomfortable for the patient, and increasing the amplitude may ultimately alter the quality to be more of a satisfying experience. Slightly withdrawing the lead may lead to appropriate fiber stimulation if high amplitude, inadequate paresthetic distribution, or pain become an issue. The procedure then concludes after lead ligation to skin, radiographic documentation, and wound dressing [45]. The outpatient trial commences once discharged and may be of variable timeframe [49]. To allow the tissue to appropriately heal from the minimal trauma of needle insertion, a waiting period of at least 72 hours is common and also helps to avoid painful stimulation after the leads are placed [42].

PNfS Permanent Implant

If satisfactory pain relief is achieved with the trial, the patient is offered a permanent implant, and placement occurs again within the operating room setting. Anchoring methods vary, but the aim is to secure the lead while mitigating the risk of erosion, migration, or lead fracture [12]. Closing the tissue in multiple planes may prevent anchor erosion [42]. All in all, the method used has no significant importance, as long as migration of the lead is not encountered, which is the most common complication [50]. Once secured, a pocket is made for the device in general proximity to the lead array. Similar to SCS, the likelihood of complication increases as the distance between the pocket and lead array increases. Fortunately, the smaller size of IPGs in the present day improves options with regard to pocket location. All wounds are irrigated prior to closure. Device programming usually stabilizes over 6 weeks as fibrosis develops around leads, further functionalizing the position [42].

Risk Mitigation

It is paramount to understand risk mitigation when pursuing PNfS as a modality. Risks are limited, but the overall health of patients comes into play and may extend to various organ systems. Therefore, the interventionalist must evaluate comorbidities prior to device trial and implantation, and medical conditions should be optimized. Nerve injury is very rare, especially with novel percutaneous techniques of lead placement. However, leads should be predominantly positioned in the proximity of the nerve and not in direct contact [13]. Patients are kept only lightly sedated during the procedure in order to maintain the ability to alert the implanter if paresthesia is experienced [45]. If so, the needle or lead should be redirected. Palpation of the skin while placing the needle promotes safe passage, and it also helps to direct the bevel downward so as to engage the lead. With regard to pocket location, the device should be located such that the patient's daily activities are not negatively affected. Typically, the pocket should receive the least amount of tissue pressure. Independent of location, it has to satisfy certain requirements: the pocket has to be deep enough to avoid hardware erosion, it should not be too deep such that reprogramming or recharging becomes a difficult task, and it should be located in a relatively immobile area since repetitive mechanical stress may have deleterious effects on device functionality [12]. If pain at the device persists, topical anesthetics, padding, or surgical revision may be considered [42].

Conclusion

PNfS is an effective technique for the management of chronic neuropathic pain and other pain syndromes. The success of therapy hinges on appropriate candidate selection and favorable positioning of leads for the most effective stimulation. Although PNfS carries less risk of complications compared to other neuromodulatory procedures, lead migration, erosion, infection, or mechanical issues with the device may occur. Unrealistic expectations with any therapy may result in suboptimal outcomes; as such, an ongoing dialogue between patient and physician may leverage expectations in the preparation process. Improvements in technology are expected within the field of interventional pain medicine, and the resurgence of PNfS as a treatment modality encourages further innovation.

Supplemental Images

References

1. Keller T, Krames ES. On the shoulders of giants: a history of the understandings of pain, leading to the understandings of neuromodulation. Neuromodulation. 2009;12(2):77–84.
2. Melzack R, Wall PD. Pain mechanisms: a new theory. Science. 1965;150(699):971–9.
3. Shealy CN, Mortimer JT, Reswick JB. Electrical inhibition of pain by stimulation of the dorsal columns: preliminary clinical report. Anesth Analg. 1967;46(4):489–91.
4. Burchiel KJ, Anderson VC, Brown FD, et al. Prospective, multicenter study of spinal cord stimulation for relief of chronic back and extremity pain. Spine. 1996;21(23):2786–94.
5. Cameron T. Safety and efficacy of spinal cord stimulation for the treatment of chronic pain: a 20-year literature review. J Neurosurg. 2004;100(3):254–67.

6. Mironer YE, Hutcheson JK, Satterthwaite JR, et al. Prospective, two-part study of the interaction between spinal cord stimulation and peripheral nerve field stimulation in patients with low back pain: development of a new spinal-peripheral neurostimulation method. Neuromodulation. 2011;14(2):151–5.
7. Weiner RL, Reed KL. Peripheral neurostimulation for control of intractable occipital neuralgia. Neuromodulation. 1999;2:217–21.
8. Deer TR, Jain S, Hunter C, et al. Neurostimulation for intractable chronic pain. Brain Sci. 2019;9:23.
9. Papuć E, Rejdak K. The role of neurostimulation in the treatment of neuropathic pain. Ann Agric Environ Med. 2013;1:14–7.
10. Chakravarthy K, Nava A, Christo PJ, et al. Review of recent advances in peripheral nerve stimulation (PNS). Curr Pain Headache Rep. 2016;20(11):60.
11. Abejón D, Krames ES. Peripheral nerve stimulation or is it peripheral subcutaneous field stimulation; what is in a moniker? Neuromodulation. 2009;12(1):1–4.
12. Slavin KV. Peripheral nerve stimulation for neuropathic pain. Neurotherapeutics. 2008;5(1):100–6.
13. Nayak R, Banik RK. Current innovations in peripheral nerve stimulation. Pain Res Treat. 2018;2018:9091216.
14. Ellrich L, Lamp S. Peripheral nerve stimulation inhibits nociceptive processing: an electrophysiological study in healthy volunteers. Neuromodulation. 2005;8(4):225–32.
15. Frahm KS, Hennings K, Vera-Portocarrero L, et al. Nerve Fiber activation during peripheral nerve field stimulation: importance of electrode orientation and estimation of area of Paresthesia. Neuromodulation. 2016;19(3):311–8.
16. Abejón D, Deer TR, Verrills P. Subcutaneous stimulation: how to assess optimal implantation depth. Neuromodulation. 2011;14:343–8.
17. Morch CD, Nguyen GP, Wacnik PW, Andersen OK. Mathematical model of nerve fiber activation during low back peripheral nerve field stimulation: analysis of electrode implant depth. Neuromodulation. 2014;17(3):218–25.
18. Krutsch JP, McCeney MH, Barolat G, et al. A case report of subcutaneous peripheral nerve stimulation for the treatment of axial back pain associated with postlaminectomy syndrome. Neuromodulation. 2008;11(2):112–5.
19. Fishman S, Ballantyne J, Rathmell J. Bonica's management of pain. Wolters Kluwer Health/ Lippincott: Williams & Wilkins; 2010.
20. Wall PD, Sweet WH. Temporary abolition of pain in man. Science. 1967;155(758):108–9.
21. Slavin KV, Weiss C. Trigeminal branch stimulation for intractable neuropathic pain: technical note. Neuromodulation. 2005;8(1):7–13.
22. Slavin KV, Nersesyan H, Wess C. Peripheral neurostimulation for treatment of intractable occipital neuralgia. Neurosurgery. 2006;58(1):112–9.
23. Oh MY, Ortega J, Belotte JB, et al. Peripheral nerve stimulation for the treatment of occipital neuralgia and transformed migraine using a C1-2-3 subcutaneous paddle style electrode: a technical report. Neuromodulation. 2004;7(2):103–12.
24. Popeney CA, Aló KM. Peripheral neurostimulation for the treatment of chronic, disabling transformed migraine. Headache. 2003;43(4):369–75.
25. Mitchell B, Verrills P, Vivian D, et al. Peripheral nerve field stimulation therapy for patients with thoracic pain: a prospective study. Neuromodulation. 2016;9:752–9.
26. Desai M, Jacob L, Leiphart J. Successful peripheral nerve field stimulation for thoracic radiculitis following Brown-Sequard syndrome. Neuromodulation. 2011;14:249–52.
27. Verrills P, Mitchell B, Vivian D, et al. Peripheral nerve stimulation: a treatment for chronic low back pain and failed back surgery syndrome? Neuromodulation. 2009;12:68–75.
28. Verrills P, Vivian D, Mitchell B, et al. Peripheral nerve field stimulation for chronic pain: 100 cases and review of the literature. Pain Med. 2011;12(9):1395–405.
29. Paicius RM, Bernstein CA, Lempert-Cohen C. Peripheral nerve field stimulation for the treatment of chronic low back pain: preliminary results of long-term follow-up: a case series. Neuromodulation. 2007;10:279–90.

30. Reverberi C, Dario A, Barolat G. Spinal cord stimulation (SCS) in conjunction with peripheral nerve field stimulation (PNfS) for the treatment of complex pain in failed back surgery syndrome (FBSS). Neuromodulation. 2013;16(1):78–83.
31. Bernstein CA, Paicius RM, Barkow SH, et al. Spinal cord stimulation in conjunction with peripheral nerve field stimulation for the treatment of low back and leg pain: a case series. Neuromodulation. 2008;11(2):116–23.
32. Yakovlev AE, Resch BE, Yakovleva VE. Peripheral nerve field stimulation in the treatment of postlaminectomy syndrome after multilevel spinal surgeries. Neuromodulation. 2011;14(6):534–8.
33. McRoberts WP, Wolkowitz R, Meyer DJ, et al. Peripheral nerve field stimulation for the management of localized chronic intractable back pain: results from a randomized controlled study. Neuromodulation. 2013;16(6):565–74.
34. Paicius RM, Bernstein CA, Lempert-Cohen C. Peripheral nerve field stimulation in chronic abdominal pain. Pain Phys. 2006;9:261–6.
35. Zhou L, Chou H, Holder E. Abdominal wall type-I complex regional pain syndrome treated effectively with peripheral nerve field stimulation: a case report. J Surg Case Rep. 2017;1:222.
36. Stinson LW Jr, Roderer GT, Cross NE, et al. Peripheral subcutaneous electrostimulation for control of intractable post-operative inguinal pain: a case report series. Neuromodulation. 2001;4(3):99–104.
37. Shaw A, Sharma M, Zibly Z, et al. Sandwich technique, peripheral nerve stimulation, peripheral field stimulation and hybrid stimulation for inguinal region and genital pain. Br J Neurosurg. 2016;30(6):631–6.
38. Lepski G, Vahedi P, Tatagiba MS, et al. Combined spinal cord and peripheral nerve field stimulation for persistent post-herniorrhaphy pain. Neuromodulation. 2013;16:84–8.
39. Al Tamimi M, Davids HR, Barolat G, et al. Subcutaneous peripheral nerve stimulation treatment for chronic pelvic pain. Neuromodulation. 2008;11(4):277–81.
40. Chan I, Brown AR, Park K, et al. Ultrasound-guided, percutaneous peripheral nerve stimulation: technical note. Neurosurgery. 2010;67:136–9.
41. Eisenberg E, Waisbrod H, Gerbershagen HU. Long-term peripheral nerve stimulation for painful nerve injuries. Clin J Pain. 2004;20(3):143–6.
42. Deer TR, Abejon D, Barolat G. Stimulation of the peripheral nervous system. In: Atlas of Implantable Therapies for Pain Management. Springer, New York, NY; 2011.
43. Huntoon MA, Burgher AH. Ultrasound-guided permanent implantation of peripheral nerve stimulation (PNS) system for neuropathic pain of the extremities: original cases and outcomes. Pain Med. 2009;10(8):1369–77.
44. Reverberi C, Bonezzi C, Demartini L. Peripheral subcutaneous neurostimulation in the management of neuropathic pain: five case reports. Neuromodulation. 2009;12(2):146–55.
45. Petersen EA, Slavin KV. Peripheral nerve/field stimulation for chronic pain. Neurosurg Clin N Am. 2014;25:789–97.
46. Campbell CM, Jamison RN, Edwards RR. Psychological screening/phenotyping as predictors for spinal cord stimulation. Curr Pain Headache Rep. 2013;17(1):307.
47. Doleys DM. Psychological factors in spinal cord stimulation therapy: brief review and discussion. Neurosurg Focus. 2006;21(6):E1.
48. Falco FJ, Berger J, Vrable A, et al. Cross talk: a new method for peripheral nerve stimulation. An observational report with cadaveric verification. Pain Physician. 2010;13(1):99.
49. Deer TR, Naidu R, Strand N, et al. A review of the bioelectronic implications of stimulation of the peripheral nervous system for chronic pain conditions. Bioelectron Med. 2020;6:9.
50. Stevanato G, Devigili G, Eleopra R, et al. Chronic post-traumatic neuropathic pain of brachial plexus and upper limb: a new technique of peripheral nerve stimulation. Neurosurg Rev. 2014;37(3):473–9.

Ultrasound Indications, Historical Aspects, and Devices in Peripheral Nerve Stimulation

Tiago da Silva Freitas

Indications, Historical Aspects, and Devices in Peripheral Nerve Stimulation

Introduction: Peripheral Nerve Stimulation History

The first therapeutic use of electricity to modulate the nervous system was described in the year 57 DC by the roman physician Scribonius Largus in his book Compositiones Medicae [1]. After inadvertently stepping on a torpedo (electric) fish on a beach, Anteros noticed a significant improvement in pain in his lower limbs due to gout. Scribonius realized that there could be therapeutic use, and he treated chronic pain like headache. In his descriptions, Scribonius lays the foundations for electrical neuromodulation of the central nervous system:

"Even chronic and intractable headaches are cured and remedied forever by placing a live torpedo below the pain site, until it passes. Once the numbness has been felt, the medicine must be removed. Furthermore, several torpedoes of the same type must be prepared, as the cure (which is torpor) is effective sometimes only after two or three sessions."

During the elaboration of their gate theory, in the 1960s, Wall and Sweet tried approaches with peripheral electrical stimulation in the suppression of neuropathic pain, inserting an electrode in their own infraorbital foramen. They managed to decrease the perception of pain throughout the period of stimulation on this peripheral nerve [2, 3]. Also in this period, some articles showing the use of electrical stimulation in peripheral nerves were performed [2, 4], even before Shealy's description of spinal cord stimulation in 1967.

T. d. S. Freitas (✉)
Functional Neurosurgery/Pain Treatment, Brasilia Pain Institute (INDOR), Brasília, Distrito Federal, Brazil

Functional Neurosurgery Department Hospital Sírio Libanês, Brasília, Distrito Federal, Brazil

T. d. S. Freitas et al. (eds.), *Neuromodulation Techniques for Pain Treatment*,
https://doi.org/10.1007/978-3-030-84778-4_9

Even after describing the spinal cord stimulation referred to above, several reports have been described in the literature using PNS. Most of these articles published in the 1970s and 1990s showed peripheral nerve implants involved in localized neuropathic pain syndrome or regional complex pain syndrome, with an approach using open surgical techniques [5–21]. The results of these studies showed few promising results, and this contributed to the decline in the use of PNS compared to the use of spinal cord stimulation as a form of neuromodulation in the treatment of pain.

The decline in the use of peripheral neurostimulation was also reflected in the industry's little interest in the development of specific materials related to this surgical technique, as well as the lack of enthusiasm to carry out registrations in regulatory bodies, such as the FDA.

The resurrection of peripheral nerve stimulation for the treatment of pain happened to Weiner and Reed in 1999, when they described the use of percutaneous electrode implants in occipital nerves for the treatment of occipital neuralgia [22]. Later, Slavin and Burchiel described the use of percutaneous techniques involving branches of the trigeminal nerve for facial pain [15–21], and from then on, a series of new articles were progressively published [23–48], increasing the efficacy evidence from this neuromodulation treatment modality.

General Indications

For reasons of cost and invasiveness, it is worth remembering that the use of neurostimulation in the peripheral nervous system is generally not the first option in the treatment of most pain syndromes, being reserved in cases where the initial conservative treatments do not achieve effectiveness in controlling pain and the patient's quality of life.

There are two major groups of chronic pain diseases where the use of peripheral nerve stimulation is more indicated and more effective. The first is the pain syndromes of neuropathic origin, restricted to the innervation of a specific peripheral nerve (painful mononeuropathies). Pain in these pain syndromes can have different causes, ranging from metabolic (diabetic), infectious (herpes zoster, leprosy), vascular (peripheral ischemic neuropathies), and traumatic (postoperative and secondary to local trauma) diseases.

The second major group of diseases that can benefit from peripheral nerve stimulation is headache. Within this large group of diseases, we can mention the ones that have the most evidence of response: occipital neuralgia, cluster headache, and migraine. However, a series of other headache modalities have progressively benefited from treatment with peripheral nerve stimulation: neuropathic facial pain (postsurgical or not), hemicrania, transformed migraine, C2-mediated headaches, and pain in occipital region pain after spine surgery.

Devices in Peripheral Nerve Stimulation

Devices used in the stimulation of peripheral nerves to treat pain have a large lag in evolution and novelties, especially when compared with the evolution of spinal stimulation systems. Much of this lag is historically due to the initial results of peripheral nerve stimulation when compared to spinal cord stimulation with studies showing worse results and a higher incidence of complications [49].

In this way, many of the studies and clinical practice in peripheral nerve stimulation are carried out with adaptations of spinal stimulation systems, which may explain the relatively high migration rates when compared to SCS.

Historically, the first description of the use of peripheral nerve stimulation happened in 1963 by Shelden [50], who performed the implantation of three patients with trigeminal neuralgia. The device was fully implantable and powered by an external radio frequency generator. The use of systems with external RF generator and nerve cuff electrodes became more common in the 1970s [51, 52, 53, 54], and this first generation of systems was quite limited as it referred to the external generator's power supply, as well as the number of contacts available to cover the painful area with tonic stimulation.

The next generations of devices for peripheral nerves were developed by Avery Laboratories and had the advantage of having electrodes with multiple contacts, as well as the existence of a flexible connection between the electrodes and the generator, which allowed better positioning of the RF receiver. On the other hand, this system only stimulated one cathode and one anode, and tests were necessary to define the best contacts for peripheral nerve stimulation. The number of migrations was also high. Numerous works were published with this system in the 1970s and 1980s [54, 55, 56, 57, 58], and although the results were promising, the RF device needed an external coil, which mitigated the correct adhesion of the device in the patient and problems such as the inability to not stimulate full-time. The fact was added to the development of fully implantable generators.

Afterward, in the 1990s, systems evolved with descriptions of the use of plate electrodes connected to fully implantable generators [59]. These systems had the same complications as hardware problems, migration, and skin sores on the systems.

The use of percutaneous electrodes in PNS became popular after the classic article by Weiner and Reed from 1999 [22], which used percutaneous electrodes in the treatment of occipital neuralgia, and from this study, several other targets were used in the treatment of different pathologies. These systems included nonspecific devices and true adaptations of the SCS electrodes, which led to the continuity of the complications arising from this adaptation: migration, system breakdown, pain at the procedure site, skin scar, and early generator depletion, among others.

New Specific Systems

In the last few years, specific devices for peripheral nerve stimulation have been developed on the market. These included percutaneous devices and fully implantable devices targeted for specific nerves.

Below there is a table with some examples of the new systems dedicated to peripheral nerve stimulation in the treatment of pain with their main characteristics of approval with respect to regulatory institutions.

Device	Approved institution	Basic description	Literature Results
StimRouter (bioness, Valencia, California) Fig. 1	FDA Under approval in ANVISA (Brazilian FDA)	This device, an implantable PNS device coupled with an external transmitter, obtained Food and Drug Administration (FDA) approval for PNS in the trunk and limbs. The differentiating feature was a small implantable tined lead, with a pickup contact that would be used with an external peripheral nerve generator	Prospective, multicenter, randomized, double-blind, partial crossover study [60] found an average pain relief at 3 months: 27.2% versus 2.3% of placebo. The percentage of patients achieving 30% or greater reduction in pain was 38% versus 10% in placebo. The attrition rate at 12 months was 51%, with only 7 explants within the first 12 months A retrospective case series [61] in axillary peripheral nerve stimulation for chronic shoulder pain (8 patients) found: Based on the ≥50% pain reduction for treatment success, 88% (7/8) were "responders." overall average pain reduction was 67% and 70% among responders; 62.5% (5/8) of patients reported that they used opioids prior to axillary PNS therapy for pain relief [61]

Device	Approved institution	Basic description	Literature Results
SPRINT (smartpatch device. Cleveland, OH, USA)	FDA	Percutaneous microlead electrodes linked to an external power source, minimally invasive, that can hold 60 days of stimulation. Indicated to shoulder pain, back pain, knee pain, and peripheral neuropathic pain	A multi-site case series with two-year follow-up for hemiplegic shoulder pain [62]: 28 patients trialed with 5 permanent implant: 50% or greater pain reduction at 6 and 12 months, and four experienced at least a 50% reduction at 24 months A prospective case series to low chronic back pain [63] with 12 months follow-up found: Twelve months after the end of PNS treatment, a majority of subjects who completed the long-term follow-up visits experienced sustained, clinically significant reductions in pain and/or disability (67%, n = 6; average, 63% reduction in pain intensity and 32-point reduction in Disability among responders)
Freedom 4 (Stimwave, USA)	FDA approved	Percutaneous electrode without a permanent implanted generator. The system uses a wireless technology, external battery	A pilot 2-phase study with 11 patients, DRG stimulation for FBSS [64] found overall pain reduction was 59.9%, with only one device placed at one location, covering only a portion of the painful areas in the majority of the subjects

Device	Approved institution	Basic description	Literature Results
Reactive8 for LBP (mainstay medical limited, Dublin, Ireland) Fig. 2	CE approved	The device consists of an implanted pulse generator (IPG) and two leads. The proximal end of each lead connects directly to the IPG, and the distal end is positioned with four stimulating electrodes in close proximity to the medial branch of the L2 dorsal ramus nerve as it crosses the L3 transverse processes. The distal end of each lead has tines designed to help fix the lead in the intertransversarii muscles between the transverse processes (Fig. 1), and the lead positioning keeps the distal ends well away from the neural foramen and the dorsal root ganglion. The IPG can be programmed to deliver stimulation between any pair of electrodes on each lead (ref. Artigo original)	A prospective, multicenter, clinical trial [65], with 1-year follow-up, for low back pain treatment found as follows: For 53 subjects with an average duration of CLBP of 14 years and average NRS of 7 and for whom no other therapies Had provided satisfactory pain relief, the responder rate was 58%. The percentage of subjects at 90 days, six months, and one Year with MCID improvement in single-day NRS was 63%, 61%, and 57%, respectively. The percentage of subjects with MCID Improvement in ODI was 52%, 57%, and 60%, while those with _MCID improvement in EQ-5D was 88%, 82%, and 81%.

Device	Approved institution	Basic description	Literature Results
Lightpulse for PNS in extremities (Neurimpulse, Rubano, PD, Italy)	CE approved	The device consists of a cylindrical quadripolar lead (Lightline, Neurimpulse, Rubano, PD, Italy) was placed on the nervous structure(s). The lead has a 1.2 mm diameter. There are two models, one with a 4 mm intercontact length (for nerve placement) and one with a 6 mm intercontact length (for brachial plexus implantation). The spiral configuration of the conductive filaments provides both stiffness and elasticity to the lead. After some centimeters, the lead came in contact with the epineurium and was fixed with a silicon ring adapter at the perineurium fascia. After successful trial: Implantation of the pulse generator (Lightpulse 100, Neurimpulse). The dimensions are volume 13 cc, thickness 7 mm, and weight 26 g. this IPG was developed with the goal of being implanted adjacent to the insertion point of the peripheral stimulation lead	A clinical case series [66] for the treatment of CRPS found: Of the 15 patients, 3 failed the trial phase, and 12 were implanted with a permanent pulse generator. After an average of 9.3 months of follow-up, the average NRS score was 3.46 ($p < 0.001$), and the The average Likert scale score at 7 points was 5.91. Nine patients were working prior to their injuries, seven of whom returned to work after receiving an implant. The average oxycodone consumption decreased to 30 mg/day, and the pregabalin dosage decreased to 75 mg/day. A multicenter observational study [67] using this device for neuropathic pain after peripheral nerve injury found: A total of 58 patients were referred to permanent IPG implantation. Stimulation failure due to lead damage or dislocation was noticed in two cases (3.4%) in six months. At the follow-up end, the relative NRS reduction averaged 258,630% ($p < 1026$) And was greater than 50% in 69% of the cases. Quality-of-life physical and mental indices were increased by 18% ($p < 0.005$) and 29% ($p < 0.0005$), respectively

Device	Approved institution	Basic description	Literature Results
HF PNS for postamputation pain (neuros medical, Willoughby Hills, Ohio, USA)	In development	This device uses a nerve cuff attached to a nerve stump. He incorporates high-frequency stimulation (10 Khz)	A pilot study [68] with 7 patients with post-amputation pain: The average pain reduction was 75% at the three-month primary end Point. These subjects were responders per predefined criterion of achieving ≥50% pain reduction in ≥50% of treatment sessions for the three-month end point. Pain medication use and interference of pain on functions were significantly reduced. The treatment efficacy was sustained through the follow-up period of up to 12 months.
SPG neurostimulatior (Sphenopalatne ganglion) (autonomic technologis-ATI, Redwood City, Calif., USA)	CE approved	This device has a lead with multiple contacts attached directly to a miniature neurostimulator and fixation plate designed specifically to stimulate the SPG for cluster headaches	Randomized, sham-controlled study found that 68% of patients had a clinically significant improvement

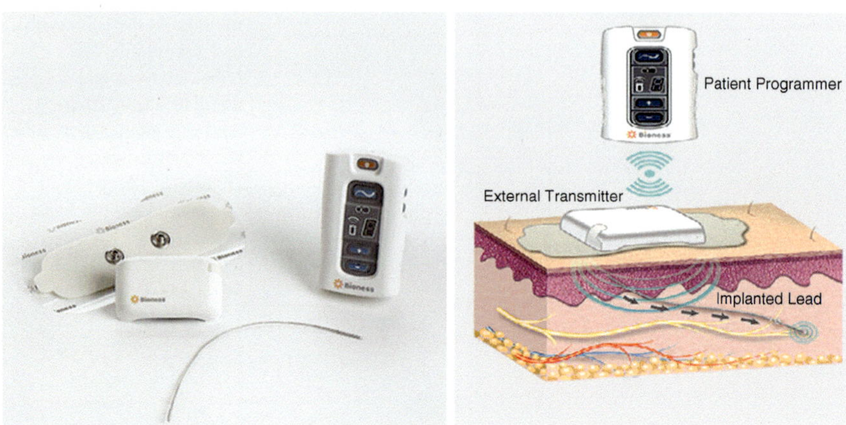

Fig. 1 StimRouter system (image printed with permission)

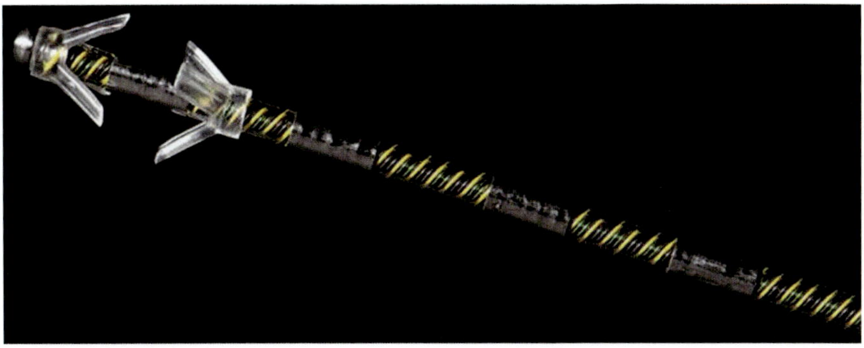

Fig. 2 Reactive8 system

Bibliography

1. Scribonius largus. Compositiones medicae.1655.696p.
2. Wall PD, Sweet WH. Temporary abolition of pain in man. Science. 1967;155:108–9.
3. White JC, Sweet WH. Pain and the neurosurgeon: a forty-year experience. Springfield, IL: Thomas; 1969. p. 894–9.
4. Shelden CH. Depolarization in the treatment of trigeminal neuralgia. Evaluation of compression and electrical methods; clinical concept of neurophysiological mechanism. In: Knighton RS, Dumke PR, editors. Pain. Boston: Little, Brown; 1966. p. 373–86.
5. Cauthen JC, Renner EJ. Transcutaneous and peripheral nerve stimulation for chronic pain states. Surg Neurol. 1975;4:102–4.
6. Kirsch WM, Lewis JA, Simon RH. Experiences with electrical stimulation devices for the control of chronic pain. Med Instrum. 1975;9:217–20.
7. Picaza JA, Cannon BW, Hunter SE, Boyd AS, Guma J, Maurer D. Pain suppression by peripheral nerve stimulation: II. Observations with implanted devices. Surg Neurol. 1975;4:115–26.
8. Campbell JN, Long DM. Peripheral nerve stimulation in the treatment of intractable pain. J Neurosurg. 1976;45:692–9.
9. Sweet WH. Control of pain by direct stimulation of peripheral nerves. Clin Neurosurg. 1976;23:103–11.
10. Nashold BS Jr, Mullen JB, Avery R. Peripheral nerve stimulation for pain relief using a multicontact electrode system: technical note. J Neurosurg. 1979;51:872–3.
11. Law JD, Sweet J, Kirsch WM. Retrospective analysis of 22 patients with chronic pain treated by peripheral nerve stimulation. J Neurosurg. 1980;52:482–5.
12. Long DM, Erickson D, Campbell J, North R. Electrical stimulation of the spinal cord and peripheral nerves for pain control: a 10-year experience. Appl Neurophysiol. 1981;44:207–17.
13. Nashold BS Jr, Goldner JL, Mullen JB, Bright DS. Long-term pain control by direct peripheral nerve stimulation. J Bone Joint Surg Am. 1982;64:1–10.
14. Waisbrod H, Panhans C, Hansen D, Gerbeshagen HU. Direct nerve stimulation for painful peripheral neuropathies. J Bone Joint Surg Br. 1985;67:470–2.
15. Long DM. Stimulation of the peripheral nervous system for pain control. Clin Neurosurg. 1986;33:323–43.
16. Iacono RP, Linford J, Sandyk R. Pain management after lower extremity amputation. Neurosurgery. 1987;20:496–500.
17. Racz GB, Browne T, Lewis R Jr. Peripheral stimulator implant for treatment of causalgia caused by electrical burns. Tex Med. 1988;84:45–50.

18. Heavner JE, Racz G, Diede JM. Peripheral nerve stimulation: current concepts. In: Waldman SD, Winnie AP, editors. Interventional pain management. 1st ed. Philadelphia: W.B. Saunders; 1996. p. 423–5.
19. Hassenbusch SJ, Stanton-Hicks M, Schoppa D, Walsh JG, Covington EC. Long-term results of peripheral nerve stimulation for reflex sympathetic dystrophy. J Neurosurg. 1996;84:415–23.
20. Stanton-Hicks M, Salamon J. Stimulation of the central and peripheral nervous system for the control of pain. J Clin Neurophysiol. 1997;14:46–62.
21. Shetter AG, Racz GB, Lewis R, Heavner JE. Peripheral nerve stimulation. In: North RB, Levy RM, editors. Neurosurgical management of pain. New York: Springer; 1997. p. 261–70.
22. Weiner RL, Reed KL. Peripheral neurostimulation for control of intractable occipital neuralgia. Neuromodulation. 1999;2:217–21.
23. Weiner RL. The future of peripheral nerve stimulation. Neurol Res. 2000;22:299–304.
24. Lou L. Uncommon areas of electrical stimulation. Curr Rev Pain. 2000;4:407–12.
25. Hammer M, Doleys DM. Perineuromal stimulation in the treatment of occipital neuralgia: a case study. Neuromodulation. 2001;4:47–51.
26. Weiner RL, Aló KM, Reed KL, Fuller ML. Subcutaneous neurostimulation for intractable C-2–mediated headaches. J Neurosurg. 2001;94:398A (abstract).
27. Dunteman E. Peripheral nerve stimulation for unremitting ophthalmic postherpetic neuralgia. Neuromodulation. 2002;5:32–7.
28. Aló KM, Holsheimer J. New trends in neuromodulation for the management of neuropathic pain. Neurosurgery. 2002;50:690–704.
29. Weiner RL. Peripheral nerve neurostimulation. Neurosurg Clin N Am. 2003;14:401–8.
30. Popeney CA, Aló KM. Peripheral neurostimulation for the treatment of chronic, disabling transformed migraine. Headache. 2003;43:369–75.
31. Jones RL. Occipital nerve stimulation using a Medtronic resume II® electrode array. Pain Physician. 2003;6:507–8.
32. Johnson MD, Burchiel KJ. Peripheral stimulation for treatment of trigeminal postherpetic neuralgia and trigeminal posttraumatic neuropathic pain: a pilot study. Neurosurgery. 2004;55:135–42.
33. Matharu MS, Bartsch WN, Frackowiak RSJ, Weiner R, Goadsby PJ. Central neuromodulation in chronic migraine patients with suboccipital stimulators: a PET study. Brain. 2004;127:220–30.
34. Oh MY, Ortega J, Bellotte JB, Whiting DM, Aló K. Peripheral nerve stimulation for the treatment of occipital neuralgia and transformed migraine using a C1-2-3 subcutaneous paddle style electrode: a technical report. Neuromodulation. 2004;7:103–12.
35. Slavin KV, Wess C. Trigeminal branch stimulation for intractable neuropathic pain: a technical note. Neuromodulation. 2005;8:7–13.
36. Kapural L, Mekhail N, Hayek SM, Stanton-Hicks M, Malak O. Occipital nerve electrical stimulation via the midline approach and subcutaneous surgical leads for treatment of severe occipital neuralgia: a pilot study. Anesth Analg. 2005;101:171–4.
37. Rodrigo-Royo MD, Azcona JM, Quero J, Lorente MC, Acín P, Azcona J. Peripheral neurostimulation in the management of cervicogenic headaches: four case reports. Neuromodulation. 2005;4:241–8.
38. Slavin KV, Nersesyan H, Wess C. Peripheral neurostimulation for treatment of intractable occipital neuralgia. Neurosurgery. 2006;58:112–9.
39. Slavin KV, Nersesyan H, Wess C. Treatment of neuropathic craniofacial pain using peripheral nerve stimulation approach. In: Meglio M, Krames ES, editors. Proceedings of the 7th INS meeting of the international Neuromodulation society: Rome, Italy, June 10–13, 2005. Bologna: Medimond International Proceedings; 2005. p. 77–80.
40. Weiner RL. Occipital neurostimulation for treatment of intractable headache syndromes. Acta Neurochir Suppl. 2007;97:129–33.

41. Schwedt TJ, Dodick DW, Trentman TL, Zimmerman RS. Occipital nerve stimulation for chronic cluster headache and hemicranias continua: pain relief and persistence of autonomic features. Cephalalgia. 2006;26:1025–7.
42. Slavin KV, Colpan ME, Munawar N, Wess C, Nersesyan H. Trigeminal and occipital peripheral nerve stimulation for craniofacial pain: a single-institution experience and review of the literature. Neurosurg Focus. 2006;21(6):E5.
43. Rogers LL, Swidan S. Stimulation of the occipital nerve for the treatment of migraine: current state and future prospects. Acta Neurochir Suppl. 2007;97(Pt 1):121–8.
44. Thimineur M, De Ridder D. C2 area neurostimulation: a surgical treatment for fibromyalgia. Pain Med. 2007;8:639–46.
45. Magis D, Allena M, Bolla M, De Pasqua V, Remacle JM, Schoenen J. Occipital nerve stimulation for drug-resistant chronic cluster headache: a prospective pilot study. Lancet Neurol. 2007;6:314–21.
46. Burns B, Watkins L, Goadsby PJ. Treatment of medically intractable cluster headache by occipital nerve stimulation: long-term follow-up of eight patients. Lancet. 2007;369:1099–106.
47. Schwedt TJ, Dodick DW, Hentz J, Trentman TL, Zimmerman RS. Occipital nerve stimulation for chronic headache: long-term safety and efficacy. Cephalalgia. 2007;27:153–7.
48. Hagen JE, Bennett DS. Occipital nerve stimulation for treatment of migraine. Practical Pain Management. 2007;7(6):43–45,56.
49. Slavin KV, editor. Stimulation of the peripheral nervous system. The Neuromodulation frontier. Basel, Karger: Prog Neurol Surg.
50. Shelden CH. Depolarization in the treatment of trigeminal neuralgia. Evaluation of compression and electrical methods; clinical concept of neurophysiological mechanism. In: Kingston RS, Dumke PR, editors. Pain. Boston: Little Brown; 1966. p. 373–86.
51. Long DM. Electrical stimulation for relief of pain from chronic nerve injury. J Neurosurg. 1973;39:718–22.
52. Campbell JN, Long DM. Peripheral nerve stimulation in the treatment of intractable pain. J Neurosurg. 1976;45:692–9.
53. Picaza JA, Cannon BW, Hunter SE, Boyd AS, Guma J, Maurer D. Pain suppression by peripheral nerve stimulation. Part II. Observations with implanted devices. Surg Neurol. 1975;4:115–26.
54. Law JD, Swett J, Kirsch WM. Retrospective analysis of 22 patients with chronic pain treated by peripheral nerve stimulation. J Neurosurg. 1980;52:482–5.
55. Waisbrod H, Panhans C, Hansen D, Gerbershagen HU. Direct nerve stimulation for painful peripheral neuropathies. J Bone Joint Surg Br. 1985;67:470–2.
56. Nashold BS Jr, Goldner JL, Mullen JB, Bright DS. Long-term pain control by direct peripheral-nerve stimulation. J Bone Joint Surg Am. 1982;64:1–10.
57. Nashold BS Jr, Mullen JB, Avery R. Peripheral nerve stimulation for pain relief using a multicontact electrode system: technical note. J Neurosurg. 1979;51:872–3.
58. Neilson KD, Watts C, Clark WK. Peripheral nerve injury from implantation of chronic stimulating electrodes for pain control. Surg Neurol. 1976;5:51.
59. Strege DW, Cooney WP, Wood MB, Johnson SJ, Metcalf BJ. Chronic peripheral nerve pain treated with direct electrical nerve stimulation. J Hand Surg. 1994;19:931–9.
60. Deer T, Pope J, Benyamin R, et al. Prospective, Multicenter, randomized, double-blinded, partial crossover study to assess the safety and efficacy of the novel Neuromodulation system in the treatment of patients with chronic pain of peripheral nerve origin. Neuromodulation. 2016;19(1):91–100.
61. Mansfield JT, Desai MJ. Axillary peripheral nerve stimulation for chronic shoulder pain: a retrospective case series [published online ahead of print, 2020 Jan 13]. Neuromodulation. 2020; https://doi.org/10.1111/ner.13096.
62. Wilson RD, Bennett ME, Nguyen VQC, et al. Fully implantable peripheral nerve stimulation for hemiplegic shoulder pain: a multi-site case series with two-year follow-up. Neuromodulation. 2018;21(3):290–5.

63. Gilmore CA, Kapural L, McGee MJ, Boggs JW. Percutaneous peripheral nerve stimulation for chronic low Back pain: prospective case series with 1 year of sustained relief following short-term implant. Pain Pract. 2020;20(3):310–20.
64. Weiner RL, Yeung A, Montes Garcia C, Tyler Perryman L, Speck B. Treatment of FBSS low Back pain with a novel percutaneous DRG wireless stimulator: pilot and feasibility study. Pain Med. 2016;17(10):1911–6.
65. Deckers K, De Smedt K, Mitchell B, et al. New therapy for refractory chronic mechanical low Back pain-restorative Neurostimulation to activate the lumbar multifidus: one year results of a prospective Multicenter clinical trial. Neuromodulation. 2018;21(1):48–55.
66. Reverberi C, Dario A, Barolat G, Zuccon G. Using peripheral nerve stimulation (PNS) to treat neuropathic pain: a clinical series. Neuromodulation. 2014;17(8):777–83.
67. Colini Baldeschi G, Dario A, De Carolis G, et al. Peripheral nerve stimulation in the treatment of chronic pain syndromes from nerve injury: a Multicenter observational study. Neuromodulation. 2017;20(4):369–74.
68. Soin A, Shah NS, Fang ZP. High-frequency electrical nerve block for postamputation pain: a pilot study. Neuromodulation. 2015;18(3):197–206.

Brachial Plexus Stimulation Using Ultrasound: New Technique Description

Thiago Frederico Nouer and Tiago da Silva Freitas

Introduction

This chapter aims to describe a recent surgical technique prescribed for ultrasound-guided implantation of peripheral brachial plexus electrodes (Ref. [1]). This technique was first described in the *Journal of Pain Medicine* by Thiago Frederic Nouer and Tiago Freitas, the authors of this chapter.

The main indication for the use of invasive neuromodulation in the brachial plexus is the treatment of chronic neuropathic pain syndromes. Nouer and Freitas described this new technique in the treatment of patients with complex regional pain syndrome in the upper limb (Ref. [1]). Historically, the use of this tool for the treatment of upper limb neuropathic syndromes has already been described in other uncontrolled series [2, 3, 4, 5, 6]. These first series described open surgical implantation techniques, involving different neuropathic pain syndromes, from CRPS to more recent neuropathies induced by leprosy [7], presenting results that varied from 60% to 83% improvement of more than 50% on neuropathic pain scales [2, 7].

The use of ultrasound in the various interventional pain techniques has added more safety, better target location, and less radiation exposure, also being used in the minimally invasive neuromodulation techniques for the treatment of pain. In the neuropathic painful upper limb syndromes, the brachial plexus has some important advantages: due to the proximity of the electrode to the nerve tissues, there is less battery consumption. There is also the possibility of better coverage of regions affected by pain. The electrode location seems to be more stable and evolve with a

T. F. Nouer
Singular Pain Clinic, Campinas, São Paulo, Brazil

T. d. S. Freitas (✉)
Brasilia Pain Institute(INDOR), Neurosurgery Department Hospital de Base de Brasília(HBDF), Functional Neurosurgery Department Hospital Sírio Libanês, Brasília, Distrito Federal, Brazil

T. d. S. Freitas et al. (eds.), *Neuromodulation Techniques for Pain Treatment*,
https://doi.org/10.1007/978-3-030-84778-4_10

lower migration rate in the plexus region than in the other peripheral nerves, as well as the possibility of rescuing the effectiveness of therapy in case of failure in the stimulation of the other peripheral nerves from the upper limb.

Descriptions of brachial plexus implants using ultrasound already exist in the literature. Goroszeniuk [8] and Bouche [2] have already described the implantation of electrodes in brachial plexus guided by ultrasound, using the interscalene technique, showing satisfactory results.

The difference between the techniques described above and the one we will now describe is the access route to the brachial plexus. In our technique, access occurs via the suclavicular space. We believe that this pathway is less prone to electrode migration, one of the main complications of peripheral nerve stimulation.

Surgical Technique

Basic Anatomy

Anatomical knowledge of the brachial plexus region and the different vascular and muscle-tendon structures is essential in performing this surgical technique. The brachial plexus usually originates from the ventral ramus of the spinal nerves of C5, C6, C7, C8, and T1 and may present variations in the contributions of C4 and T2. The anterior scalene muscle has its origin in the anterior tubercle of the transverse processes from C3 to C6, and the middle scalene muscle has its origin in the posterior tubercle of the transverse processes, from C2 to C7. Both are inserted into the first rib. Between these muscles are the intervertebral foramen from which the spinal nerves exits. **The ventral rami** follow their respective transverse processes and are oriented towards the cleft formed between the scalene muscles (interscalene cleft). Differences in the anterior orientation and sizes of the cervical transverse processes may lead to the exit of the ventral branches inside or anterior to the anterior scalene muscle. **These** anatomical variations most commonly **occur** in C5 and C6 and may or may not be related to neurological clinical symptoms, featuring neurogenic thoracic outlet syndrome. It is important to be familiar with these anatomical variations, which are easily identified through ultrasonography, because they influence the formation of the upper trunk, which may occur only after the interscalene cleft exit [9–12].

Another important anatomical variation in this region occurs with the autonomic innervation related to the upper limb, which must also be recognized by the implanter. In general, the autonomic innervation of the upper limb comes from the stellate ganglion, which can undergo anatomical variation and be bypassed by the existence of the KUNTZ nerve. This nerve is an inconstant neural structure, which originates from the second thoracic nerve or the first intercostal nerve or even from the stellate ganglion itself, having the function of contributing to the sympathetic innervation of the upper limb [14–16].

Analyzing the sympathetic and somatic anatomical aspects described above, we conclude during the elaboration of this brachial plexus neuromodulation technique that the place where these two innervations meet together is on the first rib, where the brachial plexus (somatic innervation) joins the sympathetic innervation of the upper limb, prior to its entry into the costoclavicular space towards the axilla. Thus, in this supraclavicular region, the trunks/divisions of the brachial plexus are located, with only the long thoracic and dorsal scapular nerves absent, which leave the brachial plexus passing through the scalene muscles [17, 18].

The deep cervical fascia, a dense structure of connective tissue that covers the deep cervical muscles and also the scalene muscles, is an important anatomical structure in this technique. This fascia is a continuous structure, extending from the exit of the nerves from the scalene muscles in the supraclavicular region, continuing with the subclavian artery and reaching the axillary region, where the brachial plexus is already organized into its terminal nerves, forming a structure called the sheath of the brachial plexus or axillary tunnel [13, 18]. It is through this sheath that our electrode will be inserted and conducted through the brachial plexus from the infraclavicular region to the supraclavicular region through the costoclavicular space, which allows us to directly stimulate the trunks/divisions of the brachial plexus and consequently the possibility of covering of the upper limb by neuromodulation therapy.

Surgical Technique

1. Patient positioned in supine position with the arm abducted at a 45- to 60-degree angle under slight sedation, aiming to preserve intraoperative stimulation.
2. Asepsis, antisepsis, and placement of sterile fields. The use of high-frequency linear transducer.
3. Before starting the procedure, an important step is to bend the electrode needle without a mandrel inside. This detail is important to mold the shape of the needle at an angle that allows access to the supraclavicular region under the clavicle with less risk of lung injury, overcoming the volume of the pectoral muscles and the breast. This curvature may vary according to the patient's weight and chest volume, which influence the depth of the brachial plexus in this region. Confirm that the electrode continues to pass through the needle before starting the procedure.
4. We also use a 5% nonpolar dextrose solution, connected to the needle via an extension tube, and remove all air from the system. The use of this nonpolar solution is for hydrodissection of the electrode path as well as to prevent the excessive dispersion of electric current during the intraoperative stimulation phase, a fact that can happen with polar solutions such as 0.9% saline, confusing the precise location of the electrode during the surgery. On the other hand, the volume of this nonpolar 5% dextrose solution should be kept to a minimum; ide-

ally, it should not exceed 15 ml, as the excess can make it difficult to locate the intraoperative brachial plexus.

5. We start the examination with a scanning of the proximal clavicle region until the visualization of the brachial plexus under the acoustic shadow of the clavicle (costoclavicular space), evaluating possible vascular structures in the path of our needle (thoracoacromial artery and cephalic vein). Subsequently, we start visualizing the fascicles of the brachial plexus and axillary artery in the infraclavicular region, observing their deep position in relation to the major and minor pectoral muscles and the clavipectoral fascia. We perform local anesthesia in the possible path of our target using a 22 G needle with an out-of-plane puncture, using a 2% lidocaine and adrenaline 1: 200,000 solution, always with the precaution of anesthetizing the deep portion of the pectoralis minor muscle avoiding dispersion from the anesthetic to the brachial plexus.
6. We start the out-of-plane puncture with the electrode's guide needle, navigating it distally together with the transducer to enter the brachial plexus sheath between the fascicles and the axillary artery. As the puncture is performed off-plane, we use the 5% glucose solution as hydrolocation, until the needle penetrates the sheath of the brachial plexus. We progressively administer small volumes of the solution to open the space in the sheath and advance the tip of the needle until it is hidden under the acoustic shadow of the clavicle.
7. Next, we move the transducer to the supraclavicular region and make small injections of the solution to locate the tip of the needle and always keep it in the upper direction, pointing to the brachial plexus. We remove the syringe and extensor and insert the electrode (percutaneous electrode of 8 or 16 poles) until about 3 to 5 cm of it passes through the tip of the needle. We check the position of the electrode in relation to the brachial plexus with the transducer in the supraclavicular region. We remove the needle and check the position of the electrode on the plexus again in out-of-plane and in-plane positions.
8. With the patient awake, we perform intraoperative tonic stimulation with coverage of the entire anatomical region of the upper limb, using different combinations between the electrode contacts. We generally use PW ranging between 160 and 180 μsec and amplitude ranging between 0.6 and 1.7 mA.
9. After confirmation of intraoperative stimulation, in case of a trial, we fix the electrode through the same original entry point, always in order to prevent the possibility of migration of the electrode. In the case of permanent implants, we make a small incision of 2 cm at the site of the entry point of the electrode into the skin and fix it to the fascia of the pectoralis major muscle. Subsequently, we tunnel the electrode to the subcutaneous subclavicular contralateral space, where the generator is implanted and the electrode is connected to it.

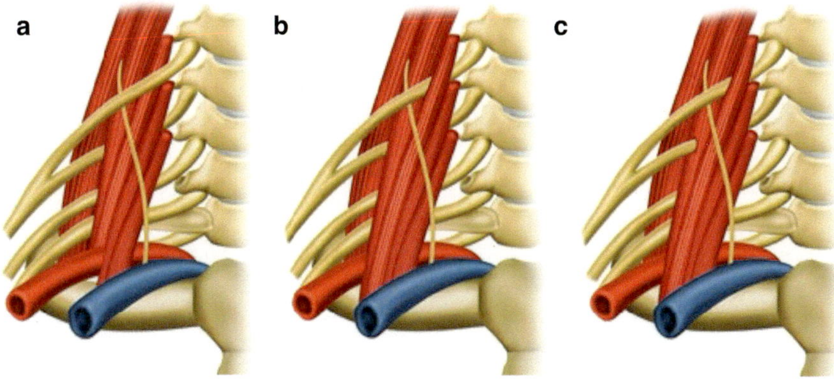

Fig. 1 (**a**) C5 root emerging anterior to the anterior scalene muscle and following its path between the anterior scalene muscle and the sternocleidomastoid muscle until it reaches the remainder of the plexus in the supraclavicular area. (**b**) C5 root emerging from its foramen, inside anterior scalene muscle, transfixing it, and following its path between the anterior scalene muscle and the sternocleidomastoid muscle until finding the remainder of the plexus in the supraclavicular area. (**c**) C-5 and C-6 roots emerging from their foramens inside anterior scalene muscle and transfixing it to find the remainder of the plexus in the supraclavicular area

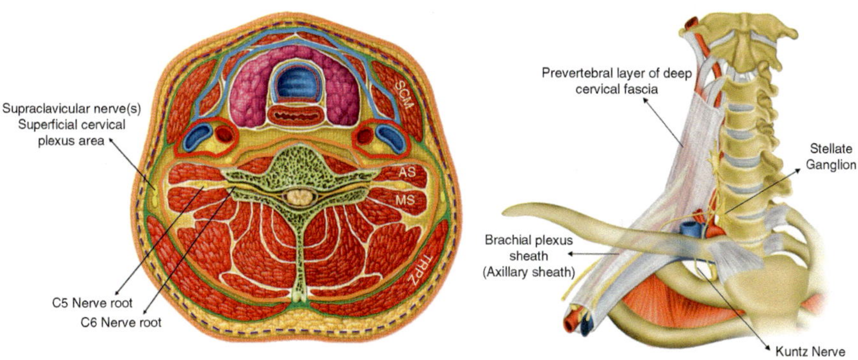

Fig. 2 TRPZ, trapezius muscle; *AS*, anterior scalene; *MS*, middle scalene; *SCM*, sternocleidomastoid. Purple dashed – superficial cervical fascia (platysma fascia), Green – investing layer of deep cervical fascia (sternocleidomastoid-trapezius fascia), Blue – middle layer of deep cervical fascia (strap muscles fascia), Orange – prevertebral layer of deep cervical fascia (vertebral muscles fascia), Red – carotid sheath, White – visceral (pretracheal) layer of deep cervical fascia

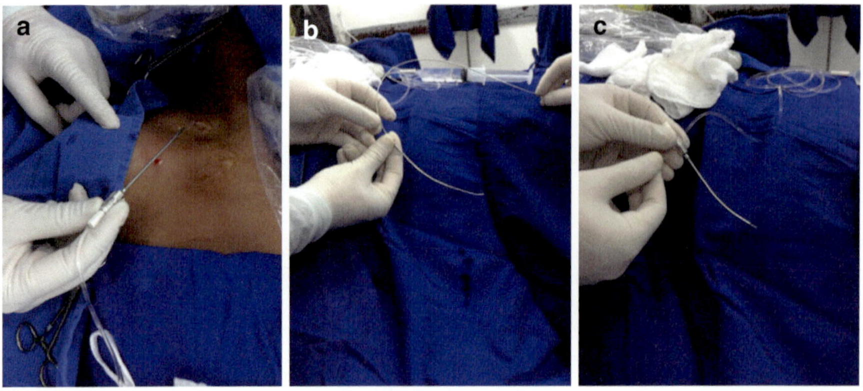

Fig. 3 (**a**) Sterile preparation and evaluation of patient anatomy, to estimate needle bent. (**b**) Test of free sliding electrode inside the bent needle. (**c**) Needle connection to extension tube and a syringe full of dextrose 5% (purge all air out of the system)

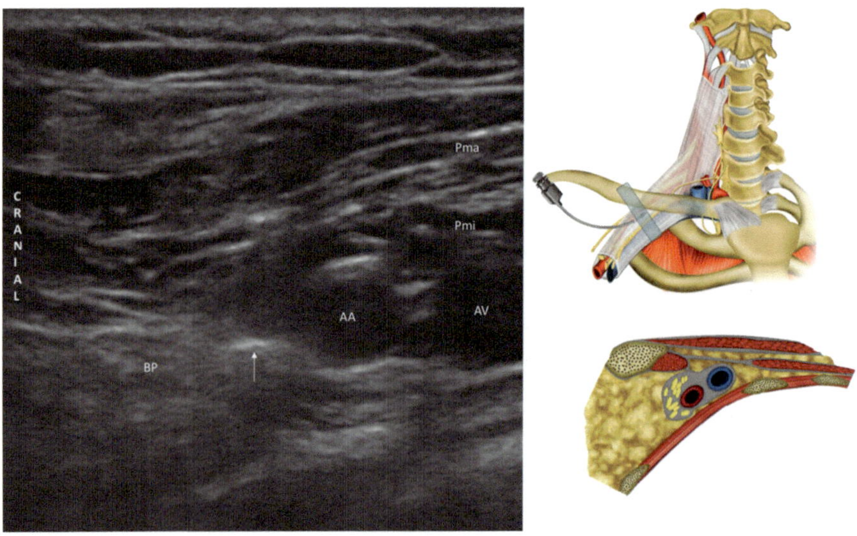

Fig. 4 Ultrasound of infraclavicular area and out of plane needle placement inside brachial plexus sheath between plexus and artery. *BP* brachial plexus; *AA* axillary artery; *AV* axillary vein; *Pma* pectoralis major; *Pmi* pectoralis minor; white arrow – needle

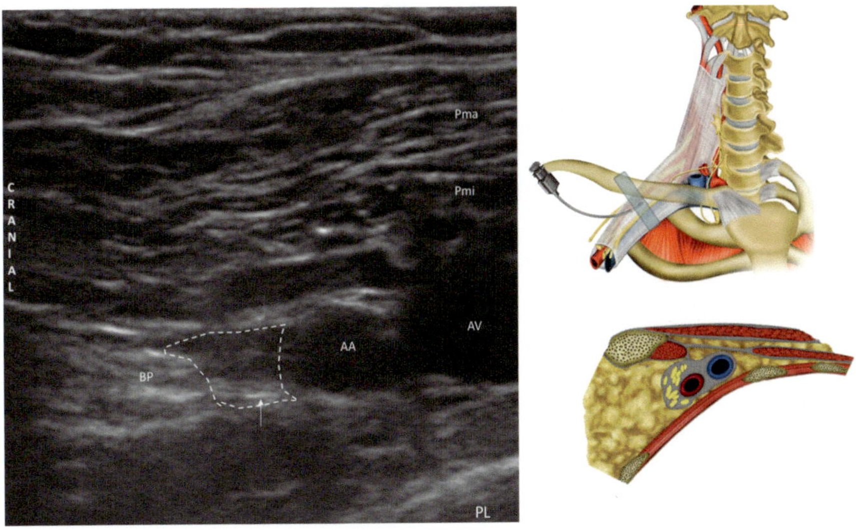

Fig. 5 Ultrasound of infraclavicular area and hydrodissection, titrated with D5W opening space and confirming positioning of needle tip between brachial plexus and axillary artery. BP – brachial plexus; AA – axillary artery; *AV* axillary vein; *Pma* pectoralis major; *Pmi* pectoralis minor; *PL* pleura; white arrow – needle; dashed line – D5W spread

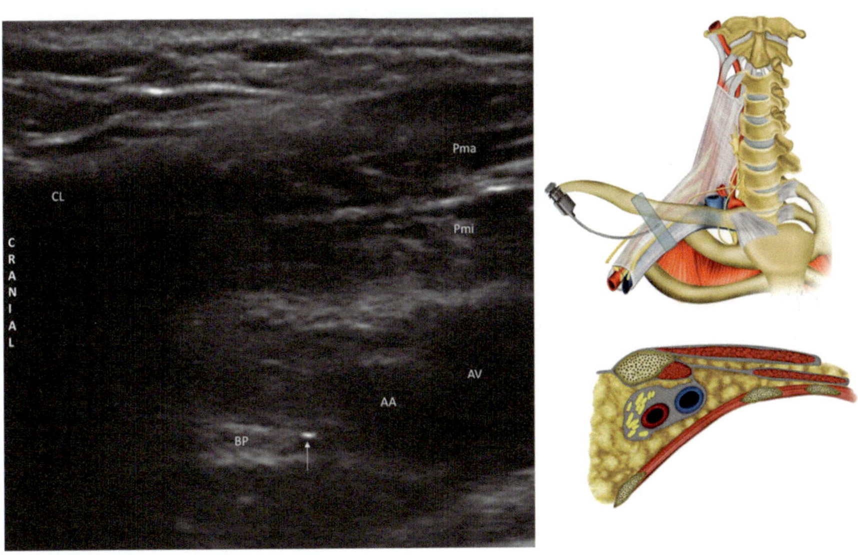

Fig. 6 Ultrasound of infraclavicular/costoclavicular progressing needle tip until it was concealed under the clavicle shadow. *BP* – brachial plexus; *AA* – axillary artery; *AV* axillary vein; *Pma* pectoralis major; *Pmi* pectoralis minor; *CL* clavicle; arrow – needle

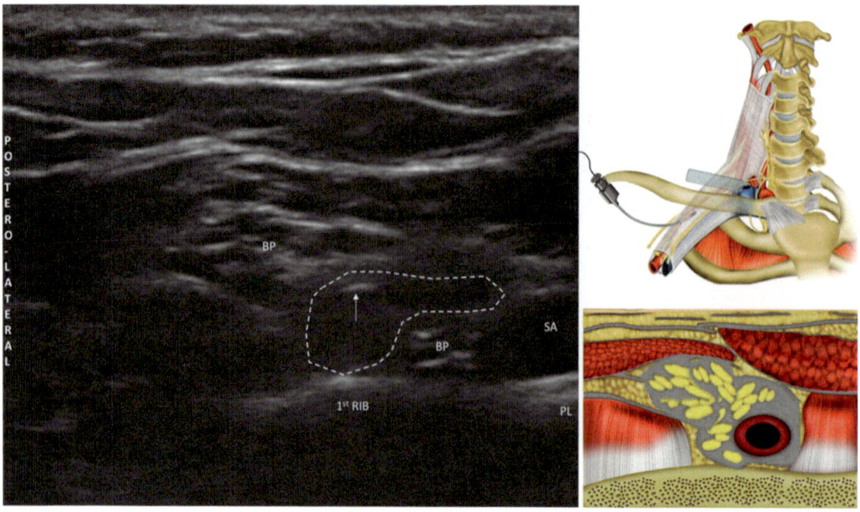

Fig. 7 Ultrasound of supraclavicular area and hydrodissection, titrated with D5W opening space and confirming the position of needle tip inside brachial plexus sheath. *BP* brachial plexus; *SA* subclavian artery; *PL* pleura; arrow – needle; dashed line – D5W spread

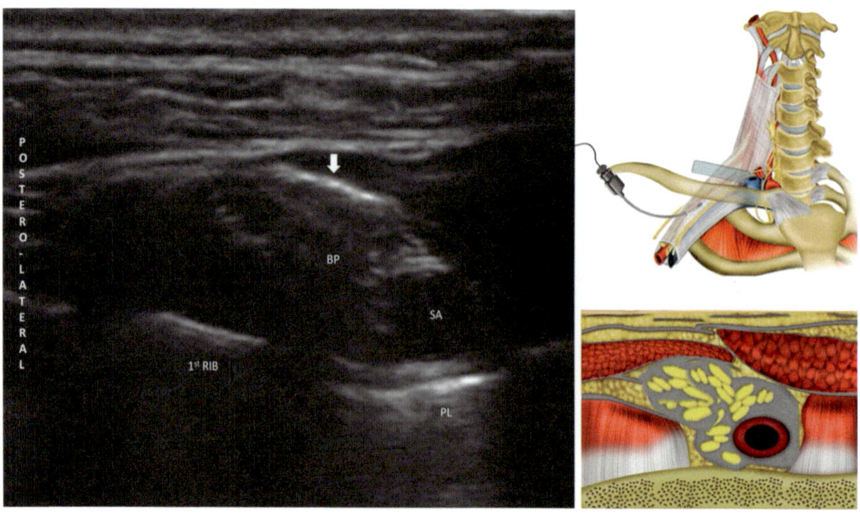

Fig. 8 Ultrasound of supraclavicular area and electrode artifact placed inside brachial plexus sheath. *BP* brachial plexus; *SA* subclavian artery; *PL* pleura; bold arrow – electrode

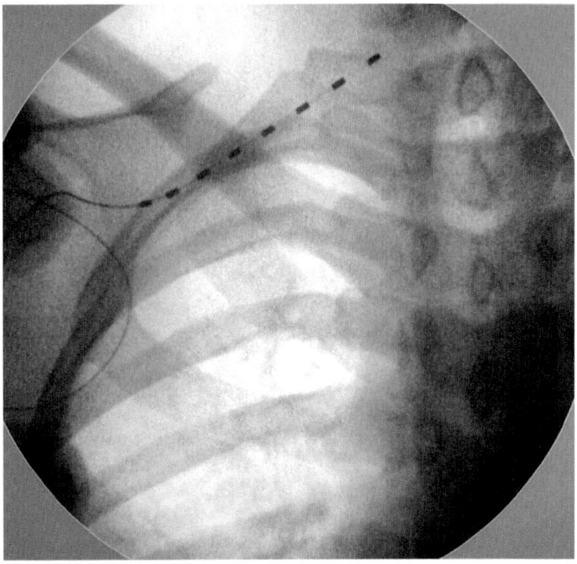

Fig. 9 Fluoroscopy control of electrode positioning

Bibliography

1. Frederico TN, da Silva Freitas T. Peripheral Nerve Stimulation of the Brachial Plexus for Chronic Refractory CRPS Pain of the Upper Limb: Description of a New Technique and Case Series.Pain Med.2020 Aug 1;21(Suppl 1):S18–S26. https://doi.org/10.1093/pm/pnaa201. PMID: 32804227.
2. Bouche B, Manfiotto M, Rigoard P, Lemarie J, Dix-Neuf V, Lanteri-Minet M, Fontaine D. Peripheral nerve stimulation of brachial plexus nerve roots and supra-scapular nerve for chronic refractory neuropathic pain of the upper limb. Neuromodulation. 2017 Oct;20(7):684–9.
3. Eisenberg E, Waisbrod H, Gerbershagen H. Long-term peripheral nerve stimulation for painful nerve injuries. Clin J Pain. 2004;20:143–6.
4. Hassenbusch S, Stanton-Hicks M, Schoppa D, Walsh J, Covington E. Long-term results of peripheral nerve stimulation for reflex sympathetic dystrophy. J Neurosurg. 1996;84:415–23.
5. Mobbs R, Nair S, Blum P. Peripheral nerve stimulation for the treatment of chronic pain. J Clin Neurosci. 2007;14:216–21.
6. Novak C, Mackinnon S. Outcome following implantation of a peripheral nerve stimulator in patients with chronic nerve pain. Plast Reconstr Surg. 2000;105:1967–72.
7. Freitas TDS, Fonoff ET, Marquez Neto OR, Kessler IM, Barros LM, Guimaraes RW, Azevedo MF. Peripheral Nerve Stimulation for Painful Mononeuropathy Secondary to Leprosy: A 12-Month Follow-Up Study. Neuromodulation. 2018 Apr;21(3):310–6.
8. Goroszeniuk T, Kothari S, Hamann W. Percutaneous implantation of a brachial plexus electrode for management of pain syndrome caused by a traction injury. Neuromodulation. 2007;10:148–55.
9. Harry WG, Bennett JDC, Guha SC. Scalene muscles and the brachial plexus: anatomical variations and their clinical significance. Clin Anat. 1997;10(4):250–2.
10. Natsis K, Totlis TTP, et al. V of the course of the upper trunk of the brachial plexus and their clinical significance for the thoracic outlet syndrome: a study of 93 cadavers. AS. 2006;72(2):188–92.

11. Natsis K, Totlis T, Tsikaras P, et al. Variations of the course of the upper trunk of the brachial plexus and their clinical significance for the thoracic outlet syndrome: a study of 93 cadavers. Am Surg. 2006;72(2):188–92. Am Surg. 2006;72(2):188-(2):188–92.
12. Leonhard V, Smith R, Caldwell G, Smith HF. Anatomical variations in the brachial plexus roots: implications for diagnosis of neurogenic thoracic outlet syndrome. Ann Anat. 2016;206:21–6.
13. Leonhard V, Caldwell G, Goh M, Reeder S, Smith H. Ultrasonographic diagnosis of thoracic outlet syndrome secondary to brachial plexus piercing variation. Diagnostics. 1927;7(3):40.
14. A. K. Distribution of the sympathetic rami to the brachial plexus: its relation to sympathectomy affecting the upper extremity. Arch Surg. 1927:15;871–7.
15. Chung IH, Oh CS, Koh KS, Kim HJ, Paik HC, Lee DY. Anatomic variations of the T2 nerve root (including the nerve of Kuntz) and their implications for sympathectomy. J Thorac Cardiovasc Surg. 2002;123(3):498–501.
16. Ramsaroop L, Partab P, Singh B, Satyapal KS. Thoracic origin of a sympathetic supply to the upper limb: the "nerve of Kuntz" revisited. J Anat. 2001;199(6):675–82.
17. McCormack AC, Jarral OA, Shipolini AR, McCormack DJ. Does the nerve of Kuntz exist? Interact Cardiovasc Thorac Surg. 2011;13(2):175–8.
18. Siegenthaler A, Curatolo M, Schliessbach J, et al. Ultrasound-guided Suprascapular nerve block, description of a novel supraclavicular approach. Reg Anesth Pain Med. 2012;37(3):325–8.

Occipital Nerve Stimulation Using an Ultrasound Surgical Technique

Tiago da Silva Freitas

History and General Indications

The purpose of this chapter is to describe the surgical technique for implanting an occipital nerve electrode using ultrasound. However, we will start with some basic considerations about history, indications, and results.

Historically, the first record with good documentation of implantation of electrodes in occipital nerves (ONS) was made by Weiner and Reed in 1999 [1]. In this study, an occipital electrode implant was performed by radioscopy in 13 patients with occipital neuralgia, and they demonstrated a good-to-excellent response (>50% pain relief) over an 18-month to 6-year follow-up.

The pathophysiology for the use of the occipital nerve in the treatment of craniofacial pain is based on the first studies developed by Goadsby [2] in 1997. In this study, he performed stimulation of the greater occipital nerve (GON) in cats resulted in increased metabolic activity of the trigeminal nucleus caudalis and cervical dorsal horn. Goadsby himself published in 2004 a study involving the use of occipital nerve stimulation to treat migraine [3].

The mechanism of action of ONS has not been fully elucidated, the main hypothesis being that of interaction in the nervous modulation of the trigeminal cervical complex by neurostimulation of this painful pathway. Anatomically, afferents from meninges terminate in the caudal trigeminal nucleus and in the medullary dorsal horn. This nucleus extends down to C2 and afferents from the back of the head travel along GON to C2.

T. d. S. Freitas (✉)
Functional Neurosurgery/Pain Ttreatment, Brasilia Pain Institute (INDOR), Brasília, Distrito Federal, Brazil

Neurosurgery Department Hospital de Base de Brasília (HBDF), Brasília, Distrito Federal, Brazil

Functional Neurosurgery Department Hospital Sírio Libanês, Brasília, Distrito Federal, Brazil

T. d. S. Freitas et al. (eds.), *Neuromodulation Techniques for Pain Treatment*, https://doi.org/10.1007/978-3-030-84778-4_11

From these first reports, several publications involving this target in the treatment of several painful pathologies of the face and skull were published. The indications have broadened, also involving cluster headaches and migraines that are difficult to control, as well as continuous hemicrania, posttraumatic, and cluster headache. Other possible indications for ONS transformed migraine, C2-mediated headaches, and occipital region pain after surgery [4–9].

As with all peripheral nerve stimulation targets, we have a lag in relation to suitable materials in the stimulation of this target. There are several lines of specific materials under development by the industry; however, we still make use of traditional percutaneous SCS electrodes for implantation in our patients, which is one of the reasons for the most common complication: migration.

The first occipital nerve implants were performed using a standard radioscopy technique; procedures involving the occipital nerves were based on identifying bony or arterial landmarks with direct palpation or fluoroscopy. Although universally accepted as an imaging technique, fluoroscopy does not provide real-time imaging of the occipital nerves or vessels. Furthermore, the therapeutic efficacy of ONS is directly related to the ability of the stimulating electrode to produce peripheral nerve dermatomal paresthesia, emphasizing the need for precision placement. In addition to the previously described, there is great variability in nerve topography. Becser et al. [10] described that the greater occipital nerve (GON) was seen between 5 and 28 mm from the midline at the level of the intermastoid line, while the lesser occipital nerve (LON) was observed between 32 and 90 mm from the midline. Due to this variability, the use of ultrasound has proven to be an effective alternative for the correct implantation of the electrode in relation to the nerve, preventing the device from becoming too superficial (leading to non-pleasure stimulation and the greater risk of bedsores) and also not very deep (leading to loss of target stimulation effectiveness and the need to use a large amount of energy, requiring high amperages and pulse widths in an attempt to capture the painful area by stimulation).

The first description in the literature with the use of USG in the occipital nerve implant was made by Sharibas et al. [11], in 2009. In this study, he demonstrated the safety and effectiveness of the technique in six patients with occipital neuralgia. From this report, several publications in the literature emerged showing the importance of using intraoperative USG, with its advantages, especially in relation to the nonuse of intra radioscopy—operative, with exposure of the interventionist and the patient. There is still no evidence in the literature that can conclude that this technique is superior to the traditional technique of radioscopy. In fact, a review of survival analysis by Pain Physician in 2017 showed the non-superiority of the ultrasound method over the radioscopic one, in a review made in the literature involving 21 patients and 52 electrodes implanted in the occipital nerve [12].

Surgical Technique

The step-by-step intraoperative simulation will be explained in the images below. Thus, as in all neuromodulation techniques, the correct diagnosis of the patient is the basic premise for correctly focusing the procedure. In the case of cranial facial pain, the diagnosis is not always simple, and confirmatory tests, as diagnostic blocks, may have to be done.

In our service, all patients who are candidates for electrode implantation undergo preoperative neuropsychological assessment, aiming to identify undertreated or mistreated psychiatric diseases and even personality disorders incompatible with the implant, as well as a history of drug or alcohol abuse.

All patients are also instructed prior to surgery on the risks of the procedure, including infection, migration, bedsores, vascular injuries, hardware-related problems (fracture, electrode breakage, problems with the generator), and pain at the generator implant site. The chances of operation and effectiveness of the procedure are also discussed.

Stimulation Trial

Although there is no strong evidence in the literature related to the real need for testing for implantation of electrodes in the occipital nerve, the trial is still used in most centers that perform this technique. In general, the parameter of minimum improvement of 50% in pain scales during a test period from 5 to 7 days is used to predict the definitive implant. However, the trial can provide us with some important additional information: it allows the patient to judge whether the paresthesias are comfortable or not for chronic and continuous use. It also allows the patient to have a realistic expectation of the therapy and possible responses to it.

Surgical Technique

First Step: Stimulation Trial Procedure

The patient's position depends on whether the stimulation will be done unilaterally or bilaterally. In the case of unilateral stimulation, the patient is placed in lateral decubitus, and in the case of bilateral stimulation, the patient is placed in a prone position, with good accommodation of the facial region (pillow). In both procedures, light sedation is performed associated with local anesthesia; be careful not to perform anesthesia of the target nerve.

Asepsis, antisepsis, placement of sterile drapes, and antibiotic prophylaxis are performed.

The puncture of the occipital nerve can be performed by two different basic routes. The first involves medial access, in the midline at the level of the posterior arch of C1, with the electrode directed laterally from this point. The second, called the lateral route, usually begins 1 cm inferior and medial to the mastoid with the electrode facing the medial region from this point, always trying to pass the electrode of the midline. According to the surgeon's experience, these two access routes can also be combined.

We then used a Tuohy needle, slightly angled, in order to adapt to the curvature of the occipital region, always remembering to test the electrode passage before starting the procedure. The passage of the needle is guided by ultrasound, based on the depth of the occipital artery, identified by its pulse in the ultrasound image, and aided, in more difficult cases, by the use of software that identifies the arterial pulse.

After the passage of the electrode, intraoperative stimulation is performed to cover the painful area with low amplitude and PW amplitudes, using tonic stimulation.

The electrodes are secured with an anchor attached to the skin. We always use double fixation, with space for the electrode to move with the cervical movement, so as not to interfere with the possibility of displacing it.

In case of a positive test, our advice is to remove the test system with a new definitive implant procedure. There is a description in the literature of implantation of permanent neurostimulation systems using the same test electrodes, with an important economic and position advantage of the ideal implant for occipital stimulation. This approach clearly presents an increased risk of infection.

Permanent Implant

Regardless of the access path chosen for the electrode (lateral or medial), an incision should always be made at the needle entry site for the correct fixation of the electrode, which will be looped and anchored. The use of ultrasound allows the surgeon to estimate in real time and precise the ideal depth for the implantation of the electrode, that is, in the subcutaneous fat, minimizing the complications of very deep electrodes (direct stimulation of musculature and fascia, causing pain) or very superficial (risk of erosion on the skin).

In the definitive implant, the ideal scenario is also to perform the test with the patient awake enough to provide information about the ideal coverage of the painful area by stimulation. There are reports in the literature of implants with the patient and general anesthesia, which in the radioscopic technique could cause an increased incidence of poorly positioned electrodes. The use of ultrasound could also minimize this risk, although there are no consistent studies that prove the difference between these techniques.

Once the electrode is installed in the correct location, it is anchored using a non-absorbable suture and a silicone anchor fixing the electrode to the fascia plane. A loop is also made at the fixation site in order to mitigate its migration. Some reports in the literature also use silicone glue in an attempt to reduce migration.

Subsequently, the electrode is tunneled to the IPG pocket. An extension is not usually used, but in cases of locations very distant from the electrode, its use may be necessary. Tunneling of the electrode and/or extensions can be done under local or general anesthesia. After connecting the electrode to the generator, the generator is fixed according to the same molds for SCS.

There are numerous possible sites described for the placement of the definitive generator: buttock, the low abdomen, and infrascapular, infraclavicular, and midaxillary line. The location must be previously defined with the patient, taking into account electrode migration and cosmetic aspects of the patient.

Complications and how to Avoid Them

There are different possibilities for complications in the ONS. The most common include electrode migration, infection, localized pain after the surgical procedure, skin erosion at the electrode site, muscle spasms, loss of stimulation effect, and hardware problems (breakage, malfunction, etc.).

As a way to try to mitigate migration, notably the most common complication of this procedure, we recommend performing a good electrode fixation, with looping and anchoring using nonabsorbable stitches; the use of silicone glue may reduce failure of the anchor/electrode interface. Minimizing the movement of the cervical region is also a valid strategy: we recommend that patients do not drive for 6 weeks and avoid flexion and rotation of the neck during this period [13]. There are descriptions in the literature using a cervical collar 10 days after surgery. Another important factor that can influence the possibility of migration is the distance from the IPG site: a distance of less than 1 meter is recommended.

A very interesting in vitro model has been described by Trentmann et al. [14] with respect to the ideal position of the IPG website. They concluded that the retromastoid to infraclavicular pathway was associated with the least electrode pathway length change and that this may result in fewer electrode migrations. The low abdominal IPG site was also an acceptable alternative, while the buttock site was associated with the greatest electrode pathway length change.

Regarding the complication of skin erosion (very superficial electrode) or undesirable muscle contractions (deep electrodes), we believe that the use of ultrasound technique by an experienced surgeon is one of the factors that can minimize the depth error during the passage of the electrode in the occipital region.

Surgical Technique (Figs. 1, 2, 3, and 4)

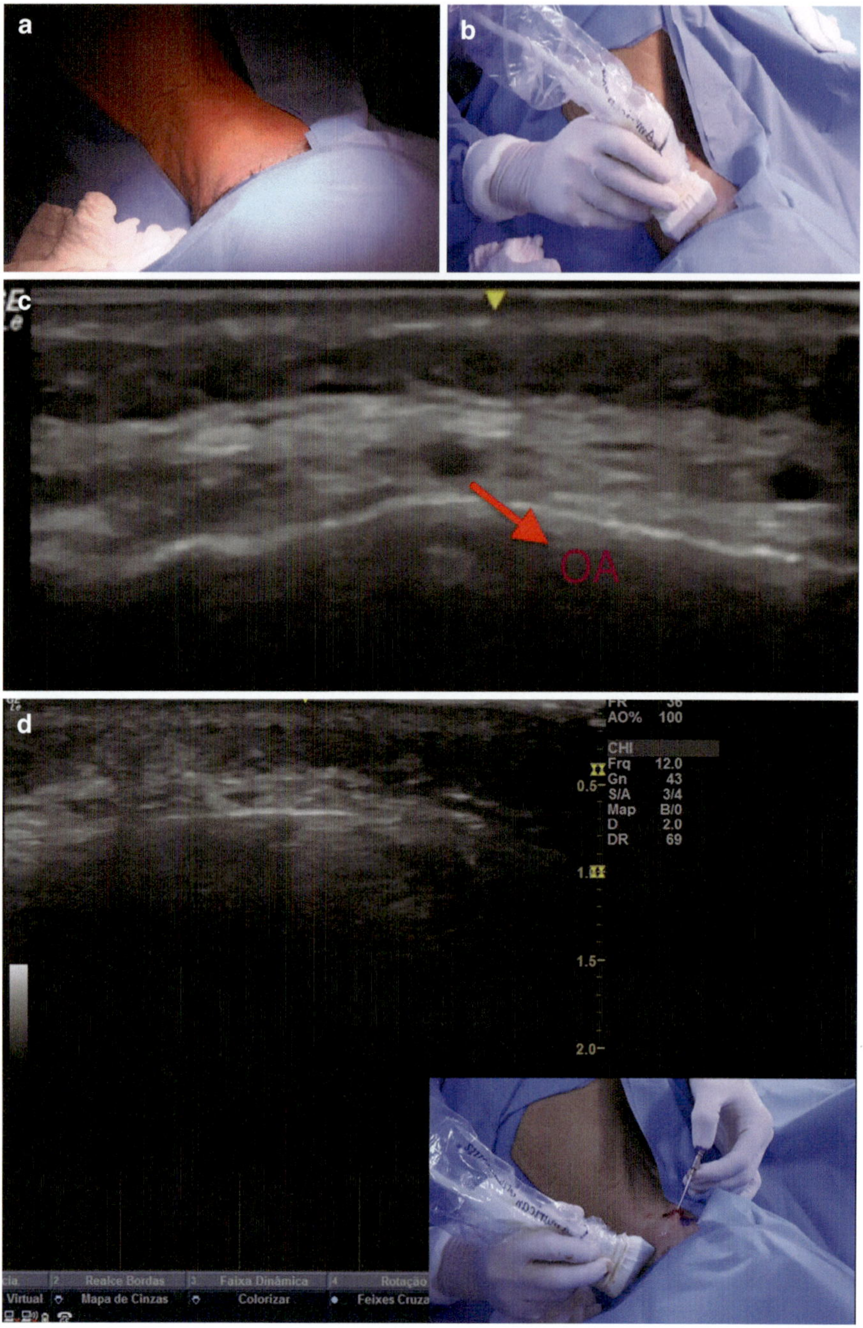

Fig. 1 (**a**) Patient positioned for testing with the occipital electrode in the right lateral decubitus position, exposing the left occipital region. (**b**) Initial insonation with the location of the occipital artery and nerves, highlighted in **c**. (**d**) Insonation and passage of the Tuohy needle in the plane of the occipital artery/nerve

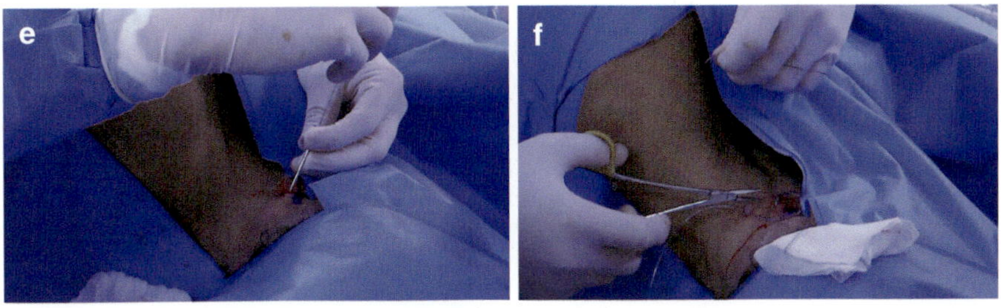

Fig. 2 (**e**) Passage of the electrode through the needle after intraoperative physiological confirmation with good coverage of the pain area. (**f**) Example of electrode fixation for trial. Using pedone anchor, nonabsorbable wires over the electrode and loop for better movement and prevention of migration

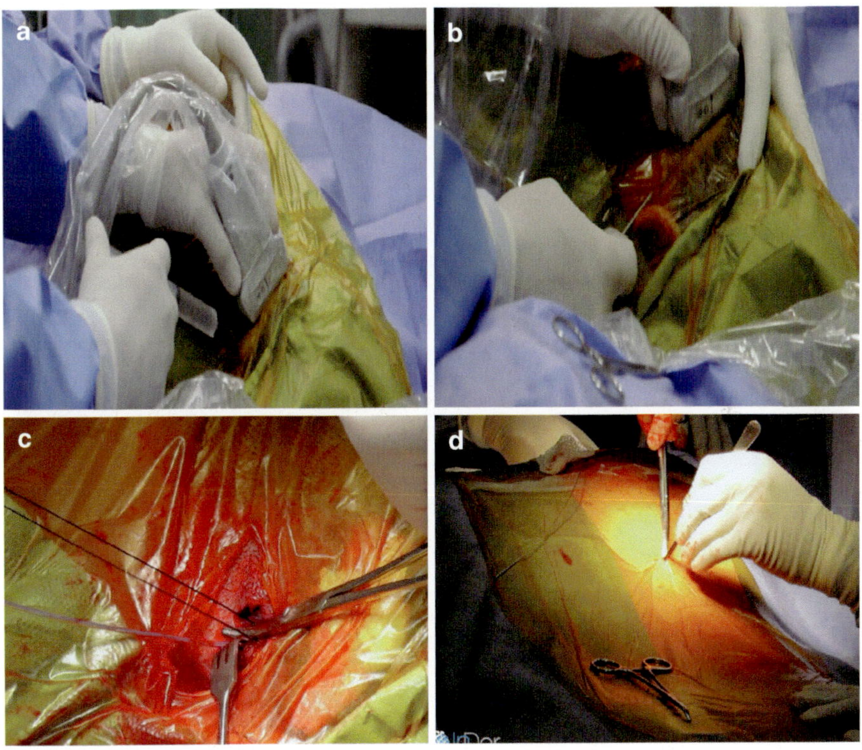

Fig. 3 (**a**) Patient positioned in the prone position for occipital nerve electrode under general anesthesia and guided by ultrasound. (**a**) Skin anesthesia. (**b**) Tuohy needle passage from lateral to medial. (**c**) Electrode fixation using silicone anchor in the fascial plane. (**d–f**) Electrode tunneling from occipital to IPG pocket in the buttock. (**g–h**) IPG extension connection and skin closing

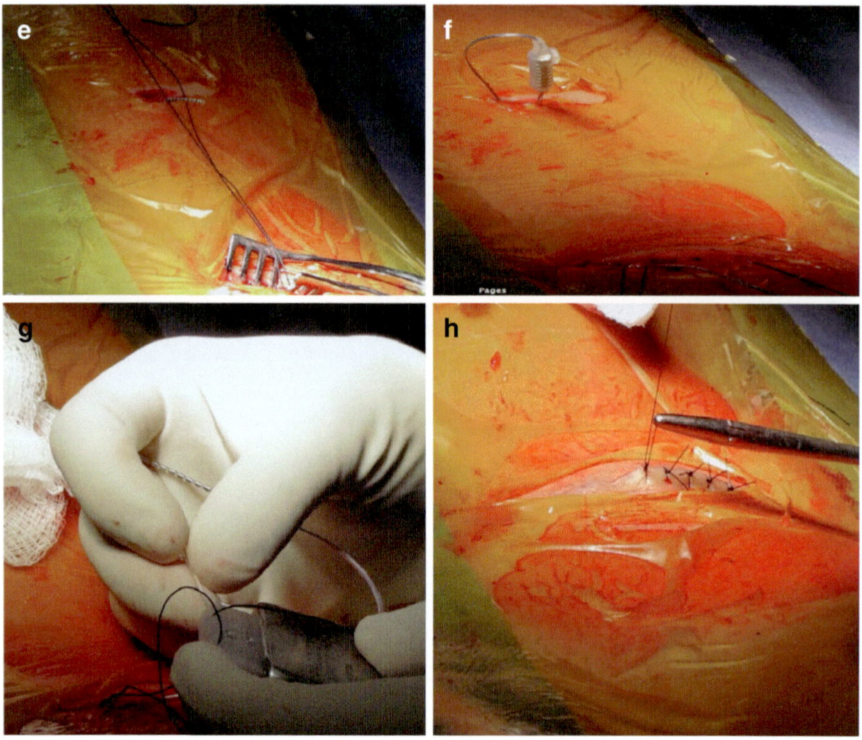

Fig. 11.3 (continued)

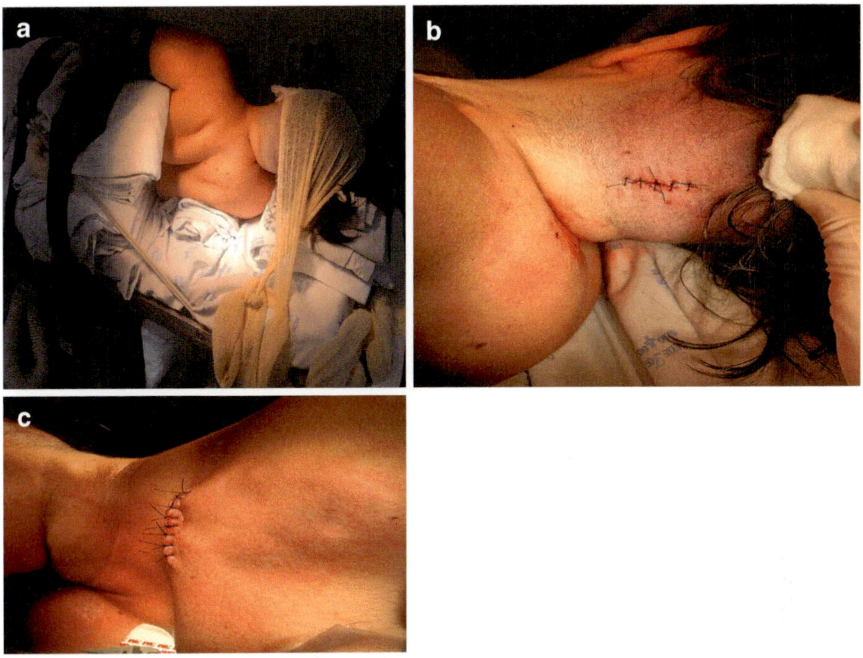

Fig. 4 (**a**) Patient positioned in the right lateral position exposing the left side for definitive implantation. (**b**) Place of definitive electrode fixation in the midline, with an electrode fixed in the fascial plane. (**c**) IPG pocket located in the left subclavicular region

Bibliography

1. Weiner RL, Reed KL. Peripheral neurostimulation for the control of intractable occipital neuralgia. Neuromodulation. 1999;2:217–21.
2. Goadsby PJ, Knight YE, Hoskin KL. Stimulation of the greater occipital nerve increases metabolic activity in the trigeminal nucleus caudalis and cervical dorsal horn of the cat. Pain. 1997;73(1):23–8.
3. Matharu MS, Bartsch T, Ward N, Frackowiak RSJ, Weiner RL, Goadsby PJ. Central neuromodulation in chronic migraine patients with suboccipital stimulators: a PET study. Brain. 2004;127:220–30.
4. Melvin EA Jr, Jordan FR, Weiner RL, Primm D. Using peripheral stimulation to reduce the pain of C2- mediated occipital headaches: a preliminary report. Pain Physician. 2007;10:453–60.
5. Slavin KV, Colpan ME, Munawar N, Wess C, Nersesyan H. Trigeminal and occipital peripheral nerve stimulation for craniofacial pain: a single institution experience and review of the literature. Neurosurg Focus. 2006;21:E6.
6. Johnstone CS, Sundaraj R. Occipital nerve stimulation for the treatment of occipital neuralgia – eight case studies. Neuromodulation. 2006;9:41–7.
7. Rodrigo-Royo MD, Azcona JM, Quero J, Lorente MC, Acin P, Azcona J. Peripheral neurostimulation in the management of cervicogenic headache: four case reports. Neuromodulation. 2005;8:241–8.
8. Popeney CA, Alo KM. Peripheral neurostimulation for the treatment of chronic, disabling transformed migraine. Headache. 2003;43:369–75.

9. Slavin KV, Nersesyan H, Wess C: Peripheral neurostimulation for treatment of intractable occipital neuralgia. Neurosurgery. 2006;58:112–9; discussion 112–119.
10. Becser N, Bovim G, Sjaastad O. Extracranial nerves in the posterior part of the head. Anatomic variations and their possible clinical significance. Spine. 1998;23:1435–41.
11. Skaribas I, Aló K. Ultrasound imaging and occipital nerve stimulation. Neuromodulation. 2010;13(2):126–30. https://doi.org/10.1111/j.1525-1403.2009.00254.x. Epub 2009 Oct 29.
12. Jones JH, Brown A, Moyse D, Qi W, Roy L. Survival analysis of occipital nerve stimulator leads placed under fluoroscopic guidance with and without ultrasonography. Pain Physician. 2017;20(7):E1115–21.
13. Trentman TL, Zimmerman RS, Dodick DW. Prog Neurol Surg. 2011;24:96–108. https://doi.org/10.1159/000323043. Epub 2011 Mar 21.
14. Trentman TL, Mueller JT, Shah DM, Zimmermann RS, Noble BM. Occipital nerve stimulator lead pathway length changes with volunteer movement: an in vitro study. Pain Pract. 2010;10:42–8.

Peripheral Nerve Stimulation in Upper Limb Using Ultrasound Technique

Tiago da Silva Freitas

General Instructions to Understand the USG Legends

The general instructions were based on the classification system used by Hannes Gruber, Alexander Loizides, and Bernhard Moriggl in their book *Sonographic Peripheral Nerve Topography, A Landmark-based Algorithm* [1].

On the left side on the upper half page, there is the following (standardized) table.

ELM	External landmark(s)
IPOP	Initial positioning of probe
ILM	Internal landmark(s)
POV	Point of optimal visibility
VAR	Relevant variations
AP	Alternative plan (if worth mentioning!)
C	Comments – if helpful/of interest regarding surgical technique
PAT	Pathology
Confirmation of the target	Neurophysiology regarding the peripheral nerve target
Notes	Any additional important information

Following the table we will have the figures with the step-by-step technique. We also used exactly the same description in the ultrasound images done by Hans Gruber in the book above cited (made with permission).

T. d. S. Freitas (✉)
Brasilia Pain Institute(INDOR), Neurosurgery Department Hospital de Base de Brasília(HBDF), Functional Neurosurgery Department Hospital Sírio Libanês, Brasília, Distrito Federal, Brazil

T. d. S. Freitas et al. (eds.), *Neuromodulation Techniques for Pain Treatment*,
https://doi.org/10.1007/978-3-030-84778-4_12

USG Technique for Peripheral Nerve Stimulation in Upper Limb [2–14]

Axillary Nerve (Figs. 1, 2, 3, 4, 5, and 6)

ELM	1. Palpable groove between the deltoid muscle and the long head of triceps muscle
IPOP	Nearly sagittal, at the reference line between acromion angle and the axilla
ILM	1. Posterior circumflex humeral artery 2. Teres minor muscle
POV	Distal to the inferior border of the teres minor muscle, on the humeral shaft, next to the posterior circumflex humeral artery
VAR	None
AP	None
C	Arm in a slight abduction and inner rotation (tension of the teres minor muscle). On further abduction a part of the humeral shaft (shadowing!) disappears from the US image; however the visualization of the nerve is further improved (nerve is stretched!) *Subluxation of electrode will be highly prevalent in these patients. The post-humeral C-flex artery is easily identified transitioning through QS (quadrangular space) and around humerus when viewing via US. Be sure to follow artery into QS to locate root of axillary nerve before it bifurcates*
PAT	Neuropathic shoulder pain
Confirmation of the target	Motor response of glenohumeral approximation, slight external rotation from teres minor, with *possible* abduction. Paresthesia to the lateral shoulder, C5–C6 dermatome (deltoid)
Notes	None

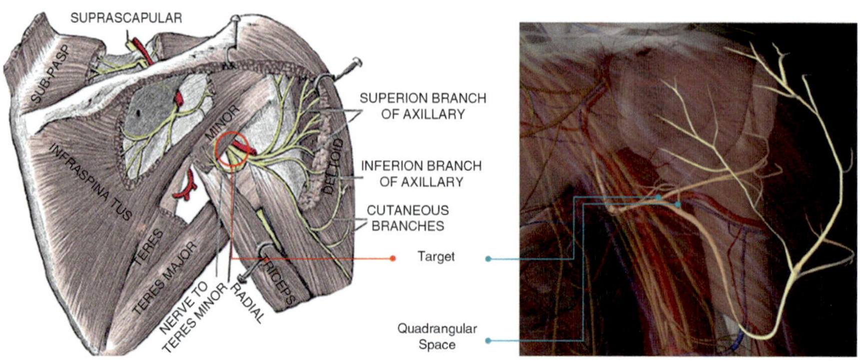

Fig. 1 Anatomical representation of the axillary nerve as a target, showing the anatomical position of the quadrangular space and the posterior circumflex artery at the neck of the humerus. (Image from StimRouter system, reprinted with permission)

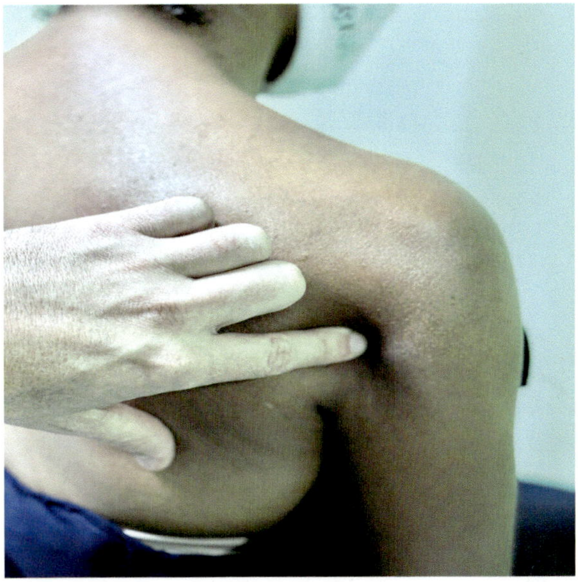

Fig. 2 Patient prone with affected UE slightly adducted. Palpate the groove between the musculus deltoideus (deltoid muscle) and the caput longum musculi tricipitis brachii (long head of triceps muscle)

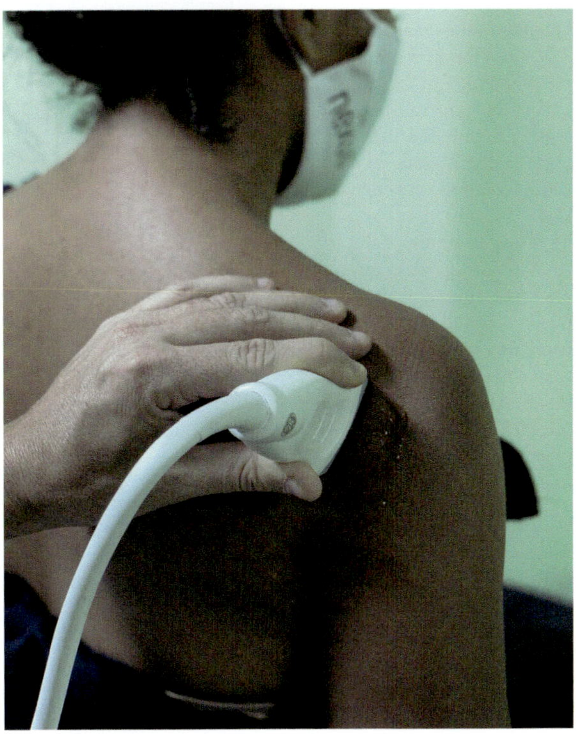

Fig. 3 Nearly sagittal probe positioning between the axilla and the angulus acromiale (acromion angle)

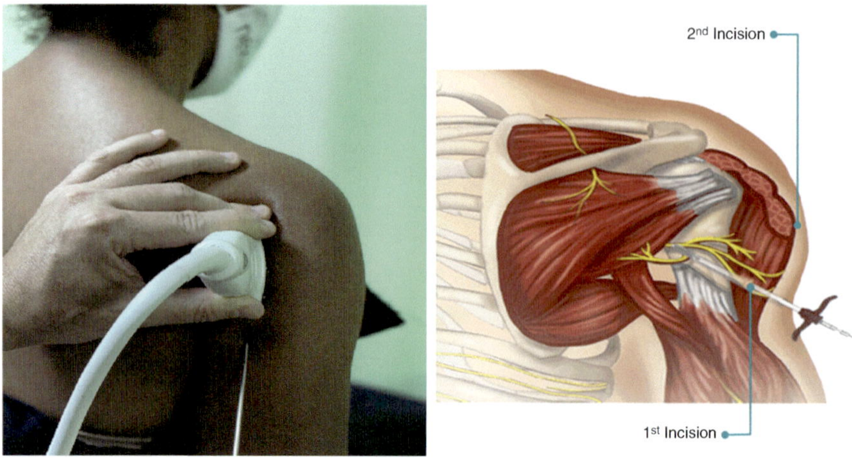

Figs. 4 and 5 Needle entry point over inferior border of posterior deltoid. Trajectory superomedial toward target in the quadrangular space. Remainder of lead tunneled across middle of deltoid muscle. In the case of Bioness system, you will have to do a second incision/excision superior and anterior to first incision/entry point (figure printed with permission)

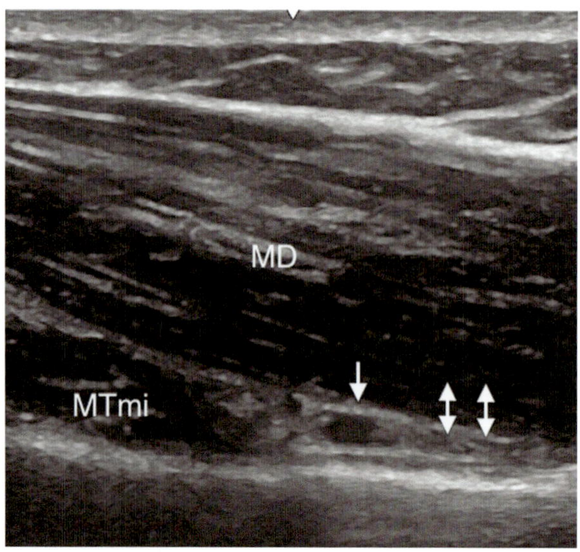

Fig. 6 Ultrasonographic imaging of the quadrilateral space. (**a**) The probe was placed parallel to the long axis of the humeral shaft, around 2 cm below the posterolateral border of the acromion on the dorsal aspect of the arm. (**b**) Ultrasonographic imaging shows tortuous posterior circumflex humeral artery (arrow) around the axillary nerve (double arrow) on the right shoulder. Also note mild thinning in the left deltoid muscle. Tm 1/4 teres minor muscle; TM 1/4 teres major muscle

Suprascapular Nerve (Figs. 7, 8, 9, 10, and 11)

ELM	1. Supraspinatus fossa 2. Upper trapezius muscle 3. Spine of scapula
IPOP	Patient prone. Entry point near medial border of scapula, superior to spine of scapula. Needle inserted inferolateral toward target in the supraspinatus fossa
ILM	1. Upper trapezius muscle 2. Supraspinatus muscle 3. Superior transverse scapular ligament
VAR	None
AP	None
C	None
PAT	Neuropathic shoulder pain
Confirmation of the target	Paresthesia in C5–C6 dermatome (shoulder)
Notes	Any additional important information

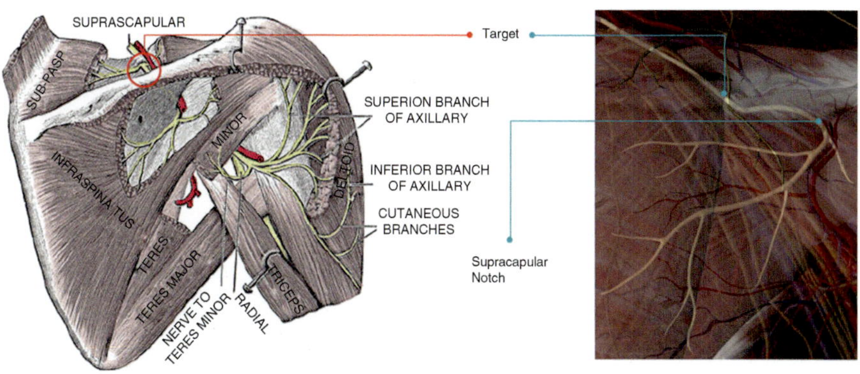

Fig. 7 Anatomical representation of the suprascapular nerve and the relevant target/anatomy: suprascapular nerve in the supraspinatus fossa, infraspinatus fossa, supraspinatus muscle, suprascapular artery, upper trapezius muscle (Image courtesy of StimRouter, reprinted with permission)

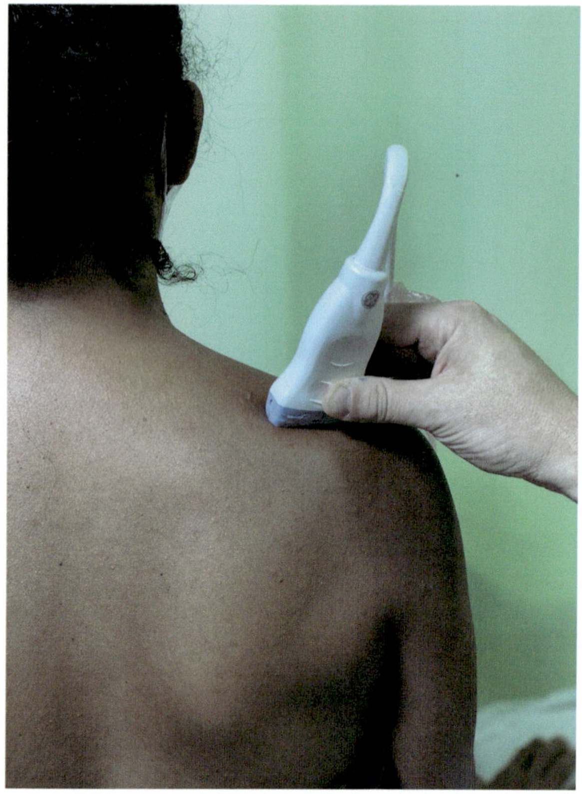

Fig. 8 Patient prone with affected UE slightly adducted, nearly transversal probe positioning over the supraspinatus fossa

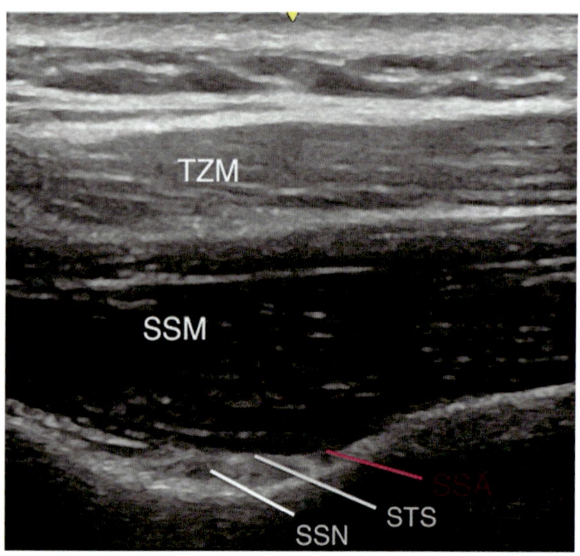

Fig. 9 Patient prone with affected UE slightly adducted, nearly transversal probe positioning over the supraspinatus fossa showing the anatomical landmarks and SSN **SSM supraspinatus muscleSSA suprascapular arterySSN suprascapular nerveTZM trapezius muscleSTS superior transverse scapular ligament**

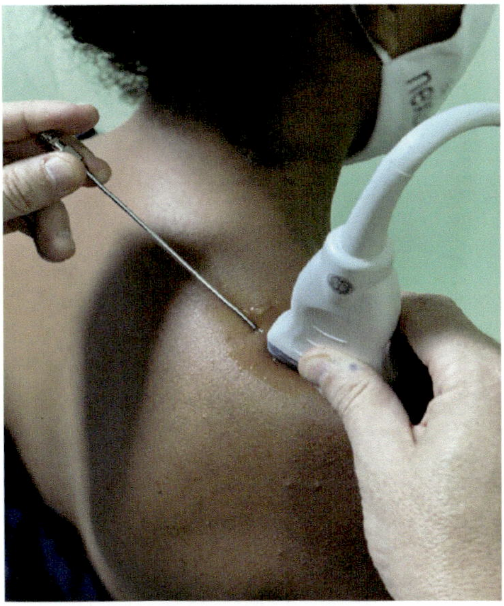

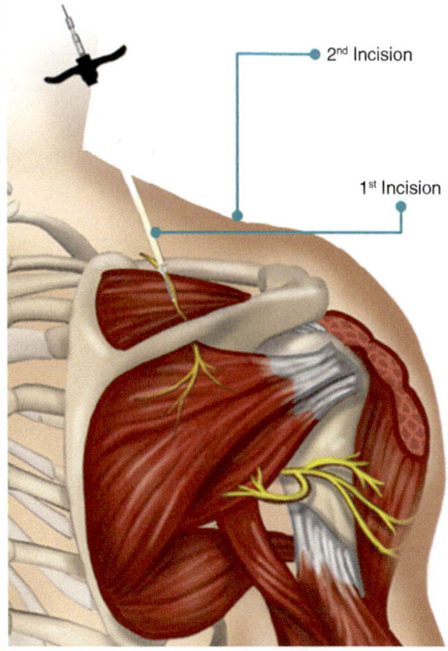

Figs. 10 and 11 Needle entry point near medial border of scapula, superior to spine of scapula. Direct inferolateral toward target in the supraspinatus fossa, after a good view from suprascapular artery and suprascapular nerve. Once you reach the target, confirm with intraoperative stimulation and paresthesias in C5–C6 dermatome (shoulder). (Fig. 11: Image from StimRouter system, reprinted with permission)

Ulnar Nerve (Figs. 12, 13, 14, 15, 16, 17, 18, 19, 20, and 21)

ELM	Proximal approach 1. Medial epicondyle of humerus Distal approach 1. Carpus ulnar flexor muscle
IPOP	Proximal Transverse, two to three fingerbreadths proximal to the medial epicondyle of the humerus Distal Transverse, at the ulnar side of the middle forearm
ILM	Proximal 1. Lateral head of the brachial triceps muscle 2. Brachial fascia Distal 1. Ulnar artery
POV	Proximal Two to three fingerbreadths proximal to medial epicondyle of the humerus Distal At the middle lower arm, ulnar to the ulnar artery
VAR	No accompanying vessels at the distal POV (ulnar artery with unusual origin and course!)

AP	None
C	As you reach the nerve in transverse approach, turn the US to sagittal view and expose the nerve to the best imaging, using it to get the correct plane to the needle
PAT	Neuropathic pain in the distal ulnar nerve distribution
Confirmation of the target	Paresthesia to C8 dermatome; medial/ulnar side of forearm, and fifth digit and medial half of fourth digit
Notes	Many patients will have undergone nerve transpositions, taking the ulnar nerve out of the ulnar groove and placing it on the other side of the medial epicondyle. Patients can become uncomfortable in these positions for long periods of time

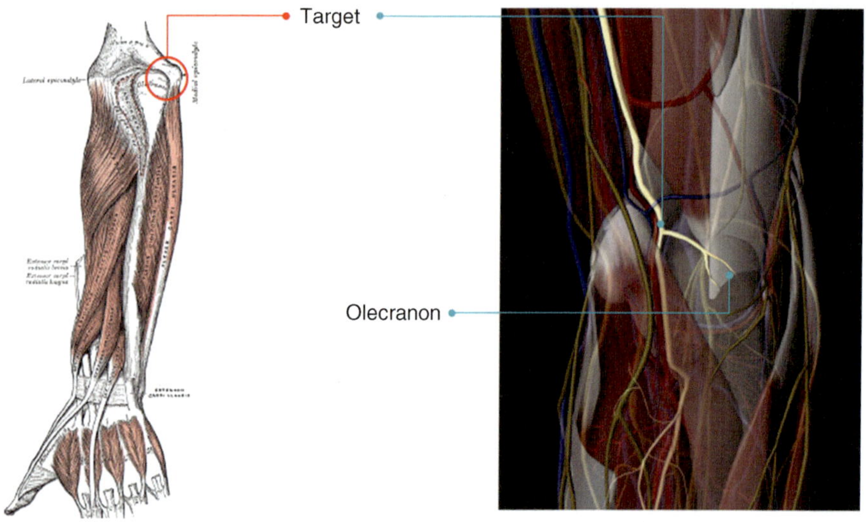

Fig. 12 Anatomical representation of the ulnar nerve as a target, showing the anatomical position in anterior and posterior view
Olecranon – bony prominence of the elbow
Medial epicondyle – lateral to olecranon, bony prominence on the interior aspect of the elbow
Ulnar groove is the space between the two. (Image from StimRouter system, reprinted with permission)

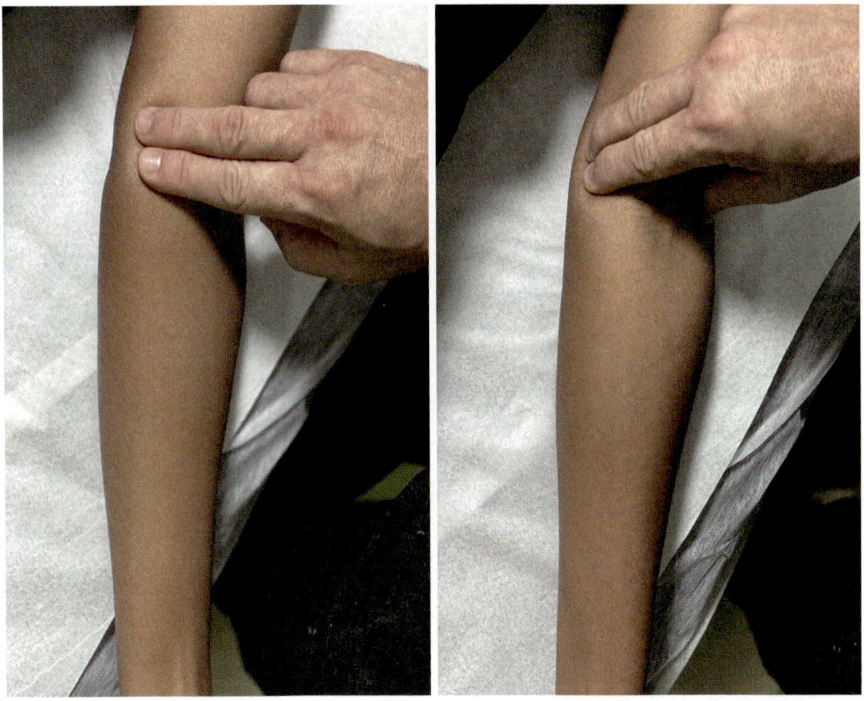

Fig. 13 Palpation of the crista supracondylaris medialis (medial supracondylar crest (MSC)) for rough distance estimation of IPOS

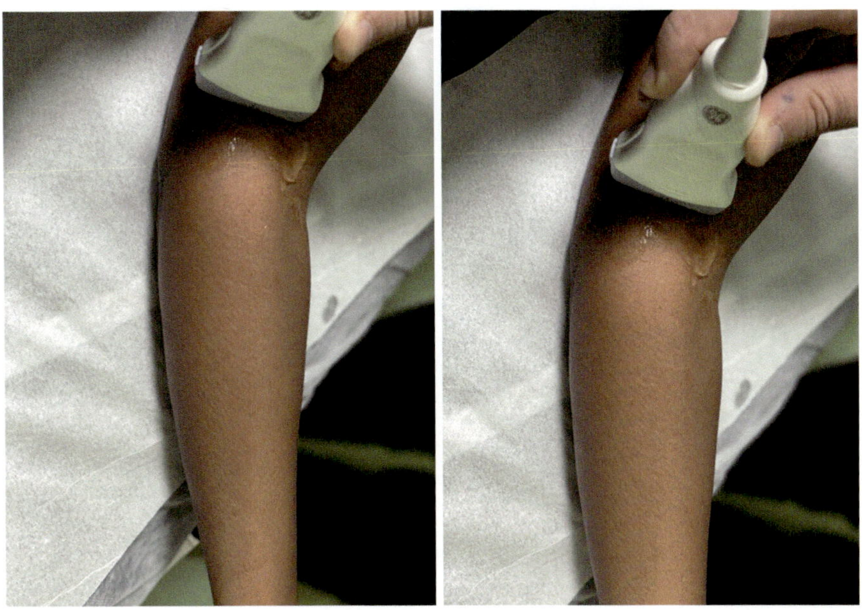

Fig. 14 Positioning of the probe in a transverse orientation two to three fingerbreadths proximal to the medial epicondyle of humerus

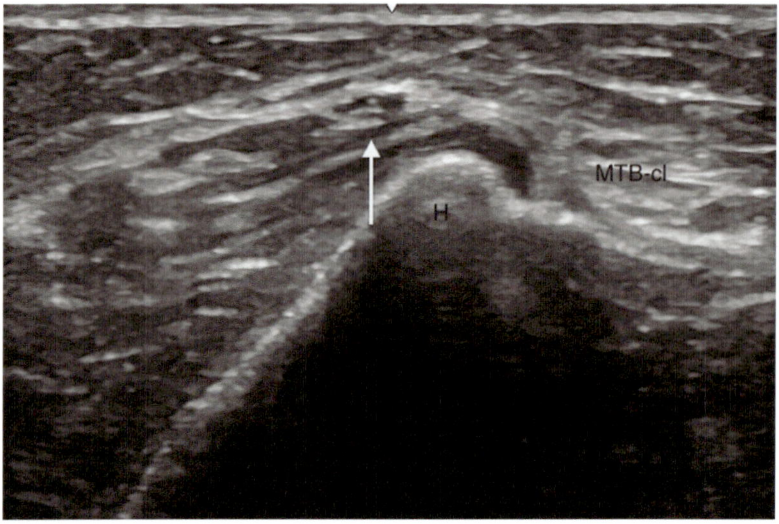

Fig. 15 Depiction of the crista supracondylaris medialis humeri (humeral medial supracondylar crest) (H) and the caput laterale musculi tricipitis brachii (lateral head of the triceps brachial muscle) MTB-CL. The ulnar nerve (arrow) lies subfascial (POV!) and adjacent to the head of the triceps brachii muscle

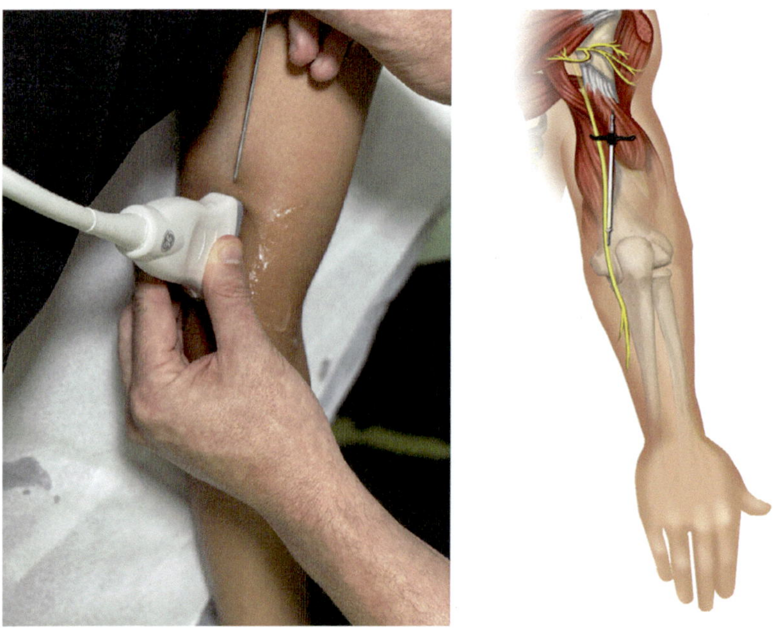

Fig. 16 As you reach the nerve in transverse approach, turn the US to sagittal view and expose the nerve to the best imaging, using it to get the correct plane to the needle.
Insert the needle from proximal to distal closer to ulnar nerve. We usually use an apolar solution (dextrose 5%) to hydrodissect the periphery of the nerve and create space to introduce the electrodes

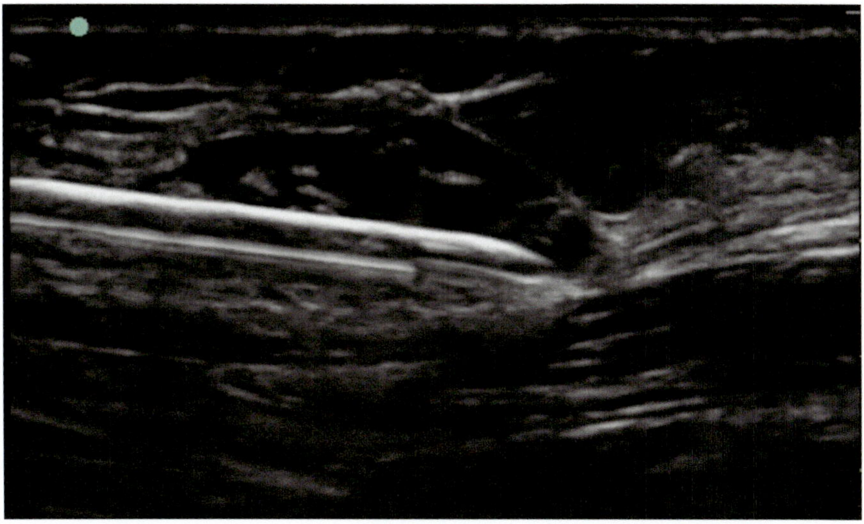

Fig. 17 Needle (N) positioned over ulnar nerve (UN) and starting hydrodissection using dextrose 5%

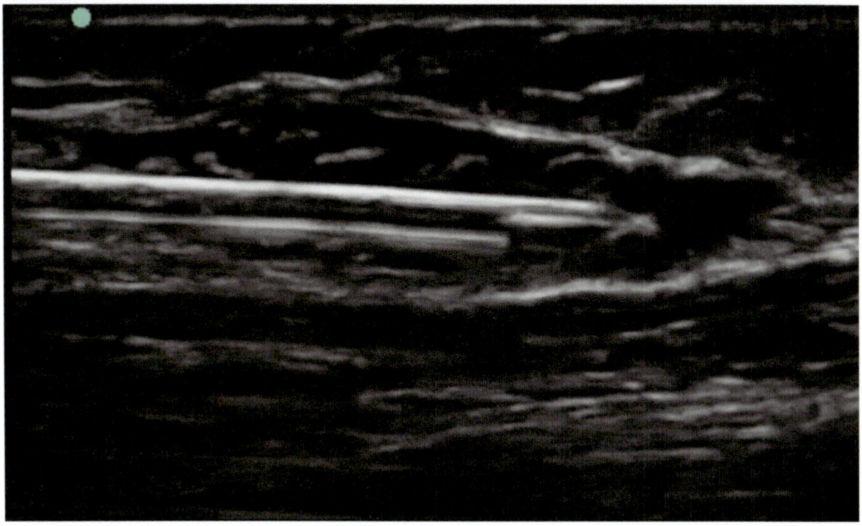

Fig. 18 More hydrodissection opening the space for the electrode

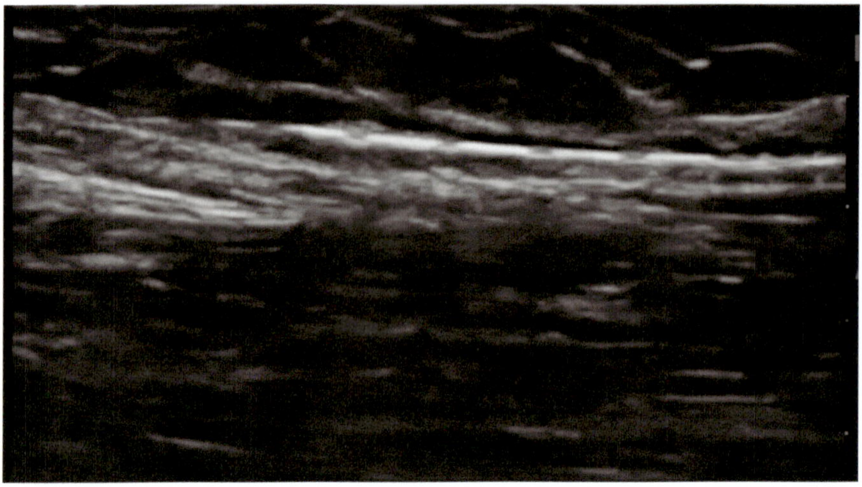

Fig. 19 Ultrasound imaging showing electrode over ulnar nerve

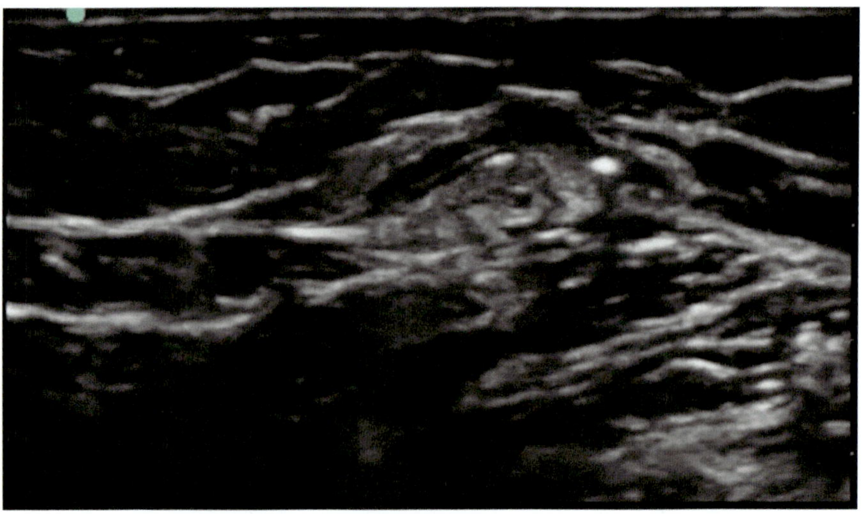

Fig. 20 A transversal image from the electrode over the ulnar nerve. E electrode, UN ulnar nerve, H hydrodissection

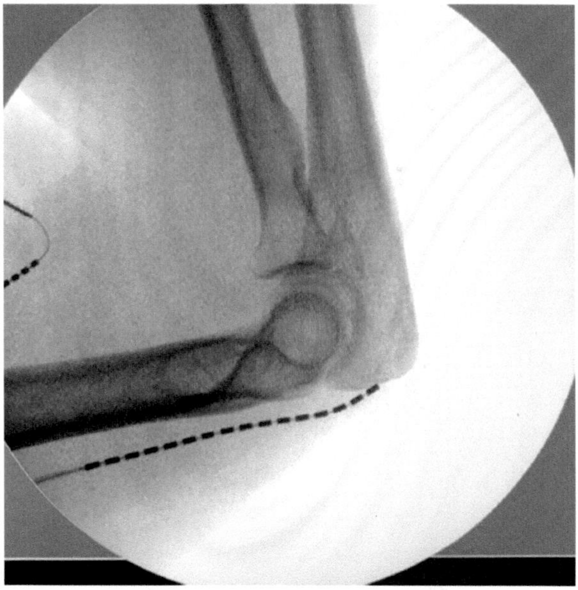

Fig. 21 Radiographic confirmation from the electrode over the ulnar nerve

Median Nerve (Nervus Medianus): Figs. 22, 23, 24, 25, and 26

ELM	Proximal approach 1. Pulsation of the A. brachialis (brachial artery) 2. Palpable epicondylus medialis humeri 3. Palpable medial border of the M. biceps brachii Distal approach 1. Middle of the forearm
IPOP	*Proximal* Oblique, center of the probe between epicondylus medialis humeri and M. biceps brachii Distal Transverse, in the middle of the forearm
ILM	Proximal 1. A. brachialis 2. M. pronator teres Distal 1. M. Fflexor digitorum superficialis 2. M. flexor digitorum profundus
POV	Proximal 1. Ulnar to the A. brachialis 2. Slightly distal as soon as the nerve "disappears" between the two heads of the M. pronator teres (orientation corresponding to the course of the nerve is a must!) Distal 1. Between M. flexor digitorum superficialis and M. flexor digitorum at the mid-forearm

VAR	Radial to the A. brachialis Dorsal to the A. brachialis A. radialis superficialis Clear distance of the nerve from the artery (more often ulnar sided)
AP	None
C	None
PAT	Neuropathic distal pain in the median nerve distribution
Confirmation of the target	Paresthesia in the median nerve distribution; the palmar surface of the first, second, and third digits and lateral half of the fourth digit, C7–C8 dermatomes
Notes	In case of using the Bioness system, loop or shelf of lead may be needed to fit the 15 cm lead distal to the elbow

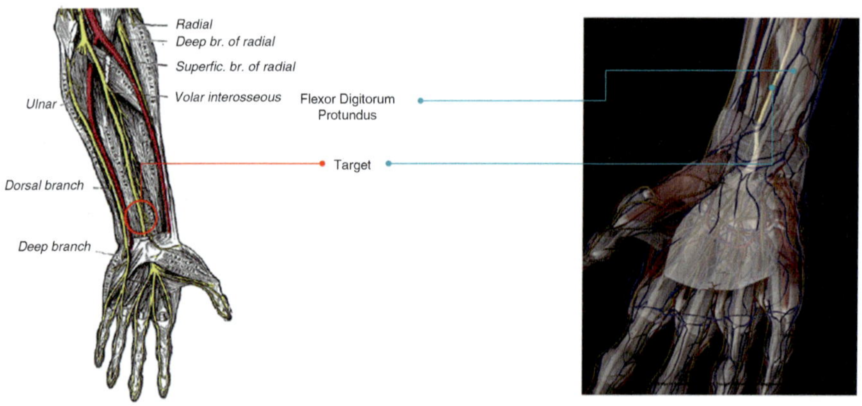

Fig. 22 Anatomical representation of the median nerve as a target, showing the anatomical position related to distal target for peripheral nerve implants. (Image from StimRouter. Printed with permission)

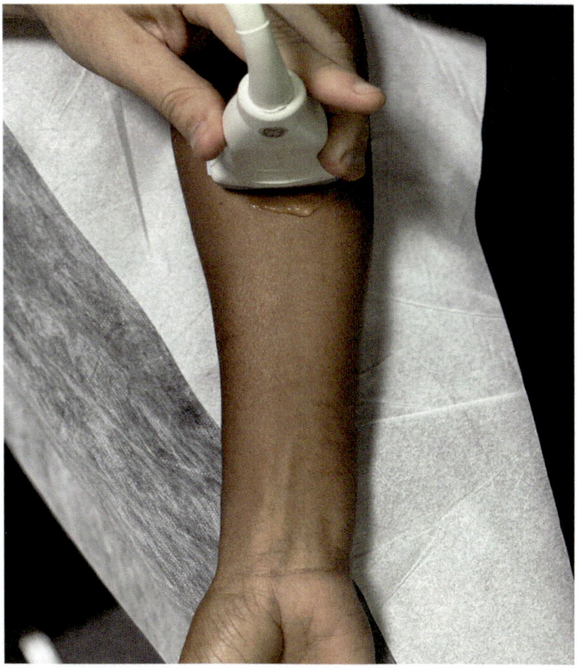

Fig. 23 Figures showing the proximal approach to localize the median nerve: palpation of the epicondylus medialis humeri, the medial border of the musculus biceps brachii, and the arteria brachialis, following the probe position in an oblique orientation between musculus biceps brachii and epicondylus medialis humeri

Radial Nerve (Nervus Radialis): Figs. 27, 28, 29, 30, 31, 32, and 33

ELM	1. Palpable groove between the M. biceps brachii and M. brachioradialis
IPOP	Three to four fingerbreadths proximal to the cubital crease
ILM	1. M. brachialis 2. M. brachioradialis
POV	Shortly before entering the fossa cubitalis
VAR	None
AP	None
C	None
PAT	Neuropathic distal pain in the distribution of the radial nerve
Confirmation of the target	Paresthesia in the radial distribution of the hand (back of the hand); C6–C8 dermatomes
Notes	Lead mapping is encouraged pre-op to eliminate the possibility of the lead crossing the elbow joint and for comfort/clearance during donning/doffing

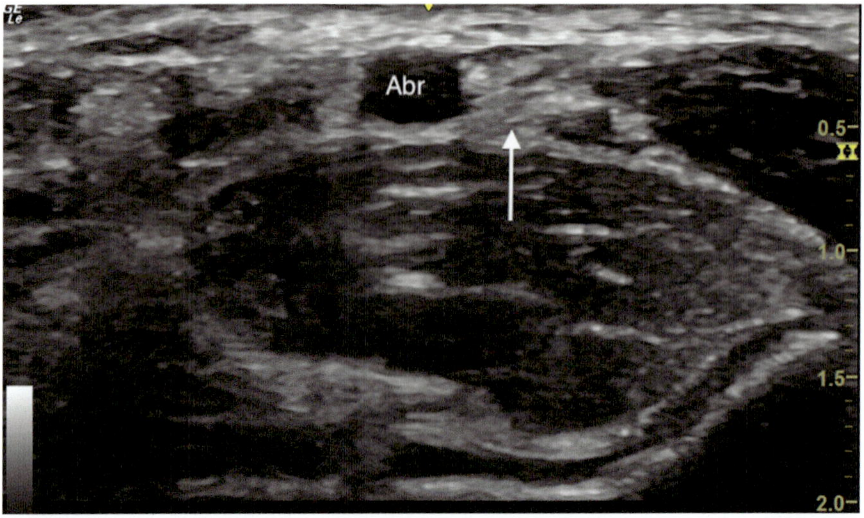

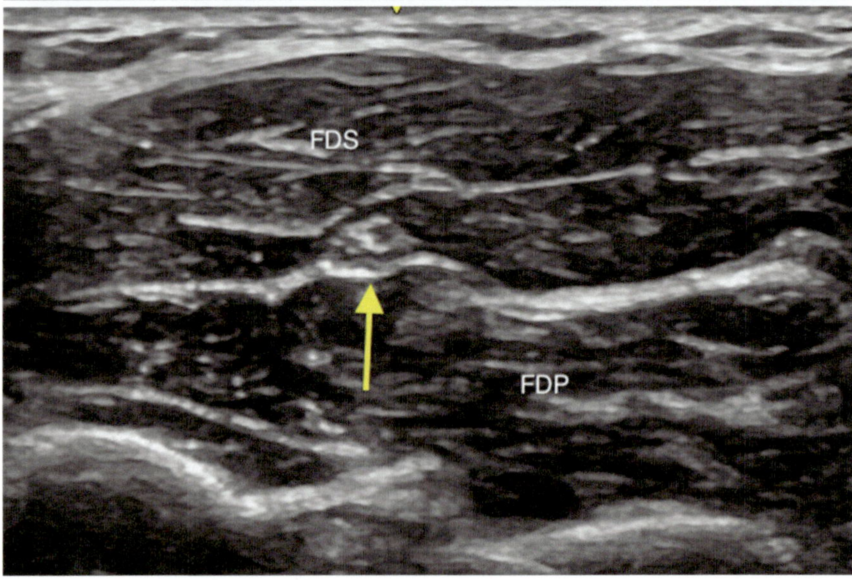

Figs. 24 and 25 Ultrasonographic imaging showing approaching the median nerve with the arteria brachialis (ABr) as internal landmark and the median nerve (arrow) is mostly found ulnar to the arteria brachialis (regular position)
Second ultrasonographic imaging showing the distal approach, US image in the mid-forearm, demonstrates that the median nerve (arrow) lies between the FDS (flexor digitorum superficialis) and the FDP (flexor digitorum profundus)

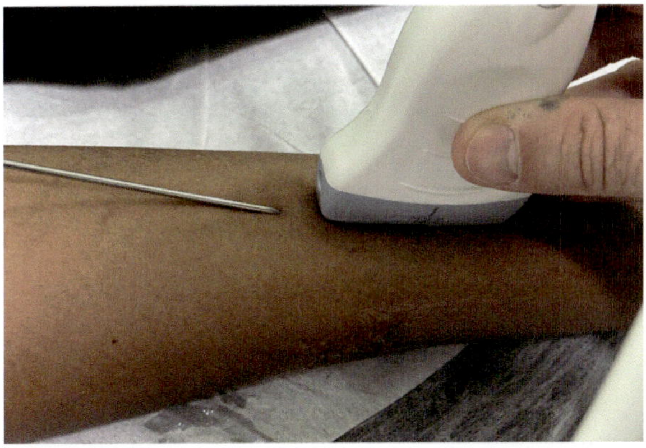

Fig. 26 Picture showing the positioning of the probe (longitudinal view to the median nerve) and needle to get the best access to the distal target

The confirmation of the target is done with paresthesia in the median nerve distribution; the palmar surface of the first, second, and third digits and lateral half of the fourth digit, C7–C8 dermatomes

For Bioness system: patient supine with UE extended and forearm supinated. The first incision is proximal to carpal tunnel/target. Insert lead distally toward the target. Tunnel remainder of lead proximally up the forearm in the same line as implanted lead.

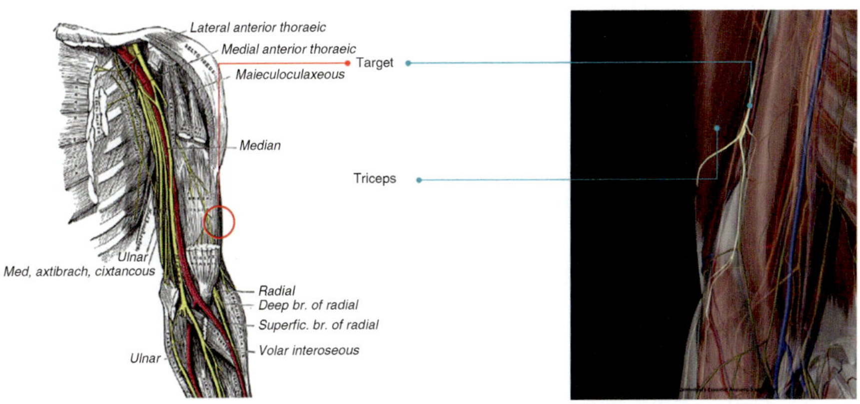

Fig. 27 Anatomical representation of the radial nerve as a target, showing the anatomical landmarks: musculospiral groove, radial sulcus/groove, located posteriorly at the center of the lateral border of the humerus bone, and olecranon process, located posterior. (Image printed with permission from StimRouter/Bioness)

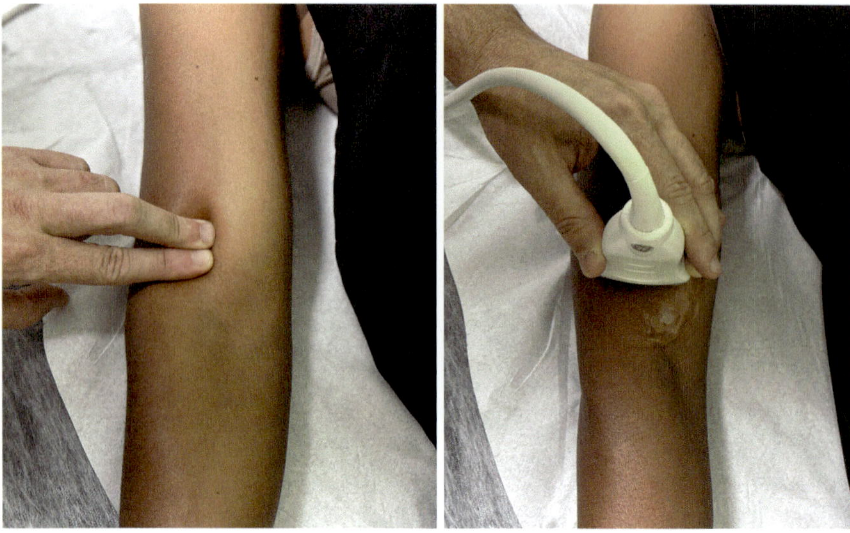

Figs. 28 and 29 Figures showing patient side-lying with affected limb on top, posterior approach: palpate the groove between the musculus biceps brachii and the musculus brachioradialis. Approach transverse probe positioning radial sided at the distal upper arm, approximately four fingerbreadths proximal to the midline of the fossa cubitalis

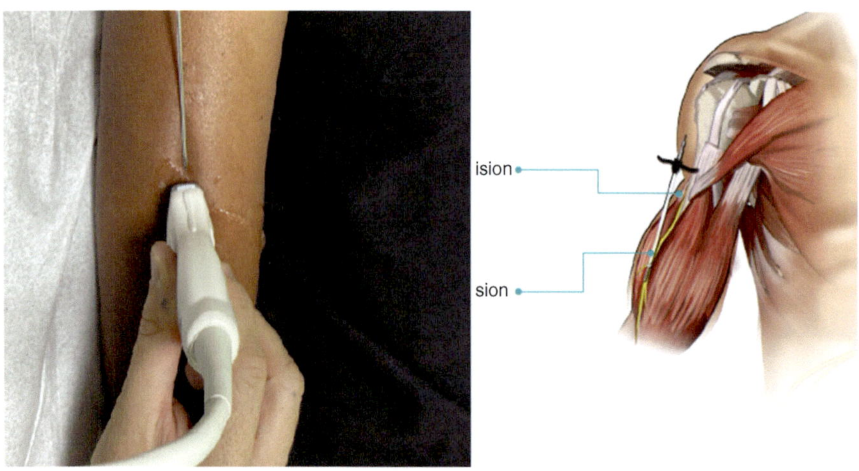

Fig. 30 Ultrasonographic imaging showing the internal landmarks: the musculus brachioradialis (MBrB) and the musculus brachialis (MBr). The radial nerve (arrow) has its POV between the musculus brachioradialis and musculus brachialis

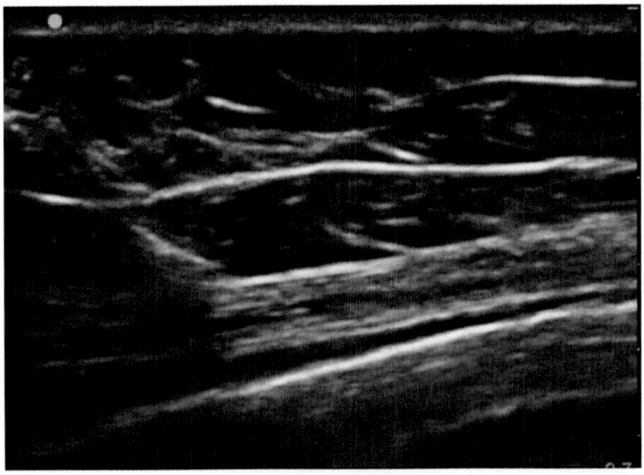

Fig. 31 Pictures showing the positioning of the probe and needle to get the best access to target 9. (Image from StimRouter. Printed with permission)

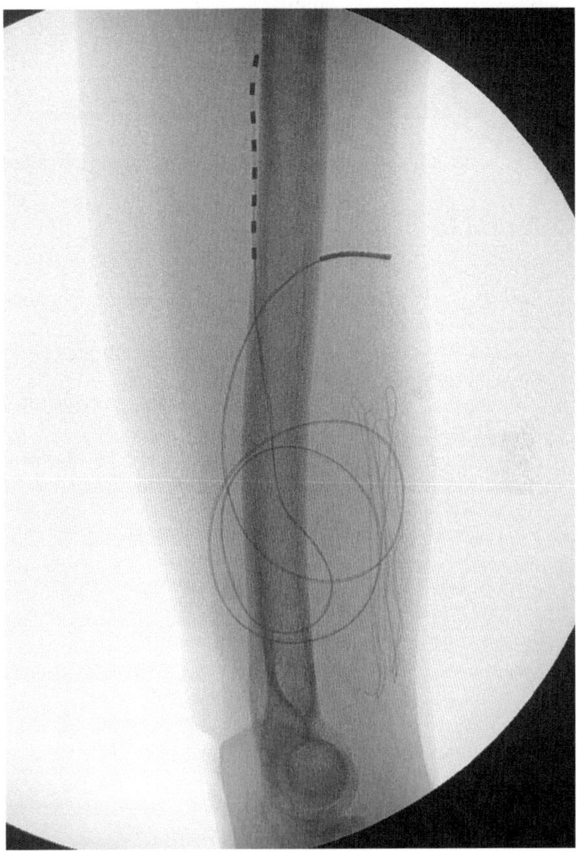

Fig. 32 Figures showing needle in the long view over radial nerve (RN), N (needle)
Ultrasonographic imaging from the electrode over radial nerve (arrows). Paresthesia in the radial distribution of the hand (back of the hand); C6–C8 dermatomes
For Bioness system: First incision proximal to the elbow and superior of the target. Stim probe inserted inferior toward the target between the long heads of the triceps and biceps. Remainder of lead is tunneled superior. Second incision/excision will be superior to the first incision

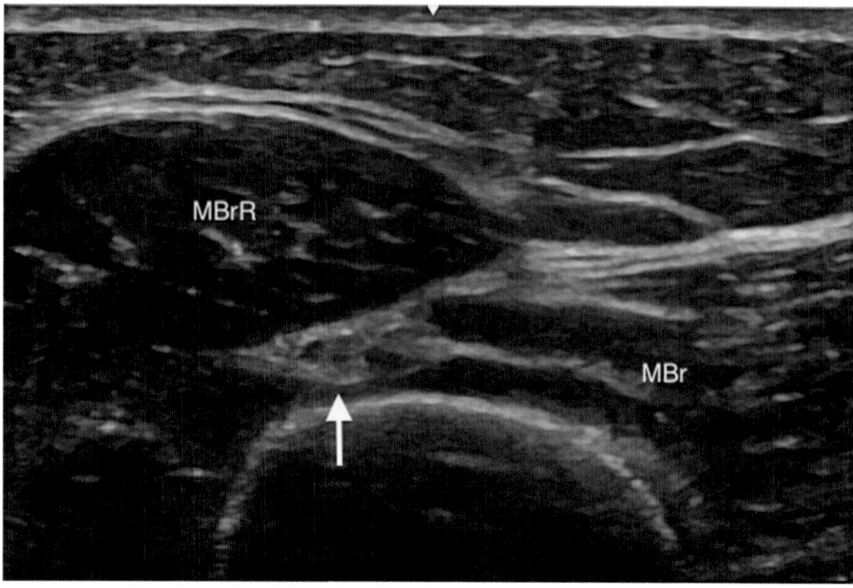

Fig. 33 Radiographic imaging showing a conventional percutaneous electrode over radial nerve

References

1. Loizides A. et al. Sonographic peripheral nerve topography. A landmark-based algorithm. Springer International Publishing; 2019.
2. Narouze S.N. et al. Atlas of ultrasound guided procedures in interventional pain management. Springer International Publishing; 2011.
3. Waldman SD. Waldman's comprehensive atlas of diagnostic ultrasound of painful conditions. Philadelphia: Wolters Kluwer; 2016.
4. Dettori N, Choudur H, Chhabra A. Ultrasound-guided treatment of peripheral nerve pathology. Semin Musculoskelet Radiol. 2018;22(3):364–74. https://doi.org/10.1055/s-0038-1641571. Epub 2018 May 23. PMID: 29791964.
5. Kaye AD, Motejunas MW, Bonneval LA, Ehrhardt KP, Latimer DR, Trescot A, Wilson KE, Ibrahim IN, Cornett EM, Urman RD, Candido KD. Ultrasound practice for chronic pain procedures: a comprehensive review. Best Pract Res Clin Anaesthesiol. 2019;33(4):465–86. https://doi.org/10.1016/j.bpa.2019.07.001. Epub 2019 Jul 18. PMID: 31791564.
6. Narouze SN. Ultrasound-guided interventional procedures in pain management: evidence-based medicine. Reg Anesth Pain Med. 2010;35(2 Suppl):S55–8. https://doi.org/10.1097/AAP.0b013e3181d24658. PMID: 20216026.
7. Chiou HJ, Chou YH, Wang HK, Lai YC. Chronic musculoskeletal pain: ultrasound guided pain control. Acta Anaesthesiol Taiwanica. 2014;52(3):114–33. https://doi.org/10.1016/j.aat.2014.08.002. Epub 2014 Oct 7. PMID: 25304316.
8. Anatomy G's. The anatomical basis of clinical practice. In: Standring S, editor. . 39th ed. Edinburgh: Elsevier Churchill Livingstone; 2005.
9. Huntoon MA, Hoelzer BC, Burgher AH, Hurdle MF, Huntoon EA. Feasibility of ultrasound-guided percutaneous placement of peripheral nerve stimulation electrodes and anchoring during simulated movement: part two, upper extremity. Reg Anesth Pain Med. 2008;33(6):558–65. https://doi.org/10.1016/j.rapm.2008.04.006. PMID: 19258971.

10. Koscielniak-Nielsen ZJ, Dahl JB. Ultrasound-guided peripheral nerve blockade of the upper extremity. Curr Opin Anaesthesiol. 2012;25(2):253–9. https://doi.org/10.1097/ACO.0b013e32835069c2. PMID: 22246462.
11. Lewis SR, Price A, Walker KJ, McGrattan K, Smith AF. Ultrasound guidance for upper and lower limb blocks. Cochrane Database Syst Rev. 2015;2015(9):CD006459. https://doi.org/10.1002/14651858.CD006459.pub3. PMID: 26361135; PMCID: PMC6465072.
12. Kowalska B, Sudoł-Szopińska I. Normal and sonographic anatomy of selected peripheral nerves. Part II: Peripheral nerves of the upper limb. J Ultrason. 2012;12(49):131–47. https://doi.org/10.15557/JoU.2012.0002. Epub 2012 Jun 30. PMID: 26674017; PMCID: PMC4579741.
13. Sohoni A, Nagdev A, Takhar S, Stone M. Forearm ultrasound-guided nerve blocks vs landmark-based wrist blocks for hand anesthesia in healthy volunteers. Am J Emerg Med. 2016;34(4):730–4. https://doi.org/10.1016/j.ajem.2016.01.020. Epub 2016 Jan 21. PMID: 26920669.
14. Rothe C, Steen-Hansen C, Lund J, Jenstrup MT, Lange KH. Ultrasound-guided block of the suprascapular nerve - a volunteer study of a new proximal approach. Acta Anaesthesiol Scand. 2014;58(10):1228–32. https://doi.org/10.1111/aas.12392. Epub 2014 Sep 3. PMID: 25186626.

Peripheral Nerve Stimulation Technique Using Ultrasound in Lower Limbs

Tiago da Silva Freitas

General Instructions to Understand the USG Legends

The general instructions were based on the classification system used by Hannes Gruber, Alexander Loizides, and Bernhard Moriggl in their book *Sonographic Peripheral Nerve Topography, A Landmark-based Algorithm* [1].

On the left side on the upper half page, there is the following (standardized) table.

ELM	External landmark(s)
IPOP	Initial positioning of probe
ILM	Internal landmark(s)
POV	Point of optimal visibility
VAR	Relevant variations
AP	Alternative plan (if worth mentioning!)
C	Comments – if helpful/of interest regarding surgical technique
PAT	Pathology
Confirmation of the target	Neurophysiology regarding the peripheral nerve target
Notes	Any additional important information

Following the table, we will have the figures with the step-by-step technique. We also used exactly the same description in the ultrasound images done by Hans Gruber in the book above (cited with permission).

T. d. S. Freitas (✉)
Brasilia Pain Institute(INDOR), Neurosurgery Department Hospital de Base de Brasília(HBDF), Functional Neurosurgery Department Hospital Sírio Libanês, Brasília, Distrito Federal, Brazil

T. d. S. Freitas et al. (eds.), *Neuromodulation Techniques for Pain Treatment*,
https://doi.org/10.1007/978-3-030-84778-4_13

USG Technique for Peripheral Nerve Stimulation in Lower Limbs [2–18]

Saphenous Nerve (Figs. 1, 2, 3, and 4)

ELM	1. Spina iliaca anterior superior (ASIS) 2. Basis patellae
IPOP	Transverse probe position in the distal third of the thigh medial to the anterior iliac spine and superior-basis patellae
ILM	1. A. femoralis (femoral artery) 2. M. sartorius (sartorius muscle) 3. M. vastus medialis (vastus medialis muscle) 4. M. adductor magnus (adductor longus muscle) 5. Membrana vastoadductoria Saphenous nerve as it exits the adductor canal. Vastus medialis muscle, sartorius muscle, semimembranosus muscle, adductor longus muscle, femoral vessels
POV	In the proximal segment of the canalis adductorius (adductor canal), anterolateral to the artery
VAR	N. saphenous (saphenous nerve) medial to the A. femoralis
AP	None
C	None
PAT	Chronic neuropathic knee pain
Confirmation of the target	Paresthesia to knee via patellar branch; L3 dermatome
Notes	None

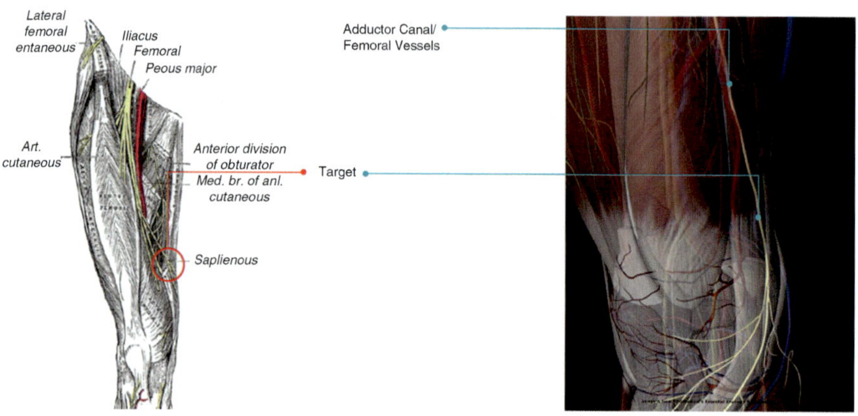

Fig. 1 Anatomical representation of saphenous nerve and the anatomical landmarks: semimembranosus muscle – most medial hamstring muscle, vastus medialis, sartorius, femoral artery, femoral vein, adductor longus (Image from StimRouter, printed with permission)

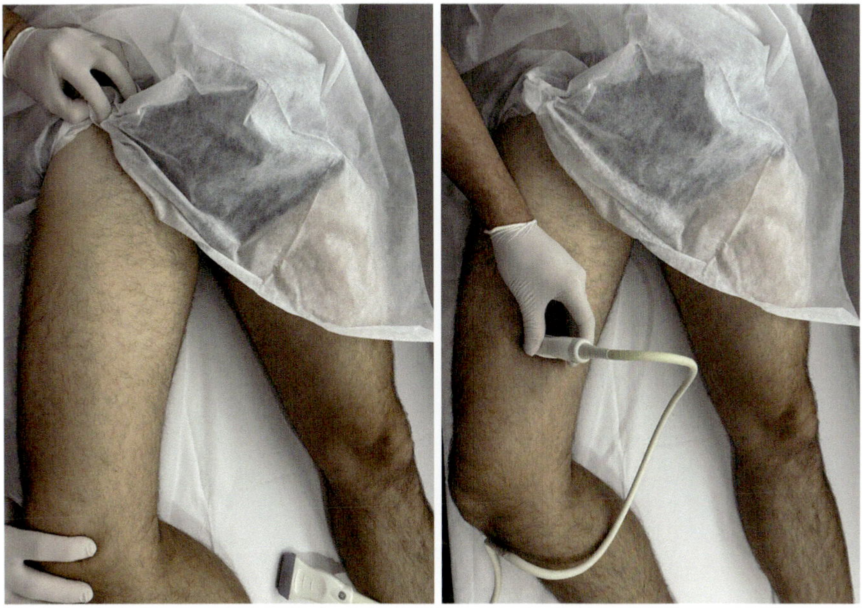

Fig. 2 Definition of the length of the thigh: from the anterior iliac spine anterior to the basis patellae. Transverse probe position at the beginning of the inner aspect of the distal third of the thigh

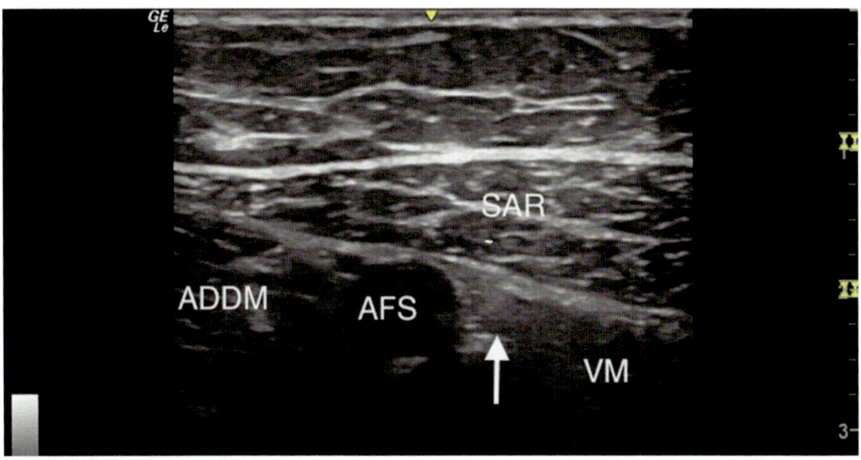

Fig. 3 US image shows the saphenous nerve (arrow) in the femoral triangle, lateral to the superficial femoral artery *(AFS)* and vein. The femoral triangle is bordered by the sartorius *(SAR)* superiorly, the vastus medialis *(VM) anterior and lateral*, and the adductor longus *(ADDM)* posterior and medial
The nervus saphenous (arrow) runs within the canalis adductorius and is clearly visible ventrolateral to the artery

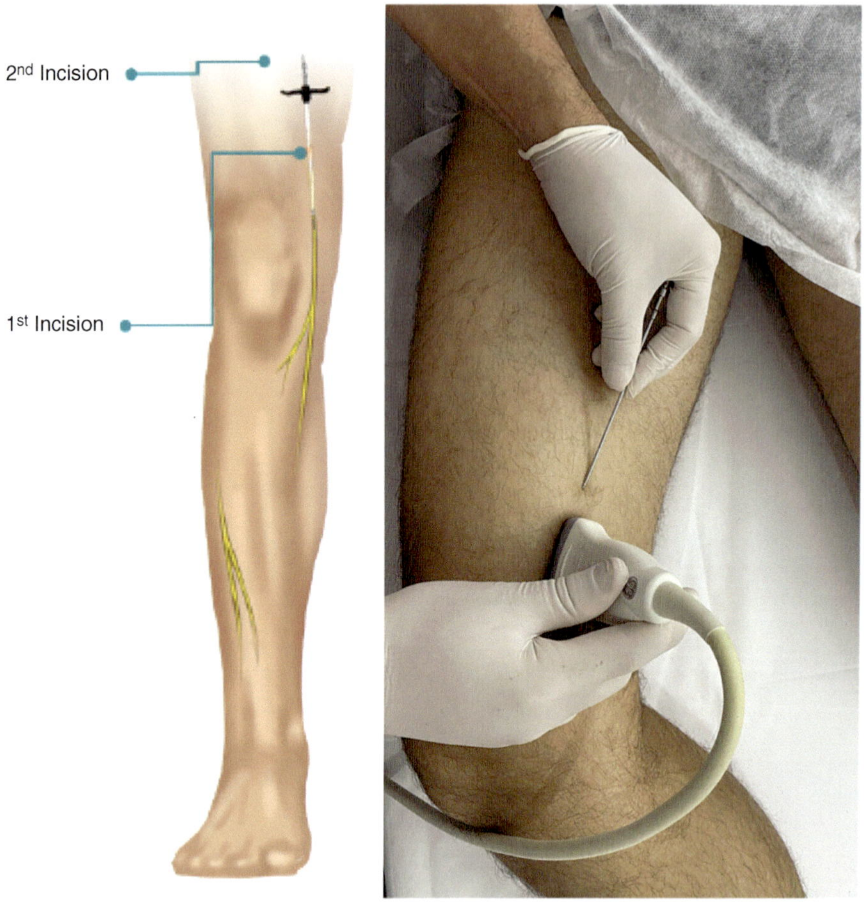

Fig. 4 Image showing the position of the needle entry point and probe direction in a patient

Tibial Nerve (Figs. 5, 6, 7, and 8)

ELM	1. Deep flexors: M. flexor digitorum longus (flexor digitorum muscle) and M. tibialis posterior (tibialis posterior muscle) 2. Palpable M. soleus (distal end)
IPOP	Transverse, about six fingerbreadths proximal to the malleolus medialis
ILM	1. M. soleus at its transition into the Achilles tendon 2. A. tibialis posterior (posterior tibial artery) and Vv. comitantes
POV	Beginning with the IPOP until some centimeters further distal

VAR	None
AP	None
C	"Even" surface (=better coupling> > less artifacts) than more distal
PAT	Neuropathic foot pain
Confirmation of the target	Paresthesia in the S1, S2, L4, and L5 dermatomes; Medial calcaneal (heel), medial plantar (sole), and lateral plantar branches (pinky toe). Motor response of toe curling
Notes	Posterior tibial nerve; approx. 3–5 cm superior of medial malleolus, 2 cm posterior to tibia; *t*ibialis posterior muscle, flexor *d*igitorum muscle, tibial *a*rtery, tibial *n*erve, flexor *h*allucis longus muscle (**TDANH**) Mixed nerve; may need to loop or shelf lead layout to fit the 15 cm lead distal to the calf. Use spinal needle (EPIMED) to go through crural fascia that is in the lower leg

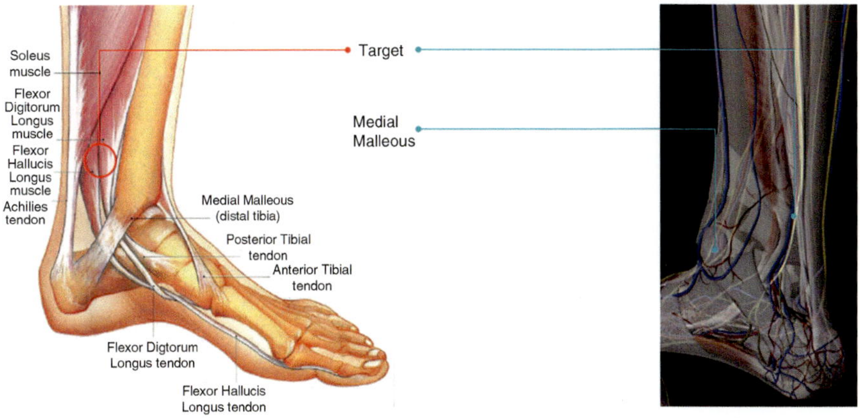

Fig. 5 Anatomical representation of tibial nerve and the anatomical landmarks: using the anachronous Tom, Dick, and Nervous Harry. Anterior to posterior are the ligaments of the tibialis posterior, flexor digitorum longus (posterior tibial artery and posterior tibial nerve), and flexor hallucis longus (Image from StimRouter, printed with permission)

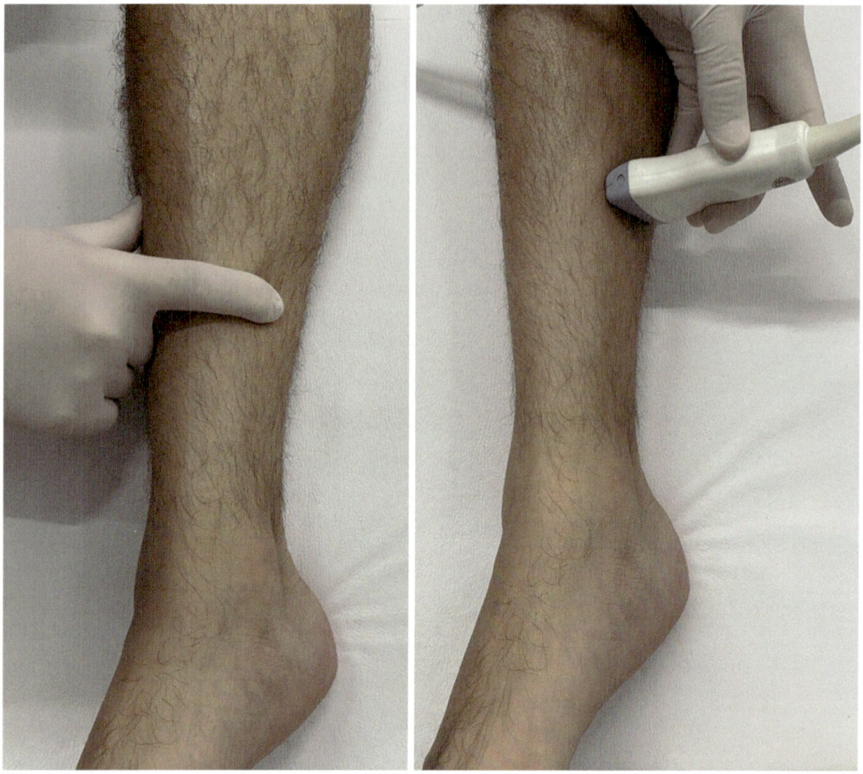

Fig. 6 Palpation of the dorsal surface of the calf between the musculus tibialis posterior and the musculus flexor digitorum longus anterior, musculus soleus, and the Achilles tendon posterior, respectively. Center of the transversely oriented probe in the area of the aforementioned indentation

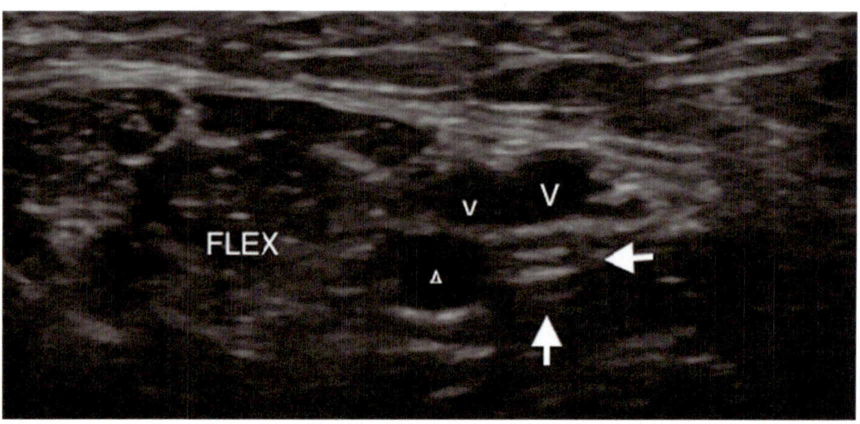

Fig. 7 The bellies of the deep flexors (FLEX) at the transition of the M. soleus into the Achilles tendon as well as the accompanying arteria tibialis posterior and venae tibialis posteriors (A/V) are guides to the nerve (arrows)

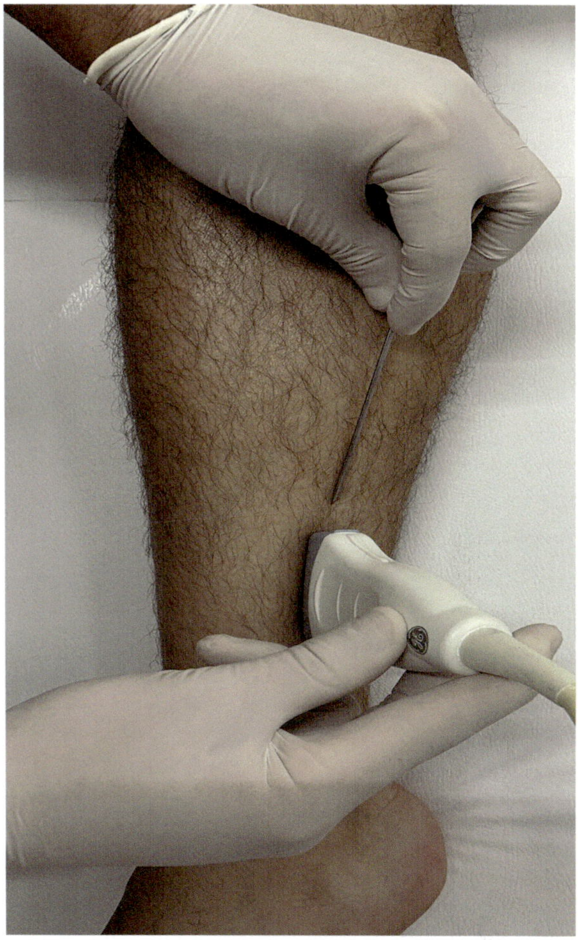

Fig. 8 Image showing the position of the needle entry point in a patient (in plane with the ultrasound probe)

Common Peroneal Nerve (Nervus Peroneus Communis): Figs. 9, 10, and 11

ELM	1. Common fibular/common peroneal nerve at the fibular neck 2. Anterior tibialis muscle 3. Evertor muscle group 4. Popliteal fossa
IPOP	Oblique (=perpendicular to the course of the bicep tendon!), with the center of the probe at the tibial border of the M. biceps femoris, three fingerbreadths proximal to the caput fibulae
ILM	1. M. biceps femoris 2. M. gastrocnemius, caput laterale
POV	Direct at or one fingerbreadth distal to the IPOP at the dorsal surface of the M. gastrocnemius and caput laterale
VAR	None
AP	None

C	None
PAT	Neuropathic pain in the lower extremity
Confirmation of the target	Paresthesia conducting down to the top (dorsum) of the foot, L5 dermatome
Notes	There are two different approaches: primary, distal to the knee = common peroneal, and secondary, proximal to the knee = common fibular. Secondary approach presented for patients that may not be able to tolerate implant distal to the knee

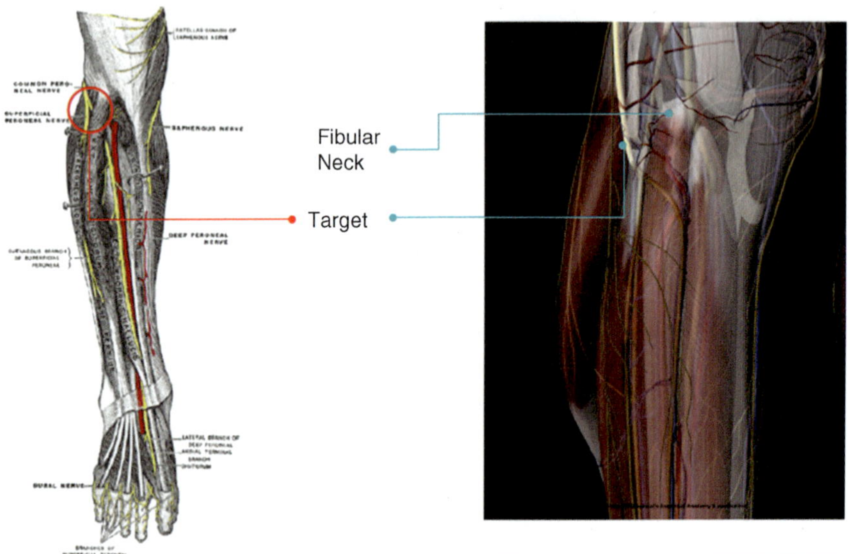

Fig. 9 Anatomical representation of the common peroneal nerve and the anatomical landmarks: popliteal fossa – back of the knee
Evertor muscle group – perone bros, posterior to anterior, superior to inferior; peroneus (fibularis) longus, peroneus (fibularis) brevis, peroneus (fibularis) tertius (image from StimRouter, printed with permission)

Fig. 10 Echography with indication of the anatomical landmarks of the common peroneal nerve (Image from StimRouter, printed with permission)
PL peroneus longus
F fibular head
US image shows the CPN (arrow) deep to the peroneus longus muscle *(PL)* and the fibular head *(F)* in the fibular tunnel

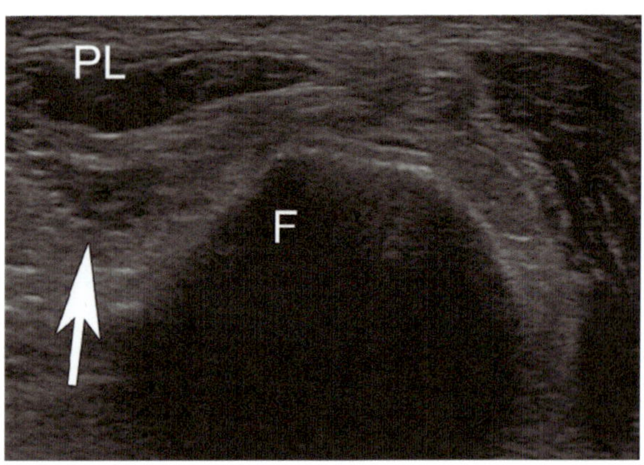

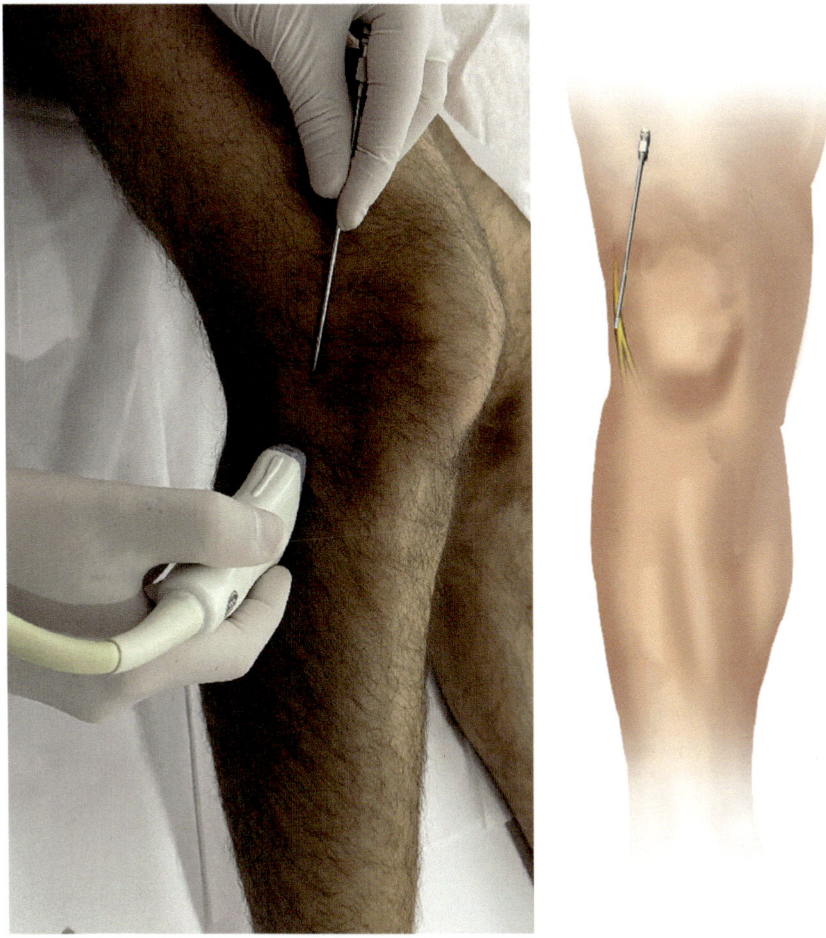

Fig. 11 Schematic image showing one of the approaches to the common peroneal nerve: Entry point inferolateral of the knee. Needle inserted superiorly toward target/outside of the knee

Superficial Peroneal Nerve (Nervus Peroneus Superficialis): Figs. 12, 13, 14, and 15

ELM	1. Palpable anterior border of the fibula (in its distal segment) 2. Palpable M. extensor digitorum longus 3. Palpable M. fibularis longus (and brevis)
IPOP	Slightly oblique*, center of probe between ELM (2) and (3)
ILM	1. Fibula** 2. M. extensor digitorum longus 3. M. fibularis longus

POV	Subfascial between M. extensor digitorum longus and M. fibularis longus within a fat-filled flat tunnel ***
VAR	Two nerves, which perforate the fascia cruris at different levels
AP	None
C	* Remember the course of the nerve ** The nerve lies on a perpendicular through its anterior border *** Common concept: all large nerves use such tunnels; thus, these nerves show good contrast
PAT	Neuropathic pain in the lower extremity
Confirmation of the target	Paresthesia conducting down to the top (dorsum) of the foot, L5 dermatome
Notes	Superficial peroneal nerve mid-shin lateral to the extensor digitorum. Fibularis longus, deep fibular nerve, anterior tibial artery Important to stay anterior to avoid gastrocnemius

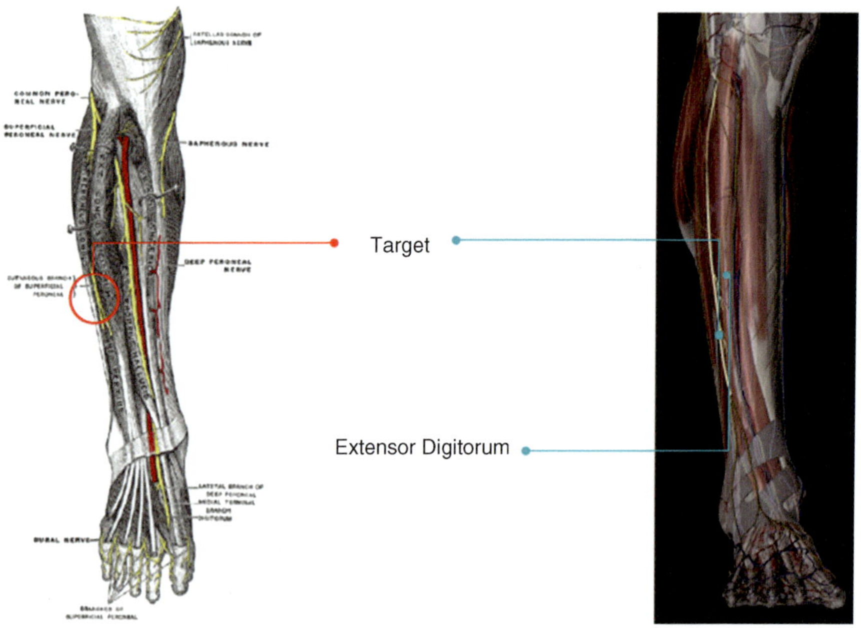

Fig. 12 Anatomical representation of the superficial peroneal nerve and the anatomical landmarks: superficial peroneal nerve mid-shin lateral to the extensor digitorum. Fibularis longus, deep fibular nerve, anterior tibial artery. (Image from StimRouter, printed with permission)

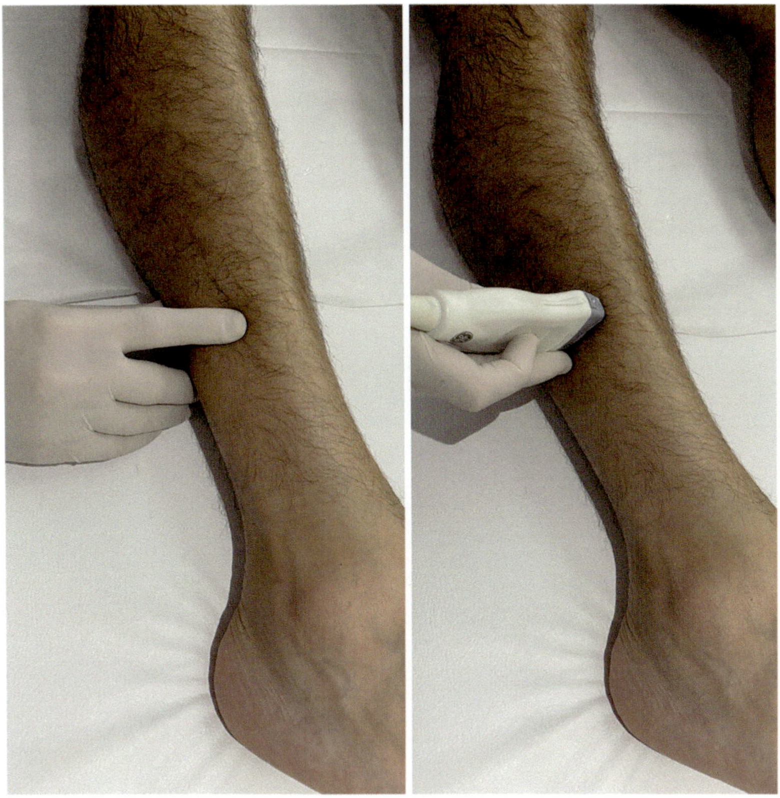

Fig. 13 Palpation of the anterior border of the fibula in a groove between the musculus extensor digitorum longus and musculi fibulares. According to the known course of the nervus fibularis superficialis (probe position perpendicular)

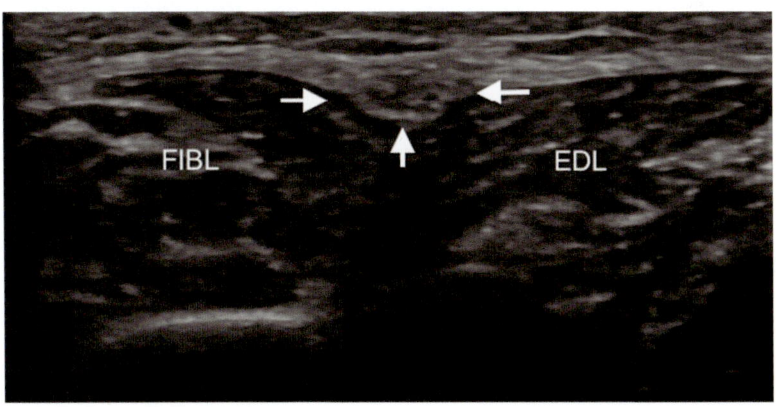

Fig. 14 US image shows the SPN (arrows) running in the fascial plane between the extensor digitorum longus *(EDL)* and the musculus fibularis longus (FIBL)
EDL extensor digitorum longus
FIBL musculus fibularis longus

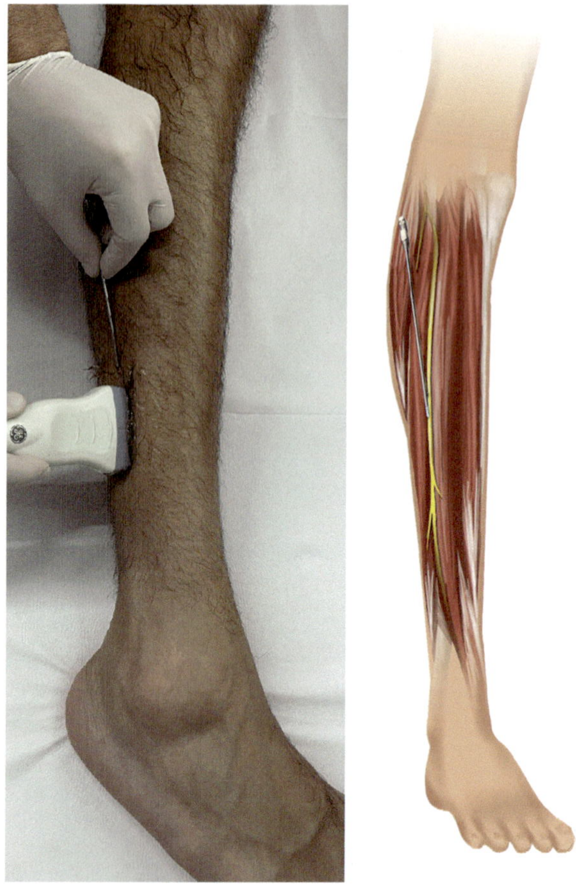

Fig. 15 After correct localization of nervus fibularis superficialis, turn the probe to the long view and set your needle entry point: superior to the target. Needle inserted inferolateral toward the target

Lateral Femoral Cutaneous Nerve (Nervus Cutaneus Femoris Lateralis): Figs. 16, 17, 18, and 19

ELM	1. Spina iliaca anterior superior (ASIS) 2. Palpable groove between M. sartorius (Sartorius muscle) and M. tensor fasciae latae
IPOP	Transverse about three to four fingerbreadths distal to the anterosuperior iliac spine, center of the probe at the palpable groove *
ILM	1. M. sartorius 2. M. tensor fasciae latae 3. Fascia latae 4. Fat-filled flat tunnel (FFFT)***
POV	Within the FFFT between the M. sartorius and M. tensor fasciae latae, about four fingerbreadths distal to the anterosuperior iliac spine
VAR	The transition of the N. cutaneous femoris lateralis concerning its course proximal to the ligamentum inguinale and on the iliac crest, respectively, is very variable! It is additionally often split

AP	None
C	* Patient should "lift the leg" * ** No compression *** There is a general rule: all big sensory nerves run through such tunnels; here they are easy to find being contrasted by surrounding fat
PAT	Neuropathic thigh pain
Confirmation of the target	Paresthesia to superior, lateral compartment of the thigh (gun holsters), L4–L5 dermatomes
Notes	Make sure patch placement is not so lateral that it becomes a clearance issue and/or so medial that it gets covered when patient is seated. Best results capture LFC proximal to bifurcation of the nerve

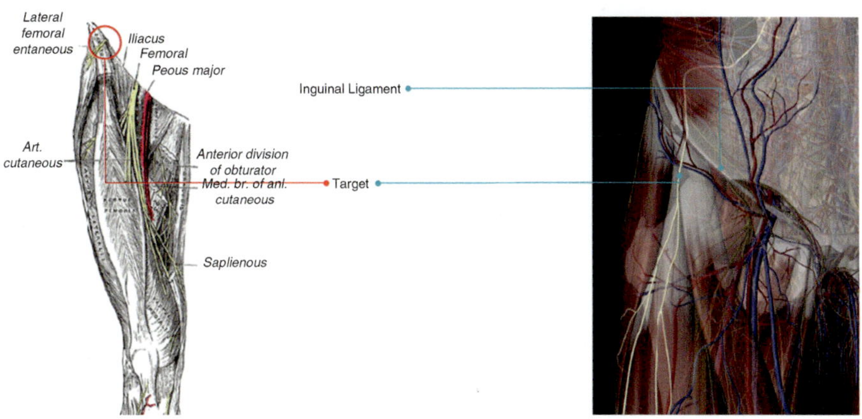

Fig. 16 Anatomical representation of the lateral femoral cutaneous nerve and the anatomical landmarks: lateral femoral cutaneous nerve inferior to the ASIS. Inguinal ligament, sartorius muscle, quadriceps muscle group. (Image from StimRouter, printed with permission)

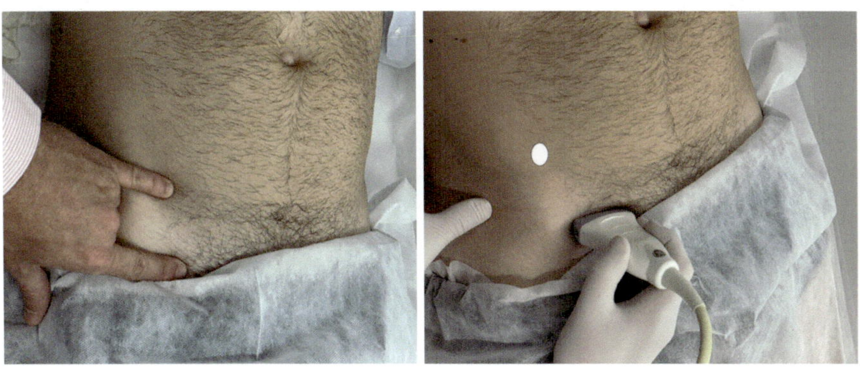

Fig. 17 Simultaneous palpation of the anterosuperior iliac spine and the groove caudal to that (in some subjects even visible) between the musculus tensor fasciae latae and the musculus sartorius Transverse probe position distal to the anterosuperior iliac spine (dotted oval), center of the probe over the identified grove

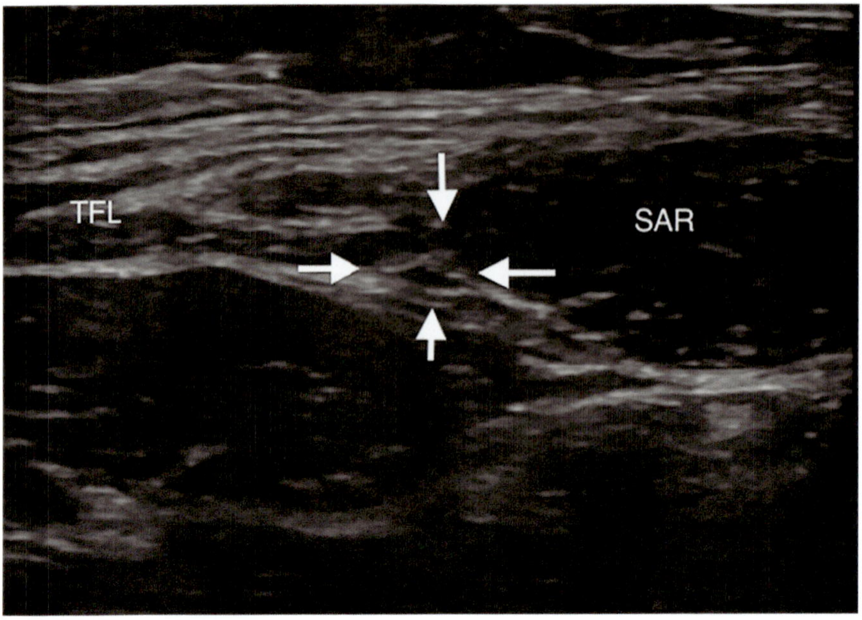

Fig. 18 The musculus tensor fasciae latae (TFL), the musculus sartorius (SAR), and the fascia latae border the "fat-filled flat tunnel" (FFFT); rather hypoechogenic because mainly filled with fat. The nerve (arrows) at the POV within the FFFT (arrowheads)

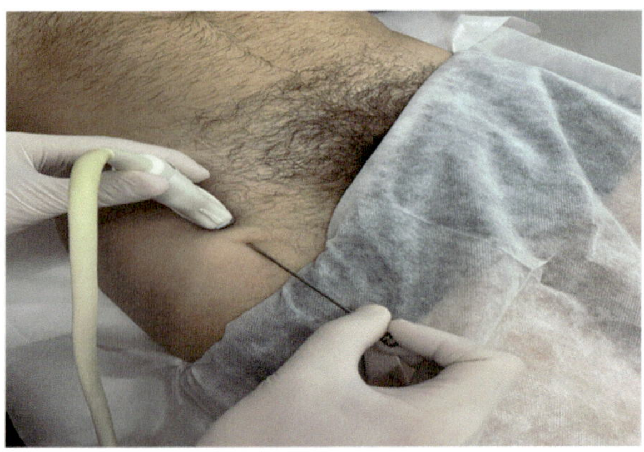

Fig. 19 After correct localization of cutaneous lateral femoral nerve, turn the probe to the long view and set your needle entry point: target will be directly inferior of the ASIS/inguinal ligament junction. Needle entry point inferior of target. Needle inserted superolateral toward the target

Femoral Nerve (Nervus Femoralis): Figs. 20, 21, 22, and 23

ELM	1. Pulsation of the A. femoralis (femoral artery) 2. Ligamentum inguinale (Inguinal ligament) or line between the spina iliaca anterior superior (ASIS) and the tuberculum pubicum
IPOP	Center of the probe a little lateral to the A. femoralis, directly below or on the ligamentum inguinale*
ILM	1. A. femoralis 2. M. iliopsoas 3. Fascia lata 4. Head of the femur (in slim people)
POV	Lateral to the A. femoralis, directly blow the ligamentum inguinale**
VAR	The distance between the nerve and artery is variable (however always lateral to it)
AP	None
C	* Important as further distal the nerve is already split into its branches ** In a typical groove of the M. iliopsoas
PAT	Neuropathic pain in the lower extremity related to the femoral nerve
Confirmation of the target	Paresthesia in femoral nerve distribution of the lower extremity; L2–L4 dermatomes
Notes	Make sure patch placement is not so lateral that it becomes a clearance issue and/or so medial that it gets covered when patient is seated. Best results capture LFC proximal to bifurcation of the nerve

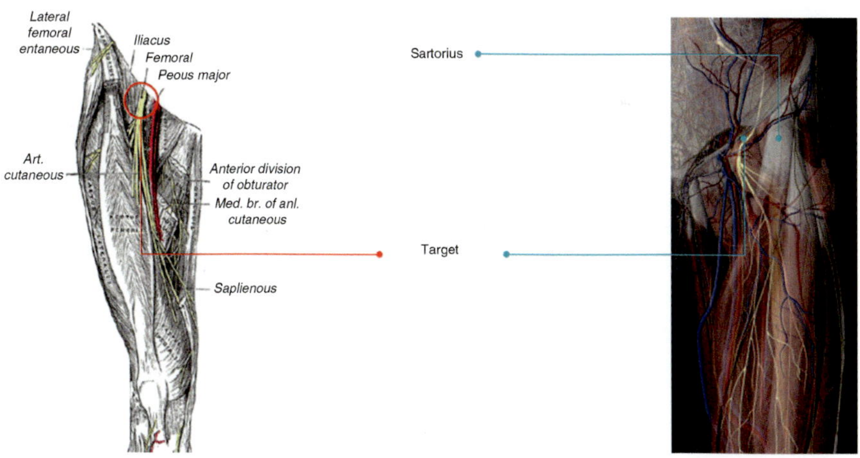

Fig. 20 Anatomical representation of the femoral nerve and the anatomical landmarks: femoral nerve inferior to the inguinal ligament. Common femoral artery and vein. Pectineus and sartorius muscles. (Image from StimRouter, printed with permission)

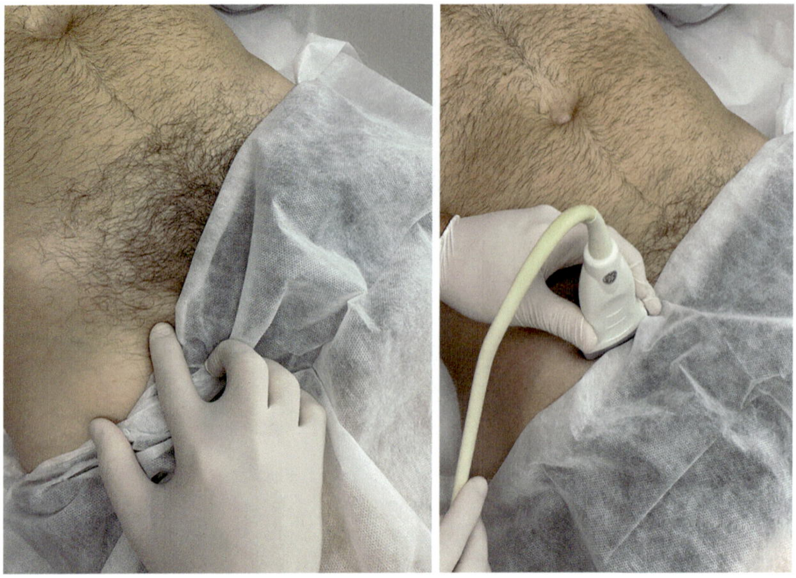

Fig. 21 The pulsation of the arteria femoralis is palpable directly distal to the middle of the inguinal ligament
The probe position is more or less transverse, its center a little lateral to the pulse of the arteria femoralis

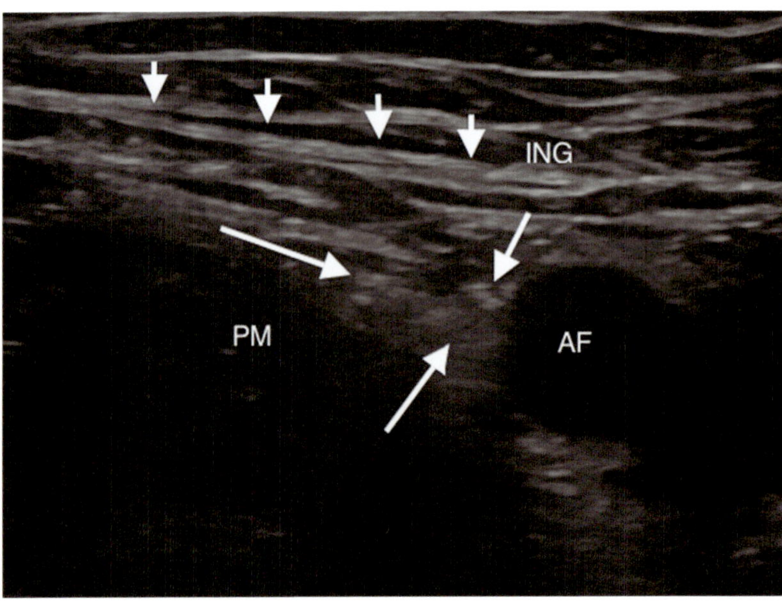

Fig. 22 In the level of the ligamentum inguinale (ING) and the arteria femoralis (AF) and the musculus iliopsoas (PM). The echogenic cross section of the nerve's main deep portion (large arrows) directly lateral to the arteria femoralis and in a groove of the musculus iliopsoas

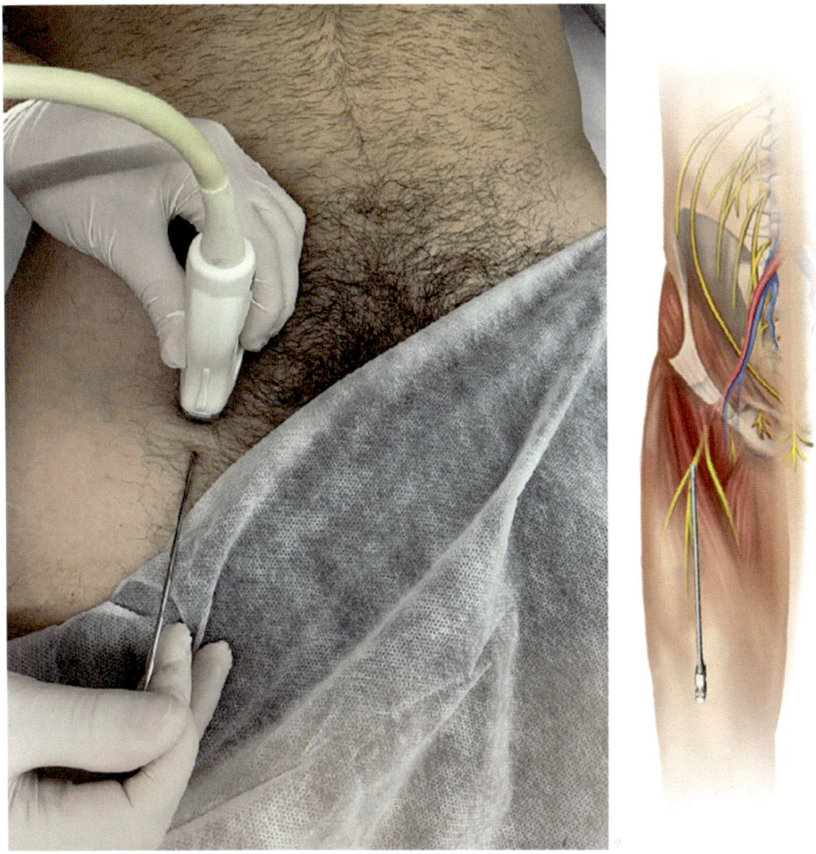

Fig. 23 After correct localization of femoral nerve: turn the probe to the long view and set your needle entry point. The first entry point inferior of the target. Needle and lead inserted in a cephalad/superior direction toward the target

Sural Nerve (Nervus Suralis): Figs. 24, 25, 26, and 27

ELM	1. Malleolus lateralis (lateral malleolus) 2. Palpable Mm. fibulares (fibularis brevis and fibularis longus muscles) 3. Palpable M. soleus (soleus muscle) 4. Shallow groove between 2 and 3
IPOP	Transverse probe position four fingerbreadths proximal to the malleolus lateralis*
ILM	1. V. saphena magna (lesser saphenous vein) 2. M. soleus 3. Mm. fibulares
POV	Exactly at IPOP **

VAR	Position relative to the V. saphena parva mirror – inverted
AP	None
C	* No compression ** Subcutaneous and usually ventral/fibular of the V. saphena parva
PAT	Neuropathic distal pain in the distribution of the sural nerve
Confirmation of the target	Paresthesia in sural distribution of the foot (heel and side; lateral calcaneal and lateral dorsal branches); S1–S2 dermatomes
Notes	None

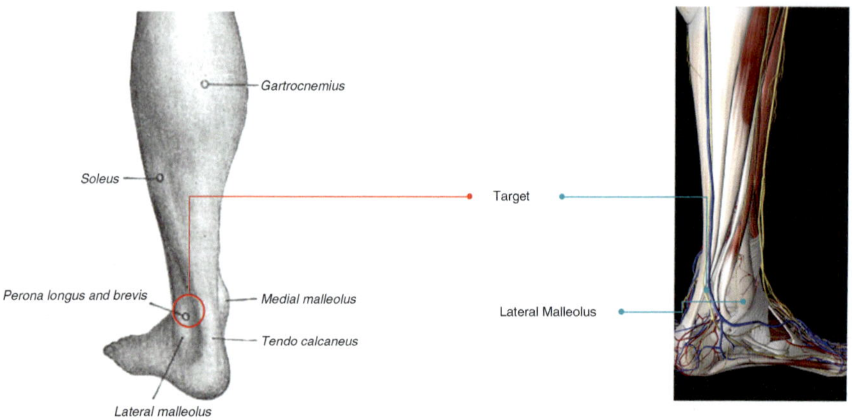

Fig. 24 Anatomical representation of the lateral femoral cutaneous nerve and the anatomical landmarks: sural nerve superior and posterior to the lateral malleolus. Fibula, the peroneus bros; fibularis brevis and fibularis longus muscles, Achilles tendon and soleus muscles. (Image from StimRouter, printed with permission)

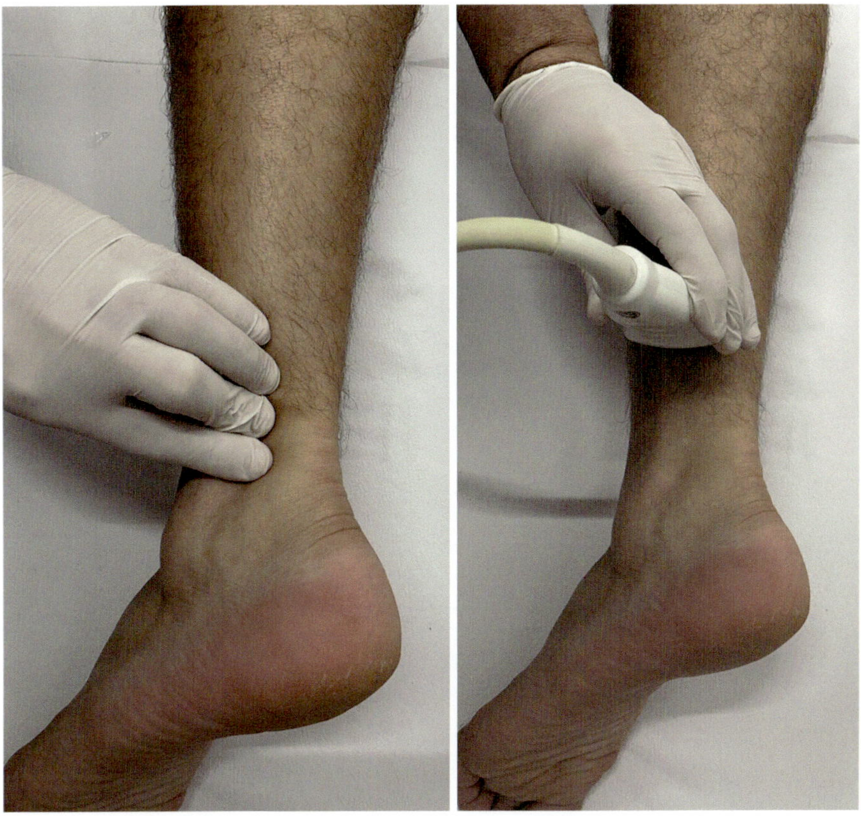

Fig. 25 Starting with the malleolus lateralis (in proximal direction), a shallow groove is palpable between the musculi fibulares and the musculus soleus
Strictly transverse position of the probe with its center on the abovementioned groove

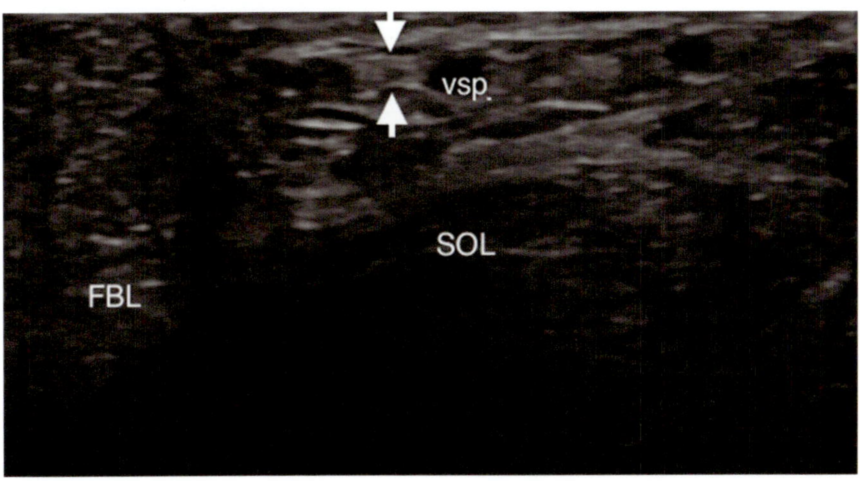

Fig. 26 The vena saphena parva (VSP) is the vascular landmark. Musculus soleus (SOL), musculus fibularis longus (FIBL). The nerve arrows) lying typically next to the epifascial vein

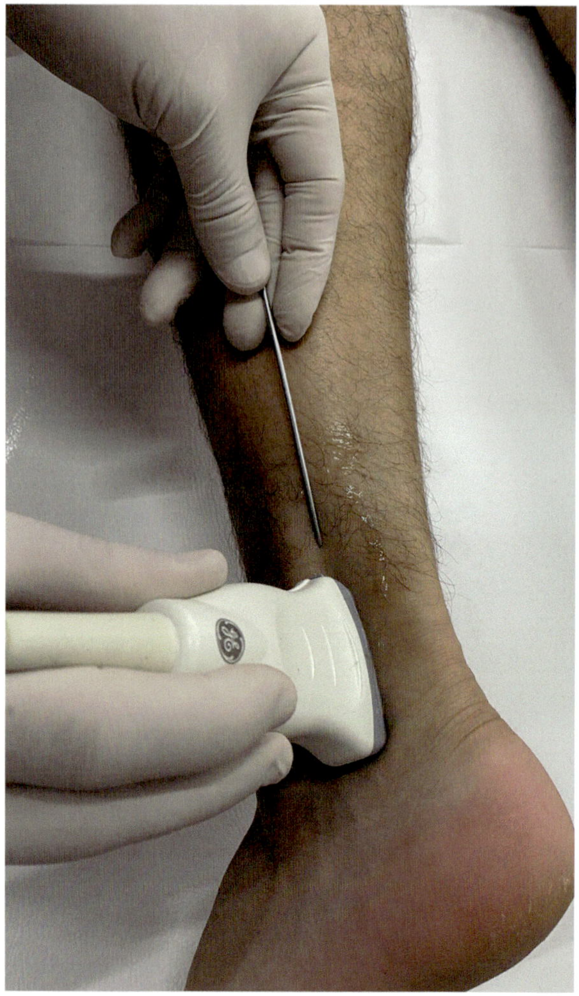

Fig. 27 After correct localization of the sural nerve, turn the probe to the long view and set your needle entry point: entry point proximal to target. Needle inserted inferior toward target. Remainder of lead is tunneled on lateral lower leg, away from calf/Achilles

Sciatic Nerve (Nervus Ischiadicus): Figs. 28, 29, 30, and 31

ELM	1. Nervus ischiadicus (sciatic nerve) proximal to the popliteal fossa 2. M. biceps femoralis (biceps femoral muscle) 3. M. Semitendinosis 4. M. semimembranosus 5. Arteria femoralis (femoral artery)
IPOP	Transverse probe position with its center in the middle of the thigh, one to maximum two fingerbreadths distal to the sulcus glutealis* [more exactly: divide the line tuber ischiadicum – tip of the trochanter major ("Tu-Tr-line") – into thirds, the perpendicular through the border between medial/middle third indicates the probe placement]
ILM	1. M. biceps femoris (caput longum) 2. M. adductor magnus
POV	Between the M. biceps femoris (caput longum, lying dorsal) and M. adductor magnus (lying ventral)
VAR	Two nerves (N. tibialis and N. fibularis communis) in case of high division
AP	None
C	None
PAT	Neuropathic pain radiating from the lower back/buttocks through the leg
Confirmation of the target	Paresthesia in sciatic distribution of the leg (lateral/posterior thigh (hamstring), anterior below the knee); S1, L4, and L5 dermatomes
Notes	None

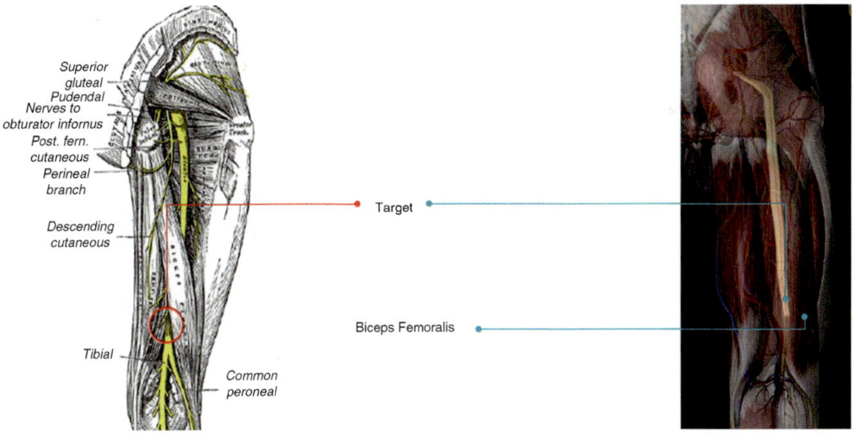

Fig. 28 Anatomical representation of the sciatic nerve and the anatomical landmarks: sciatic nerve proximal to the popliteal fossa. Biceps femoralis, semitendinosus, semimembranosus, femoral artery. (Image from StimRouter, printed with permission)

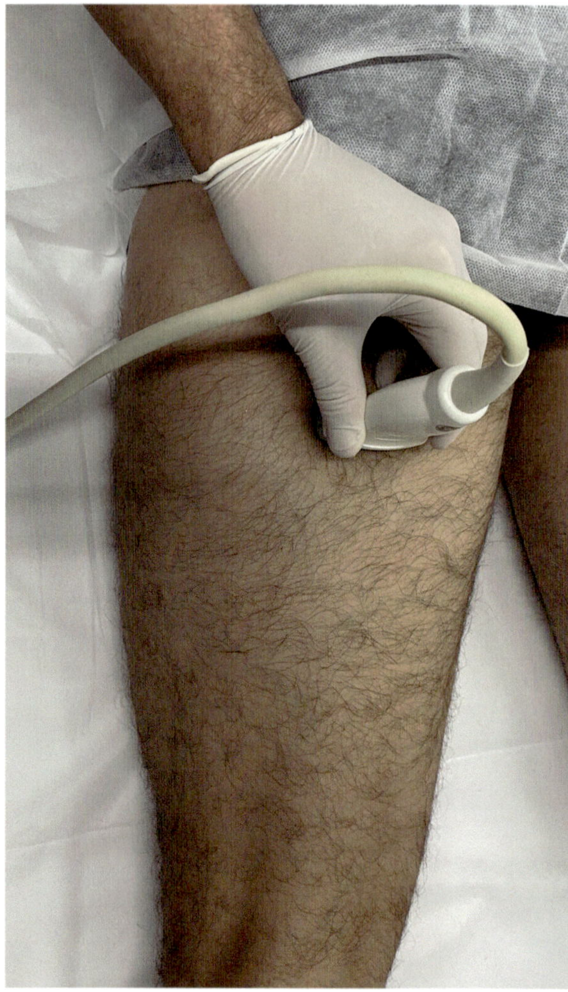

Fig. 29 Transverse probe position with its center in the middle of the thigh, just a little distal to the sulcus glutealis

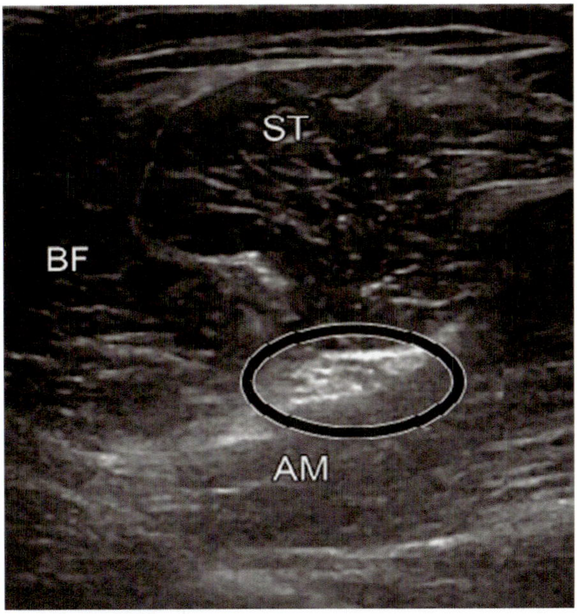

Fig. 30 Image illustrates the sciatic nerve proximal to the popliteal fossa, deep to the ST and BF, superficial to the AM. (Image from StimRouter, printed with permission)
ST semitendinosus
BF biceps femoralis
AM adductor magnus

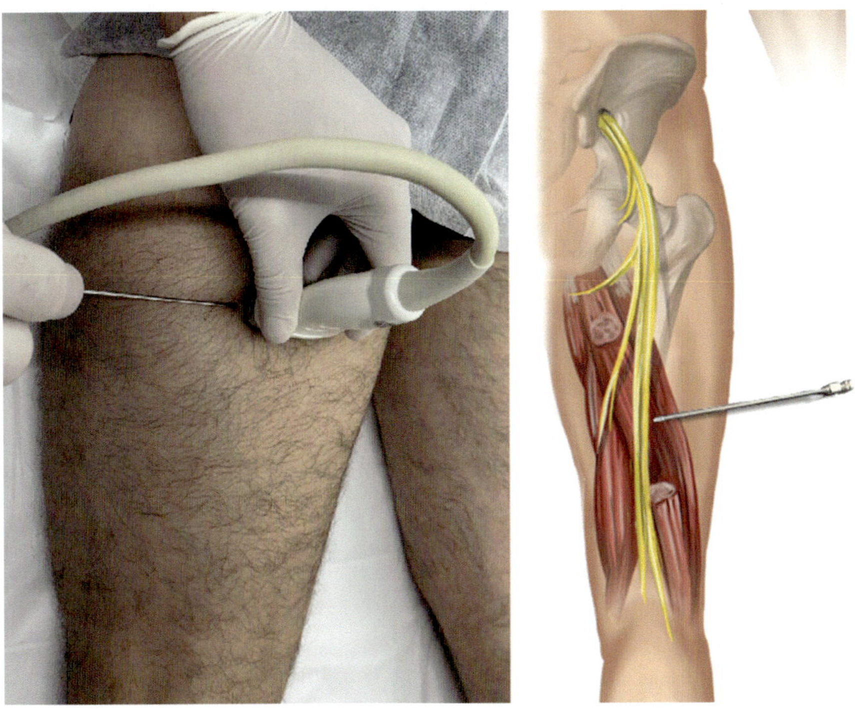

Fig. 31 After correct localization of the sciatic nerve, set your needle entry point: patient in prone position. Entry point lateral to target. Needle inserted medially toward the target. Remainder of lead is tunneled on lateral leg, away from hamstring/back of the leg

References

1. A Loizides et al. Sonographic peripheral nerve topography. A Landmark-based Algorithm. Springer International Publishing; 2019.
2. Narouze S.N. et al. Atlas of ultrasound guided procedures in interventional pain management. Springer International Publishing; 2011.
3. Waldman SD. Waldman's comprehensive atlas of diagnostic ultrasound of painful conditions. Philadelphia: Wolters Kluwer; 2016.
4. Dettori N, Choudur H, Chhabra A. Ultrasound-guided treatment of peripheral nerve pathology. Semin Musculoskelet Radiol. 2018;22(3):364–74. https://doi.org/10.1055/s-0038-1641571. Epub 2018 May 23. PMID: 29791964.
5. Kaye AD, Motejunas MW, Bonneval LA, Ehrhardt KP, Latimer DR, Trescot A, Wilson KE, Ibrahim IN, Cornett EM, Urman RD, Candido KD. Ultrasound practice for chronic pain procedures: a comprehensive review. Best Pract Res Clin Anaesthesiol. 2019;33(4):465–86. https://doi.org/10.1016/j.bpa.2019.07.001. Epub 2019 Jul 18. PMID: 31791564.
6. Narouze SN. Ultrasound-guided interventional procedures in pain management: evidence-based medicine. Reg Anesth Pain Med. 2010;35(2 Suppl):S55–8. https://doi.org/10.1097/AAP.0b013e3181d24658. PMID: 20216026.
7. Chiou HJ, Chou YH, Wang HK, Lai YC. Chronic musculoskeletal pain: ultrasound guided pain control. Acta Anaesthesiol Taiwanica. 2014;52(3):114–33. https://doi.org/10.1016/j.aat.2014.08.002. Epub 2014 Oct 7. PMID: 25304316.
8. Anatomy G's. In: Standring S, editor. The anatomical basis of clinical practice. 39th ed. Edinburgh: Elsevier Churchill Livingstone; 2005.
9. Lewis SR, Price A, Walker KJ, McGrattan K, Smith AF. Ultrasound guidance for upper and lower limb blocks. Cochrane Database Syst Rev. 2015;2015(9):CD006459. https://doi.org/10.1002/14651858.CD006459.pub3. PMID: 26361135; PMCID: PMC6465072.
10. Yurgil JL, Hulsopple CD, Leggit JC. Nerve blocks: part II. Lower extremity. Am Fam Physician. 2020;101(11):669–79. PMID: 32463641.
11. Xu J, Zhou R, Su W, Wang S, Xia Y, Papadimos T, Zhao J, Xu X. Ultrasound-guided bilateral pudendal nerve blocks of nulliparous women with epidural labour analgesia in the second stage of labour: a randomised, double-blind, controlled trial. BMJ Open. 2020;10(8):e035887. https://doi.org/10.1136/bmjopen-2019-035887. PMID: 32843515; PMCID: PMC7449485.
12. Gupta G, Radhakrishna M, Tamblyn I, Tran DQ, Besemann M, Thonnagith A, Elgueta MF, Robitaille ME, Finlayson RJ. A randomized comparison between neurostimulation and ultrasound-guided lateral femoral cutaneous nerve block. US Army Med Dep J. 2017;2–17:33–8. PMID: 28853117.
13. Head SJ, Leung RC, Hackman GP, Seib R, Rondi K, Schwarz SK. Ultrasound-guided saphenous nerve block--within versus distal to the adductor canal: a proof-of-principle randomized trial. Can J Anaesth. 2015;62(1):37–44. https://doi.org/10.1007/s12630-014-0255-1. Epub 2014 Oct 22. PMID: 25337966.
14. Kowalska B, Sudoł-Szopińska I. Normal and sonographic anatomy of selected peripheral nerves. Part III: Peripheral nerves of the lower limb. J Ultrason. 2012;12(49):148–63. https://doi.org/10.15557/JoU.2012.0003. Epub 2012 Jun 30. PMID: 26674560; PMCID: PMC4579744.
15. Taha AM. Brief reports: ultrasound-guided obturator nerve block: a proximal interfascial technique. Anesth Analg. 2012;114(1):236–9. https://doi.org/10.1213/ANE.0b013e318237fb40. Epub 2011 Oct 24. PMID: 22025494.
16. Huntoon MA, Huntoon EA, Obray JB, Lamer TJ. Feasibility of ultrasound-guided percutaneous placement of peripheral nerve stimulation electrodes in a cadaver model: part one, lower extremity. Reg Anesth Pain Med. 2008;33(6):551–7. https://doi.org/10.1016/j.rapm.2008.04.007. PMID: 19258970.

17. Yablon CM, Hammer MR, Morag Y, Brandon CJ, Fessell DP, Jacobson JA. US of the peripheral nerves of the lower extremity: a landmark approach. Radiographics. 2016;36(2):464–78. https://doi.org/10.1148/rg.2016150120. Epub 2016 Feb 12. PMID: 26871986.
18. Rha DW, Lee SH, Lee HJ, Choi YJ, Kim HJ, Lee SC. Ultrasound-guided injection of the adductor longus and pectineus in a cadaver model. Pain Physician. 2015;18(6):E1111–7. Erratum in: Pain Physician. 2016 Feb;19(2):101. PMID: 26606024.

Peripheral Nerve Stimulation (PNS) Using Ultrasound: Trunk and Pelvic Regions

Tiago da Silva Freitas

General Instructions to Understand the USG Legends

The general instructions were based on the classification system used by Hannes Gruber, Alexander loizides, and Bernhard Moriggl in their book *Sonographic Peripheral Nerve Topography, A Landmark-based Algorithm* [1].

On the left side on the upper half page, there is the following (standardized) table.

ELM	External landmark(s)
IPOP	Initial positioning of probe
ILM	Internal landmark(s)
POV	Point of optimal visibility
VAR	Relevant variations
AP	Alternative plan (if worth mentioning!)
C	Comments – if helpful/of interest regarding surgical technique
PAT	Pathology
Confirmation of the target	Neurophysiology regarding the peripheral nerve target
Notes	Any additional important information

Following the table we will have the figures with the step-by step technique. We also used exactly the same description in the ultrasound images done by Hans Gruber in the book above cited (made with permission).

T. d. S. Freitas (✉)
Brasilia Pain Institute(INDOR), Neurosurgery Department Hospital de Base de Brasília(HBDF), Functional Neurosurgery Department Hospital Sírio Libanês, Brasília, Distrito Federal, Brazil

T. d. S. Freitas et al. (eds.), *Neuromodulation Techniques for Pain Treatment*, https://doi.org/10.1007/978-3-030-84778-4_14

USG Technique for Peripheral Nerve Stimulation in Trunk/Pelvis

Ilioinguinal and Iliohypogastric Nerves: Figs. 1, 2, 3, 4, 5, 6, and 7

ELM	1. Spina iliaca anterior superior (ASIS) 2. Crista iliaca (iliac crest)
IPOP	About three to four fingerbreadths cranio-posterior to the spina iliaca anterior superior; the probe is coupled almost perpendicularly to the crista iliaca
ILM	1. Crista iliaca (iliac crest) 2. M. obliquus externus abdominis (external oblique muscle) 3. M. obliquus internus abdominis (internal oblique muscle) 4. M. transversus abdominis (transverse abdominal muscle)
POV	Between M. transversus abdominis and M. obliquus internus abdominis
VAR	Common trunk of both nerves
AP	None
C	The shadow of the crista iliaca must be depicted in the ultrasound image; directly next to the crista iliaca is N. ilioinguinalis, and about 1 cm medial to that is N. iliohypogastricus
PAT	Neuropathic pelvic/genital pain
Confirmation of the target	Paresthesia in pelvic/genital distribution (ilioinguinal); L1 dermatome. Paresthesia to iliohypogastric distribution (lower abdominal area); L1 dermatome
Notes	Being one of a group of nerves in the peripheral lumbar plexus, it is important to confirm with the patient that the paresthesia is distributed in the proper area

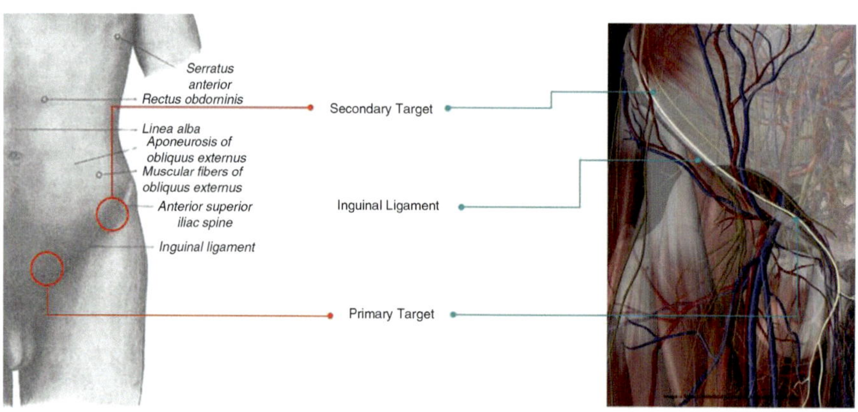

Fig. 1 Anatomical representation of ilioinguinal nerve and the anatomical landmarks: ASIS (anterior superior iliac spine) (bony prominence on the hip) and external obliques – muscle (StimRouter image, printed with permission)

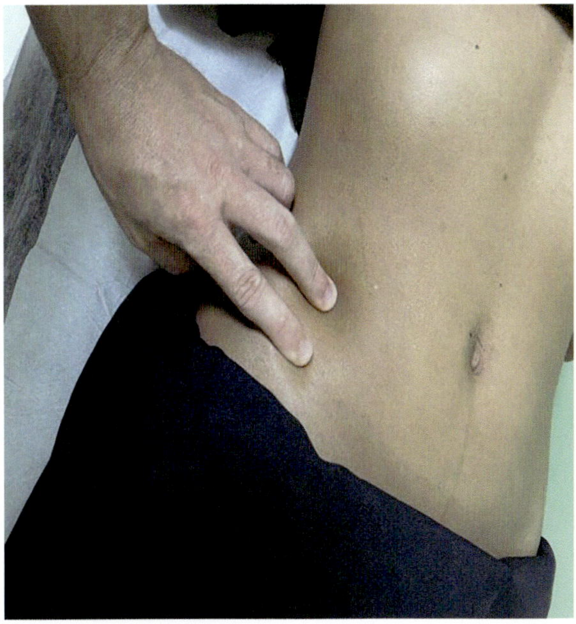

Fig. 2 Simultaneous palpation of the spina iliaca anterior superior and the crista iliaca; the middle finger indicates the optimal IPOP

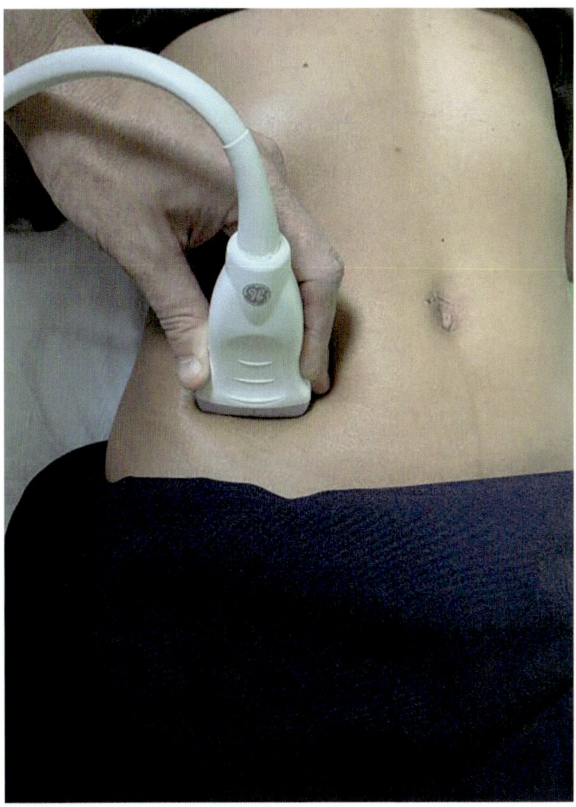

Fig. 3 The lateral end of the probe is directly over the crista iliaca; the medial end is pushed into the abdominal wall

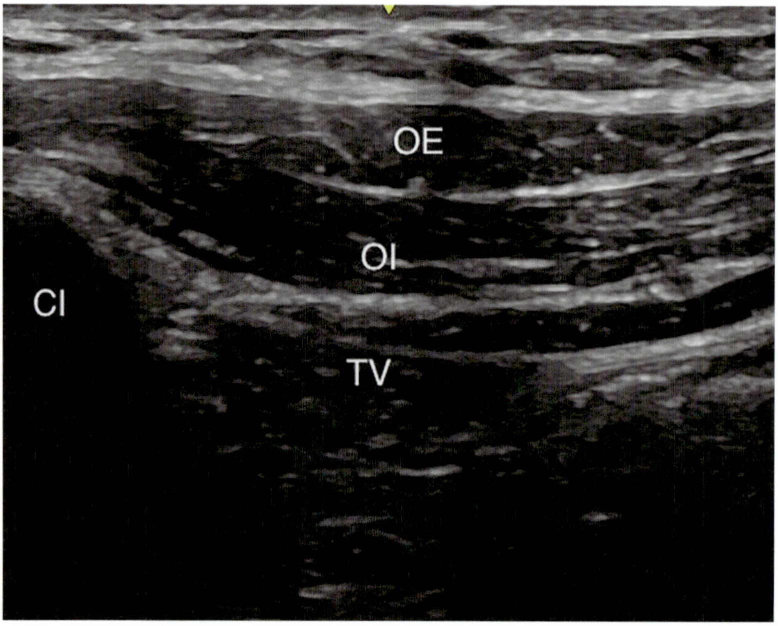

Fig. 4 Ultrasonographic imaging from the anatomical landmarks and the targets: OE external obliques muscle, OI internal obliques muscle, TV transverse abdominal muscle

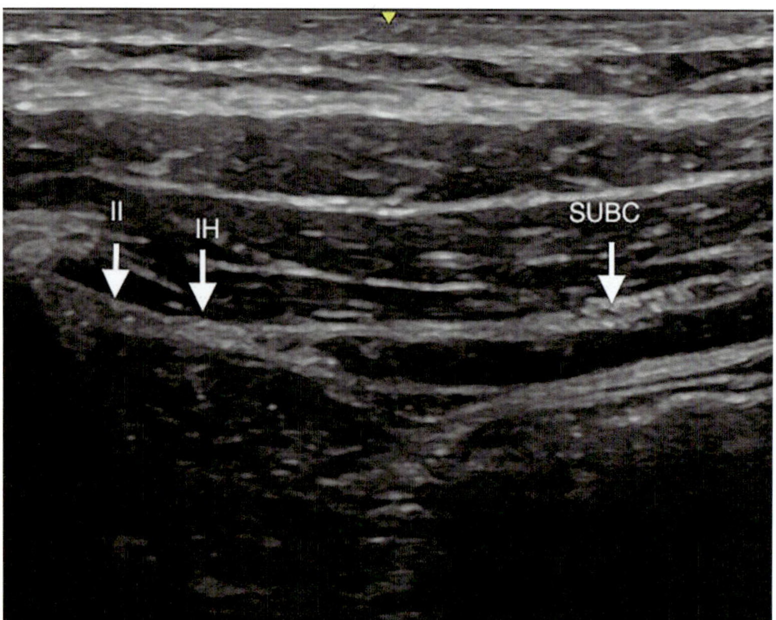

Fig. 5 Ultrasonographic imaging from the anatomical landmarks and the targets: ilioinguinal and iliohypogastric nerves (arrows)

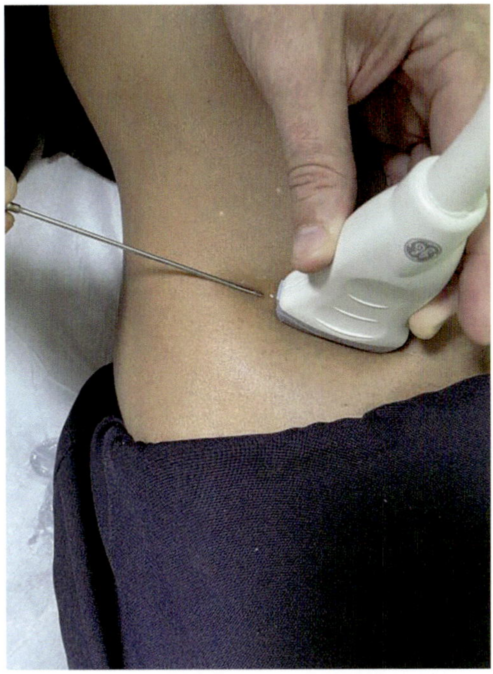

Fig. 6 Schematic figure showing needle entry point inferomedial to ASIS

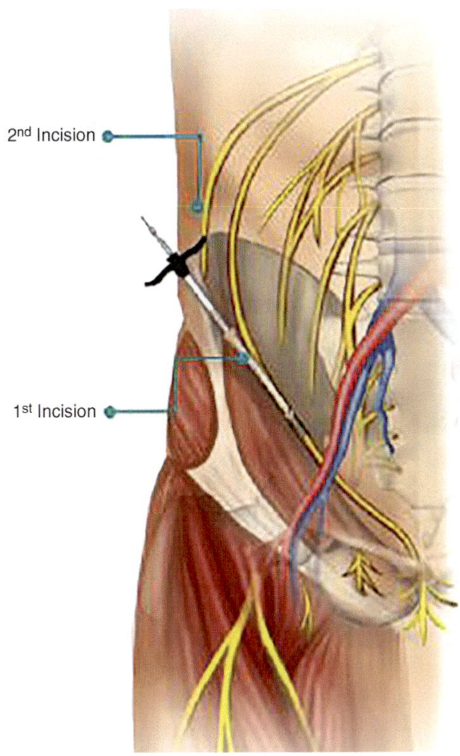

Fig. 7 Needle and electrode inserted inferomedially toward target exiting inguinal canal. (Image printed with permission from StimRouter)

Cluneal Nerve: Figs. 8, 9, 10, 11, and 12

ELM	1. Lateral border of the M. latissimus dorsi 2. Crista iliaca (iliac crest, IC)
IPOP	Medial to the lateral border of the M. latissimus dorsi, about two fingerbreadths cranial to the crista iliaca Superior cluneal nerve at the lumbar vertebrae (L3) level, superomedial to the Ilium. Multifidus, longissimus thoracis, iliocostalis, latissimus dorsi
ILM	1. Fascia thoracolumbalis (superficial lamina) 2. M. iliocostalis lumborum
POV	Within the M. iliocostalis lumborum
VAR	None
AP	None
C	From IPOP move probe repeatedly up and down to find POV
PAT	Neuropathic lower lumbar back pain related to the cluneal nerve
Confirmation of the target	Paresthesia in the cluneal nerve distribution (upper buttocks/hip); L1, L2, and L3 dermatomes
Notes	Lead mapping pre-op is highly recommended in order to arrive at a donning/doffing site that the patient can reach

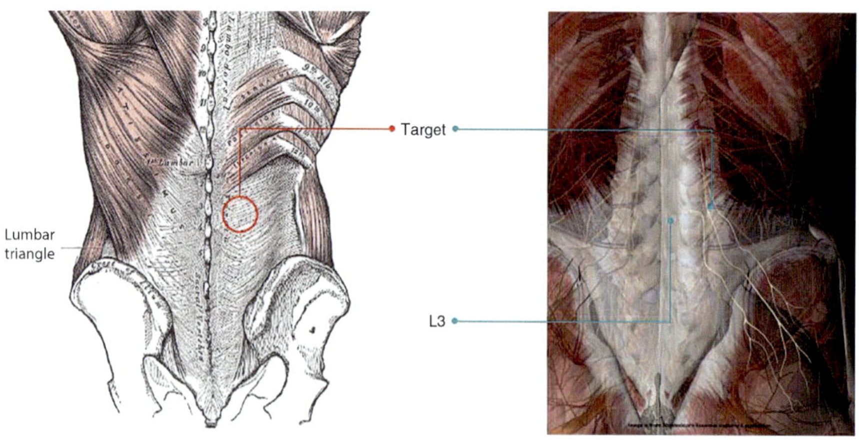

Fig. 8 Anatomical representation of the superior cluneal nerve and the anatomical landmarks: latissimus dorsi overlies the other muscle groups; iliocostalis, longissimus thoracis, and multifidus

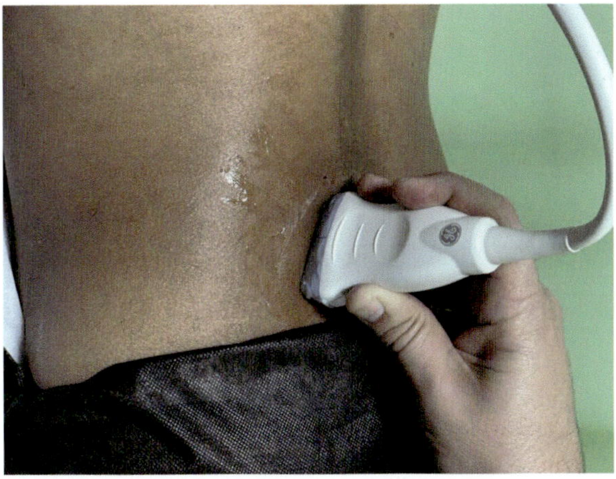

Fig. 9 After palpation of the trigonum lumbale (middle finger of the left hand) for definition of the lateral border of the musculus latissimus dorsi and simultaneous indication of the crista iliaca (thumb of the right hand). The probe is placed slightly oblique (perpendicular to the assumed course of the nerves!) about two fingerbreadths cranial to the crista iliaca and centered on the musculus iliocostalis lumborum. Index finger at the crista iliaca

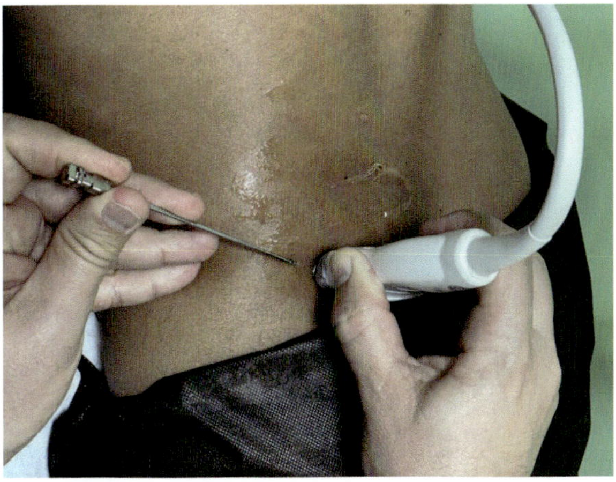

Fig. 10 Schematic figure showing patient in a prone position. Needle entry point is made superior to target at L3. Electrode inserted inferiorly toward the target

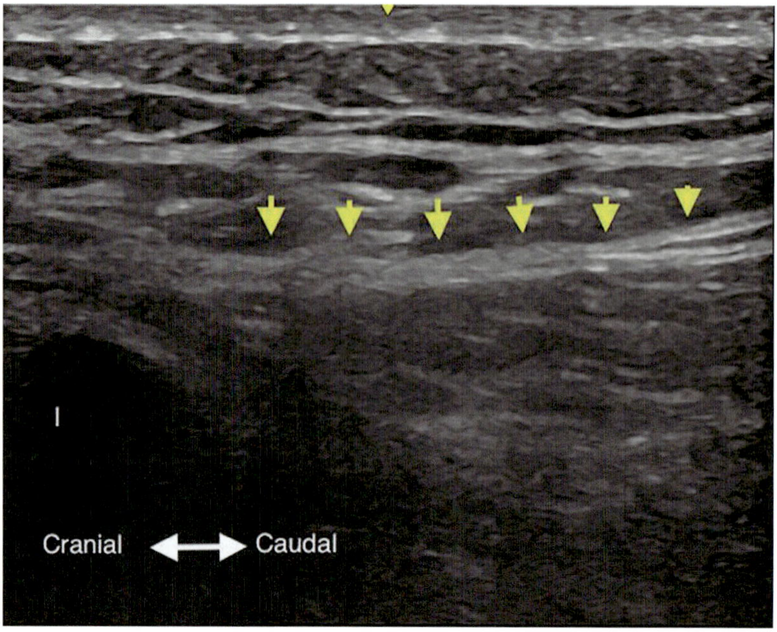

Fig. 11 The long axis view of the superior cluneal nerve
Yellow arrows indicate superior cluneal nerve

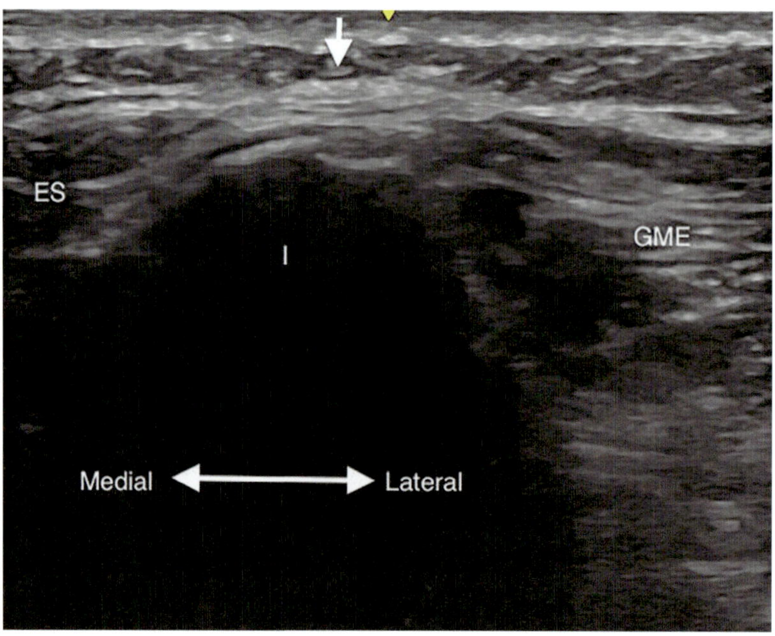

Fig. 12 The short-axis view of the superior cluneal nerve
GME gluteus medius; ES erector spinae

Genitofemoral Nerve: Genital Rami (Figs. 13, 14, and 15)

ELM	1. Palpation of the A. femoralis (femoral artery) 2. Ligamentum inguinale (inguinal ligament) or baseline between spina iliaca anterior and tuberculum pubicum
IPOP	Directly cranial and parallel to the ligamentum inguinale
ILM	1. A. iliaca externa (external iliac artery) 2. A. circumflexa ilium profunda (deep circumflex iliac artery)
POV	Ventral do the A. circumflexa ilium profunda
VAR	Course dorsal to the A. circumflexa ilium profunda
AP	None
C	The artery must be depicted longitudinally R. femoralis (femoral rami) already divided into at least two branches in most cases
PAT	Neuropathic lower inguinal/abdominal pain
Confirmation of the target	Paresthesia to genital distribution; L1 dermatome
Notes	Pre-op patch placement will be necessary to ensure comfort and to address any pubic hair, garment issues, or extra adipose tissue or hernias in area. Pre-op stimulation to determine tolerance is recommended in this sensitive region

itals.

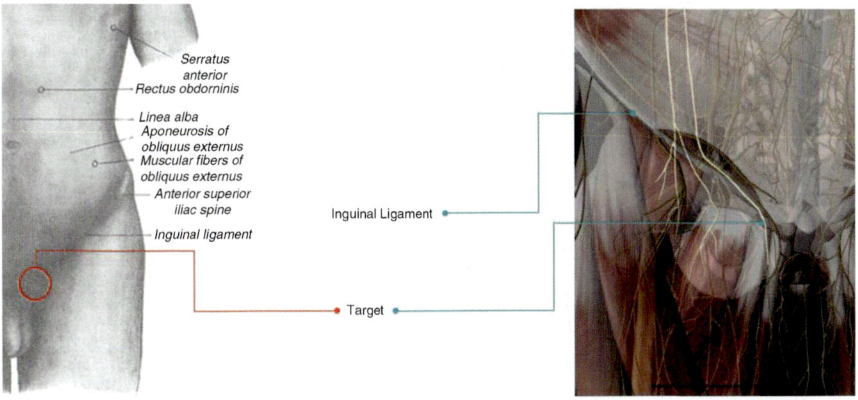

Fig. 13 Anatomical representation of the genital rami and important anatomic structures: genitofemoral nerve as it exits the inguinal canal. ASIS, pubic bone, inguinal ligament, external obliques muscle, transverse abdominal muscle. (Figure printed with permission from StimRouter)

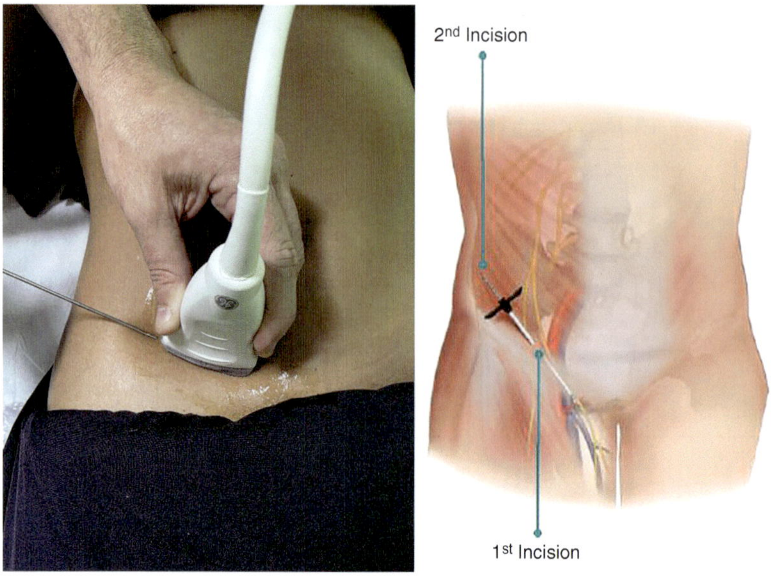

Fig. 14 Schematic figure showing genitofemoral approach: patient supine. Entry point inferomedial to ASIS. Needle inserted inferomedially toward the target/genitals. Before starting do palpation of the arteria femoralis (rough orientation to find the internal landmarks arteria iliaca externa and arteria circumflexa ilium profunda more easily) and positioning of the probe cranial to the ligamentum inguinale (or the abovementioned baseline) for assessing the internal landmarks

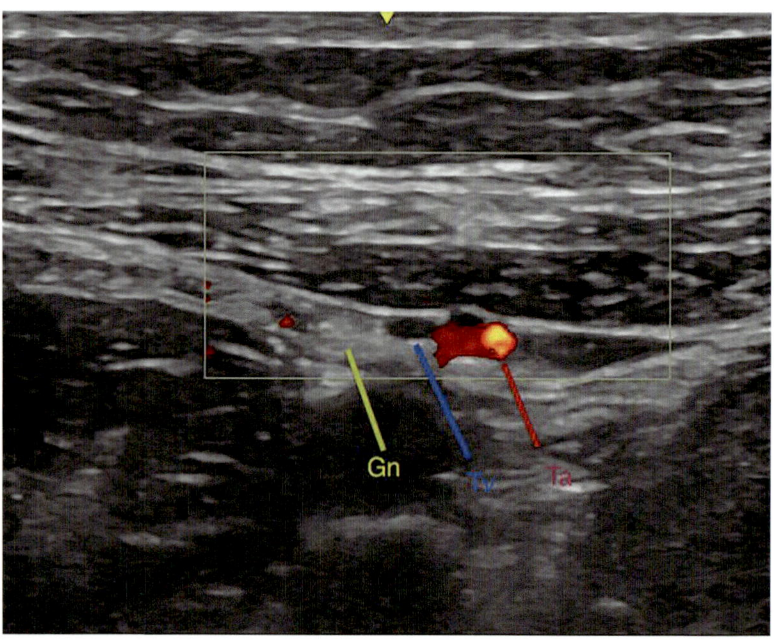

Fig. 15 Localizing the (right [R]) genital branch of the genitofemoral nerve. Gn: genital nerve; Ta, testicular artery; Tv, testicular vein; Dd, vas deferens duct; Sp, symphysis pubis; red circle, spermatic cord (external spermatic fascia)

Pudendal Nerve (Nervus Pudendus): Figs. 16, 17, 18, 19, and 20

ELM	1. Palpable tuber ischiadicum (ischial tuberosity)
IPOP	Transverse, about one fingerbreadth cranial to the upper border to the tuber ischiadicum Pudendal nerve at junction of sacrospinous and sacrotuberous ligaments. Sciatic nerve, sacrum, piriformis muscle, gluteus maximus muscle
ILM	1. M. obturatorius internus (internal obturator muscle) 2. OS ischii (bone ischium) 3. A. pudenda interna (internal pudendal artery)
POV	Next and medial to the M. obturatorius internus
VAR	Branching proximal to the Alcock channel> > two nerve cross sections Lacking of the A. pudenda interna (at IPOP) Nerve is perforated by the A. pudenda interna (or a branch)
AP	None
C	Use a curved array probe "Waterfall sign" Cave: do not mix up with the resembling but more laterally found ligamentum sacrotuberale
PAT	Neuropathic pelvic/genital pan
Confirmation of the target	Paresthesia in the buttocks, external genitals, perineum and/or anus; S2, S3, and S4 dermatomes
Notes	Difficult procedure but successful in the past when done with proper planning. Consider patch placement outside of the beltline when mapping lead pathway PTNS and tibial implants in the upper leg have been successfully used to resolve pudendal and chronic pelvic pain. Approaches to the tibial nerve in the upper and lower leg eliminate many of the difficulties arising from directly targeting the pudendal nerve

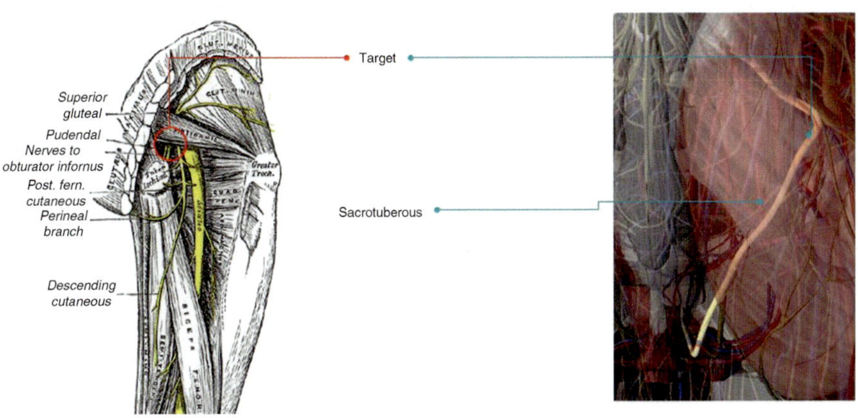

Fig. 16 Anatomical representation of the genital rami and important anatomic structures: pudendal nerve at junction of sacrospinous and sacrotuberous ligaments. Sciatic nerve, sacrum, piriformis muscle, gluteus maximus muscle

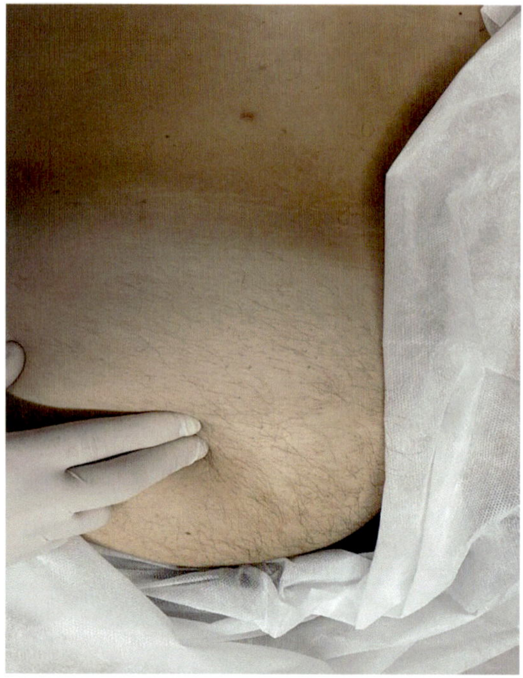

Fig. 17 Palpation of the whole tuber ischiadicum (use two fingers!)

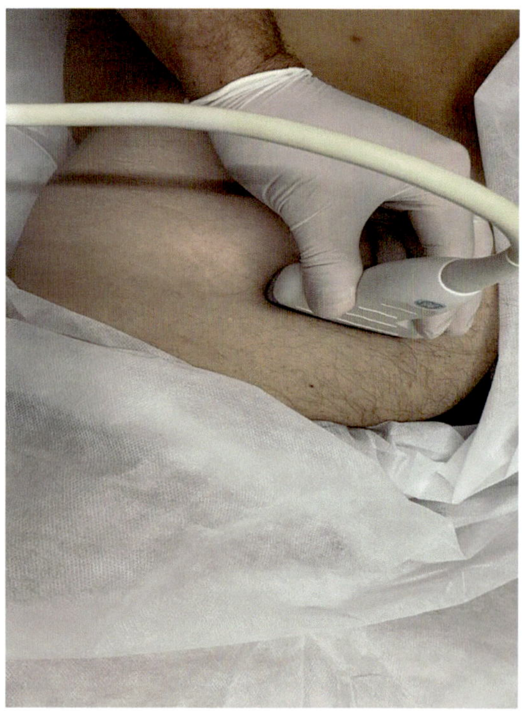

Fig. 18 Palpation of the whole tuber ischiadicum (use two fingers!)
Strict transverse probe position, center of the probe a little medial to aforementioned lan**dmark**

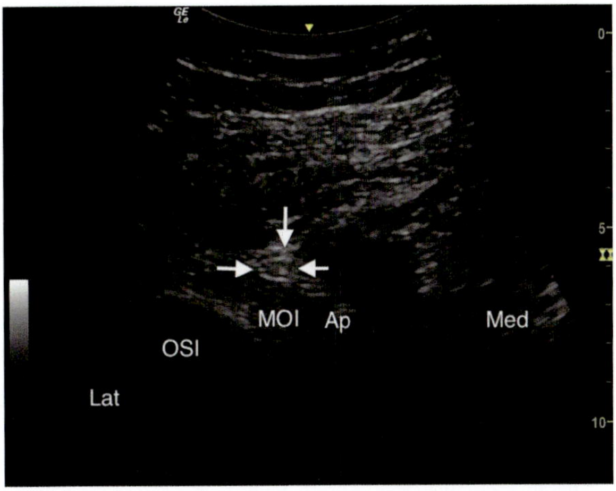

Fig. 19 The internal landmarks are the arched course of the musculus obturatorius (MOI, "waterfall sign") around the OS ischii (OSI, incisura ischiadica minor). Neighboring arteria pudenda interna (AP), lateral (LAT), and medial (MED) Optimal delineated nerve (arrows) as its entry into the "Alcock channel" (next and medial to the musculus obturatorius internus)

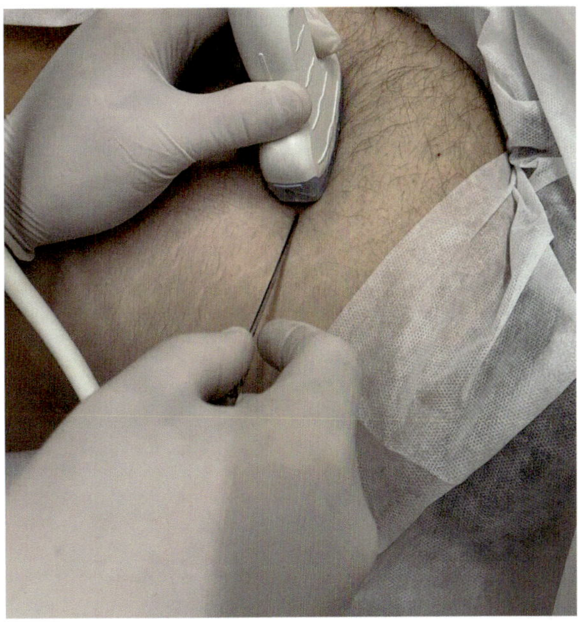

Fig. 20 Schematic figure showing pudendal approach

References

1. A. Loizides et al. Sonographic peripheral nerve topography. A Landmark-based Algorithm. Springer International Publishing; 2019.
2. Narouze S.N. et al. Atlas of ultrasound guided procedures in interventional pain Management. Springer International Publishing; 2011.
3. Waldman SD. Waldman's comprehensive atlas of diagnostic ultrasound of painful conditions. Philadelphia: Wolters Kluwer; 2016.
4. Dettori N, Choudur H, Chhabra A. Ultrasound-guided treatment of peripheral nerve pathology. Semin Musculoskelet Radiol. 2018;22(3):364–74. https://doi.org/10.1055/s-0038-1641571. Epub 2018 May 23. PMID: 29791964.
5. Kaye AD, Motejunas MW, Bonneval LA, Ehrhardt KP, Latimer DR, Trescot A, Wilson KE, Ibrahim IN, Cornett EM, Urman RD, Candido KD. Ultrasound practice for chronic pain procedures: a comprehensive review. Best Pract Res Clin Anaesthesiol. 2019;33(4):465–86. https://doi.org/10.1016/j.bpa.2019.07.001. Epub 2019 Jul 18. PMID: 31791564.
6. Narouze SN. Ultrasound-guided interventional procedures in pain management: evidence-based medicine. Reg Anesth Pain Med. 2010;35(2 Suppl):S55–8. https://doi.org/10.1097/AAP.0b013e3181d24658. PMID: 20216026.
7. Chiou HJ, Chou YH, Wang HK, Lai YC. Chronic musculoskeletal pain: ultrasound guided pain control. Acta Anaesthesiol Taiwanica. 2014;52(3):114–33. https://doi.org/10.1016/j.aat.2014.08.002. Epub 2014 Oct 7. PMID: 25304316.
8. Anatomy G's. In: Standring S, editor. The anatomical basis of clinical practice. 39th ed. Edinburgh: Elsevier Churchill Livingstone; 2005.
9. Herring AA, Stone MB, Nagdev AD. Ultrasound-guided abdominal wall nerve blocks in the ED. Am J Emerg Med. 2012;30(5):759–64. https://doi.org/10.1016/j.ajem.2011.03.008. Epub 2011 May 12. PMID: 21570238.
10. Daniels SP, Xu HS, Hanna A, Greenberg JA, Lee KS. Ultrasound-guided microwave ablation in the treatment of inguinal neuralgia. Skelet Radiol. 2021;50(3):475–83. https://doi.org/10.1007/s00256-020-03618-2. Epub 2020 Sep 30. PMID: 33000286.
11. Shian B, Larson ST. Abdominal Wall pain: clinical evaluation, differential diagnosis, and treatment. Am Fam Physician. 2018;98(7):429–36. PMID: 30252418.
12. Droghetti A, Fusco P, Marini M, Harizai F, Scimia P. Ultrasound-guided serratus anterior plane block and parasternal block in cooperative sedation for S-ICD implantation. Pacing Clin Electrophysiol. 2019;42(7):1076–8. https://doi.org/10.1111/pace.13727. Epub 2019 Jun 4. PMID: 31116436.
13. Chin KJ, Versyck B, Pawa A. Ultrasound-guided fascial plane blocks of the chest wall: a state-of-the-art review. Anaesthesia. 2021;76(Suppl 1):110–26. https://doi.org/10.1111/anae.15276. PMID: 33426660.
14. Hebbard P, Fujiwara Y, Shibata Y, Royse C. Ultrasound-guided transversus abdominis plane (TAP) block. Anaesth Intensive Care. 2007;35(4):616–7. PMID: 18020088.
15. Daniels SP, Xu HS, Hanna A, Greenberg JA, Lee KS. Ultrasound-guided microwave ablation in the treatment of inguinal neuralgia. Skelet Radiol. 2021;50(3):475–83. https://doi.org/10.1007/s00256-020-03618-2. Epub 2020 Sep 30. PMID: 33000286.

Abdominal and Pancreatic Pain: Sites and Techniques in Neuromodulation

Leonardo Kapural, Simran Dua, and Priodarshi Roychoudhury

Introduction

Abdominal pain is a common symptom reported in up to 25% of the adult population at any one time [1, 2]. Abdominal pain lasting 3 months or longer is defined as chronic abdominal pain (CAP) [3]. CAP affects about 1–2% of the adult population, with women being affected more frequently [3, 4]. CAP can originate from either the abdominal wall or the viscera. In about 35% to 51% of patients, the cause for abdominal pain remains a mystery [5, 6]. Chronic pancreatitis (CP) has an annual incidence of 5 to 8 and prevalence of 42 to 73 cases per 100,000 adults in the United States [7, 8]. Abdominal pain is reported in more than 80% of CP patients [9].

The pain is classically reported as a dull epigastric pain radiating to the back which worsens after meals; the pattern, character, and severity of pain can vary [10]. This does not always correlate with the extent of pathological changes of CP [9, 11–13].

Etiology

CAP can be associated with inflammatory disorders like chronic pancreatitis and inflammatory bowel disease or functional disorders like functional abdominal pain syndrome, functional dyspepsia, gastroparesis, and irritable bowel syndrome [14]. Surgical procedures like herniorrhaphy, adhesiolysis, cholecystectomy, and

L. Kapural (✉) · S. Dua
Chronic Pain Research Institute, Winston-Salem, NC, USA

P. Roychoudhury
Department of Anesthesia and Pain, Toronto General Hospital, University of Toronto, Toronto, ON, Canada

T. d. S. Freitas et al. (eds.), *Neuromodulation Techniques for Pain Treatment*,
https://doi.org/10.1007/978-3-030-84778-4_15

open contaminated procedures (postsurgical adhesions) are strongly associated with CAP. Abdominal pain is reported in up to 48% of chronic postsurgical pain cases [14]. Apart from visceral pain and abdominal wall pain, central pain generated in the spinal cord and/or brain might lead to CAP. Chronic abdominal wall pain (CAWP) is defined as pain of more than 1 month of focal tenderness (less than 2.5 cm in diameter). Approximately 10–30% CAP patients may have CAWP. The most common cause of abdominal wall pain is entrapment of the branches of the cutaneous abdominal nerves due to surgery or anatomical variations.

Pathophysiology

CAP occurs due to derangement of adaptive and protective functions performed by normal physical, emotional, and perceptual integration. Maladaptive neuroplastic changes and peripheral and central sensitization may result in hyperalgesia and allodynia. Nociceptive pain occurs due to localized inflammation in abdominal chronic pain syndromes, where the degree of inflammation correlates with the severity of the pain [15]. However, certain CAP syndromes occur without any gross tissue injury or structural disease. Gastrointestinal inflammation leads to acute and chronic pain in inflammatory bowel disease, celiac disease, and acute infectious gastroenteritis, leading to increased expression of transient receptor potential vanilloid type-1 (TRPV-1). Visceral hypersensitivity via central and peripheral mechanisms and lack of structural changes is a characteristic of dysmotility disorders like irritable bowel syndrome (IBS; 14).

Pathophysiology of Pain in Chronic Pancreatitis (CP)

Inflammatory molecules released from damaged cells following pancreatic inflammation activate mast cells and platelets, leading to nociceptive pain signal transmission to the pain centers of the brain via dorsal root ganglia and dorsal horn of the spinal cord. Ductal obstruction with stones or stricture leads to ductal hypertension and inflammation causing continuous pain. Though many patients with continuous pain are seen to have inflammatory head mass, pseudocyst, or pancreatic cancer, many develop continuous neuropathic pain without any structural complications or evidence of inflammation. Pancreatic nociceptive afferent injury often leads to neuronal hyperresponsiveness due to peripheral and central sensitization, which can result in a continuous pain in the absence of a nociceptive input. CP patients with chronic pain have evidence of histological changes in the pancreas including increase in the density and volume of the intrapancreatic nerves and alterations in cerebral cortical thickness, suggesting that pancreatic and central neural changes occur over a long period of time [16]. Central sensitization is associated with poor outcomes with invasive endoscopic and surgical treatment [17].

Clinical Features

Clinical presentation varies with etiology. Patients with CP often complain of boring, deep, sharp, and penetrating epigastric pain, radiating to the back, increasing after fatty food ingestion, and often associated with nausea and vomiting. Steatorrhea may occur in advanced cases when pancreatic lipase secretion is reduced. Other signs and symptoms include diabetes mellitus, jaundice, abdominal distension, dyspnea, pleural effusion, ascites, significant weight loss, and abdominal mass.

Inspection of the abdomen might give a hint regarding the chronic pain source. For example, surgical scars with allodynia or hyperalgesia raise suspicion of nerve damage or neuroma. CAWP can be diagnosed with careful physical examination, revealing a well-localized point tenderness with palpation contrary to visceral pain, which is quite diffused.

Clinical presentation varies with etiology. Patients with CP often complain of boring, deep, sharp and penetrating epigastric pain, radiating to the back, increasing after fatty food ingestion, and often associated with nausea and vomiting. Steatorrhea may occur in advanced cases when pancreatic lipase secretion is reduced. Other signs and symptoms include diabetes mellitus, jaundice, abdominal distension, dyspnea, pleural effusion, ascites, significant weight loss, or an abdominal mass.

Inspection of the abdomen might give a hint regarding the chronic pain source. For example, surgical scars with allodynia or hyperalgesia raise suspicion of nerve damage or neuroma. CAWP can be diagnosed with careful physical examination, revealing a well-localized point tenderness with palpation contrary to visceral pain, which is diffused in nature.

Diagnosis

Carnett's test is a useful physical examination to diagnose abdominal wall pain. In supine position, knees and hips are flexed to decrease abdominal wall tension, and the patient is asked to lift the head and shoulders off the bed to tighten his/her abdominal muscles. Carnett's test is deemed positive with increased pain on palpation as the patient contracts the abdominal muscles. Positive response to trigger point injections or nerve blocks might also confirm the diagnosis. Patients with visceral disease involving the peritoneum may lead to a false-positive Carnett's test [6].

Psychometric tests such as depression inventories are useful tools in addition to history and physical examinations to establish an appropriate diagnosis.

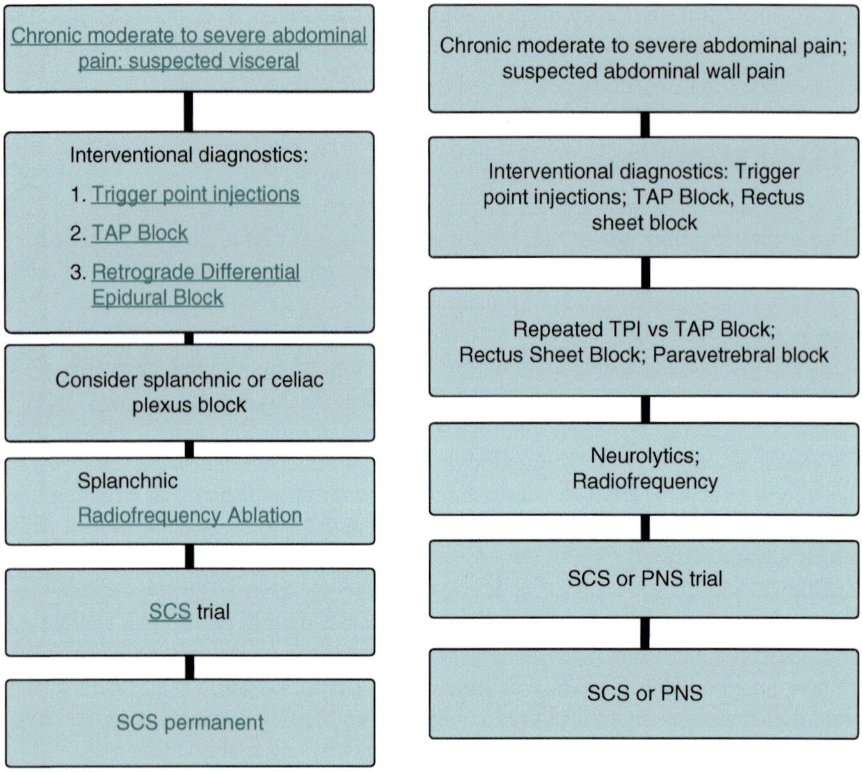

Fig. 1 Proposed pain management algorithms for an interventional diagnostics and therapy of predominantly visceral and predominantly abdominal wall pain. Please note that such step-by-step approaches were not validated in prospective studies and are mostly based on a smaller and few larger case series [40–45]

Nerve blocks may be of diagnostic or therapeutic value for abdominal pain. Sympathetic nerve blocks target the splanchnic nerves, celiac plexus, or superior hypogastric nerve plexus and help in diagnosing visceral pain. Somatic nerve blocks include intercostal nerve blocks, transversus abdominis plane (TAP) blocks, rectus abdominis sheath blocks, and ilioinguinal, iliohypogastric, and genitofemoral blocks (6; Fig. 1).

Differential retrograde epidural block (DREB) may help to differentiate between visceral and non-visceral pain. The diagnostic value of DREB relies on the sensitivity of various nerve fibers to local anesthetics. Sympathetic fibers and visceral afferents have a higher C to Aδ fiber ratio (10:1) and are more sensitive to local anesthetic blockade compared to somatic nociceptive fibers. DREB involves epidural catheter placement under fluoroscopy with injection of saline twice (placebo), followed by incremental doses of a local anesthetic with frequent neurological examinations. However, DREB cannot determine the contribution from the vagal nerves, and the sensitivity and specificity of DREB are low [6].

TAP block is both diagnostic and therapeutic for somatic pain. Ultrasound guidance for TAP block allows deposition of local anesthetics in between the internal oblique and transversus abdominis muscles around the anterior branches of the thoracolumbar ventral rami providing analgesia to the entire anterolateral abdominal wall between the costal margin and the inguinal ligament. Although the value of TAP block in determining abdominal wall pain is still debatable, the block as a single injection or continuous infusion through a catheter can be used to treat various abdominal wall pain syndromes (6; Fig. 1).

Treatment

Pharmacotherapy with H2 antagonists, proton pump inhibitors, gabapentinoids, and tricyclic antidepressants is usually the first line of management. Nerve blocks with local anesthetics with or without corticosteroids, chemical neurolysis, and surgeries are other treatment options for CAP unoptimized with pharmacotherapy and lifestyle modifications. Opioids present a potential threat of producing tolerance, addiction, and reduction of gastrointestinal motility and exacerbating symptoms of CAP. Cognitive behavioral therapy and mindfulness have been effective in patients as coping strategies.

Interventions aim at inhibiting/modulating pain transmission. Classically the greater and lesser splanchnic nerves and celiac plexus were targeted for visceral pain control. The philosophy of these blocks is to target the sympathetic innervation of the abdominal organs consisting of pre-ganglionic fibers of T5 to T12. Together with communicating rami, these fibers course in the direction of the sympathetic chain and then make synaptic contacts with post-ganglionic neurons at the celiac, aortorenal, and superior mesenteric ganglion. The splanchnic nerves are located in a relatively narrow space between the vertebra and pleura (Fig. 2a) and hence can be targeted more accurately and subjected to neurolysis and radiofrequency ablation (RFA) unlike the celiac plexus widely spread around the abdominal aorta which can only be subjected to only neurolysis. Celiac plexus blocks are classically performed ta rough a transaortic, retrocrural, or transdiscal approach without any established advantage of one over another. While celiac plexus block involves percutaneous placement of the needle through the paraspinal area of the L1 vertebral body, splanchnic plexus blocks are performed bilaterally at T11 to deliver local anesthetic to the paravertebral compartment medial to the pleural cavity, targeting the greater and lesser splanchnic nerves (posterior third of T11 vertebral body; Fig. 2b).

A. Anatomy-based schematics of the RF needle approach to splanchnic nerve block and denervation. While such denervation is most frequently conducted by placing an active tip of RF needle between posterior and middle third of T11 vertebral body width (shown as No1), at T12 level (not shown) active tip usually is placed between middle and anterior third.

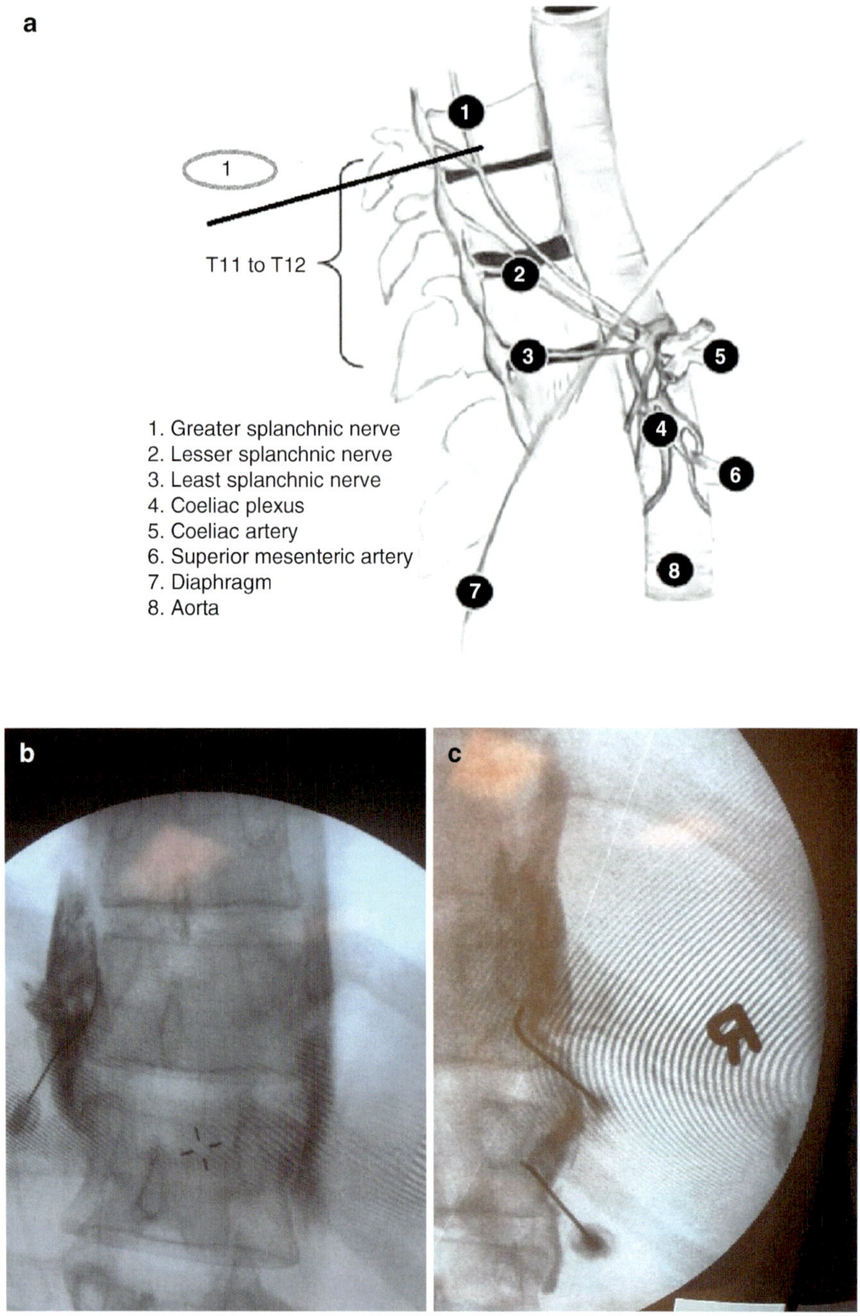

Fig. 2 (**a**) Anatomical basis for neural denervation. (**b**) Bilateral splanchnic block at T11 level. (**c**). Right-sided radiofrequency ablation of splanchnic nerves

B. For splanchnic block needle is positioned under 60 degree caudal angle to the vaste of T11 vertebral body. It is advanced to posterior to middle third of the vertebral body line. Contrast was delivered and then 15–20 cc of 0.375% bupivacaine.
C. During radiofrequency ablation, a sensory stimulation is used during RF needle advancement in order to achieve concordant abdominal pain. Frequently, RF needle is advanced to the line of posterior third/middle third width of vertebral body while another needle to middle/anterior third vertebral body line. After the contrast confirmed no vascular spread, RF ablation is conducted at 80 degrees.

RFA (Fig. 2c) is associated with longer-lasting pain relief. However, recurrence does occur following the nerve regeneration requiring a repeat procedure. These interventions are not devoid of complications. Pneumothorax, post-interventional neuritis, hypotension, or diarrhea may occur.

Role of Neuromodulation in Visceral Pain

The role of neuromodulation and electrical stimulation of the dorsal horn is established in various chronic pain syndromes [18], including radicular low back pain, post-laminectomy syndrome [19], complex regional pain syndrome [20–22], and peripheral vascular disease [23, 24]. Spinal cord stimulation (SCS) acts by delivery of low current from an implantable generator to epidural leads, creating a small electrical field into and around the spinal cord at that level. A number of hypotheses have been proposed to explain the mechanism of pain relief with SCS [18, 25]. Supraspinal activation might account for the analgesic effects [26]. SCS is also hypothesized to act by modulation of afferent signals in the dorsal horn by "closing the spinal gate" by activation of large myelinated fibers which in turn inhibit the small nociceptive fibers [27] or by the inhibitory neuromodulator release like GABA [28, 29]. SCS also has the potential to block nerve conduction by antidromic activation [30, 31].

Neurosurgical data [32–37] suggests that lesioning of the postsynaptic dorsal column pathway via midline myelotomy inhibits the generation and maintenance of chronic visceral pain by removing the ascending limb acting as the facilitatory pain loop. SCS may or may not affect/interrupt this ascending pathway. SCS also acts by downregulation of intersegmental or supraspinal sympathetic outflow [29, 38, 39].

Clinical Evidence of SCS in CAP

Evidence from our two larger published case series and national survey reported efficacy of conventional SCS (Fig. 3) for CAP due to chronic pancreatitis and other causes of chronic abdominal pain with an average pain decrease from VAS pain

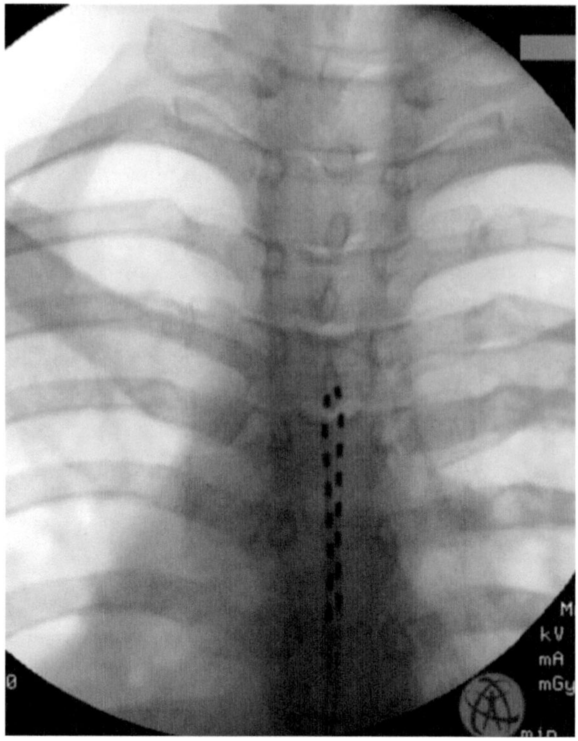

Fig. 3 Placement of two eight-contact leads into the posterior epidural space using conventional SCS. Leads were typically placed up to T4 level, and most frequently utilized contacts were around T4 and T5 levels. Paresthesia mapping is required within concordant abdominal area of patient's pain

score of about 8 to about 4 cm [40–42]. We also surveyed 76 case reports of conventional SCS used to treat CAP with varied etiologies which found significant improvement in pain scores in patients following a permanent implant [40]. Survey included a large group of patients who received SCS for the pain from chronic pancreatitis and detailed technical aspects of conventional SCS. Epidural leads in the majority of the patients were placed with tips of eight contact leads at T4, 5, or 6 and midline [40].

The first larger case series with long-term follow-up (1 year) for SCS to treat pain from chronic pancreatitis included 30 consecutive patients who received up to 14 days of SCS trial. Monitored were pain scores, functional capacity change via Pain Disability Index (PDI), and change in patients' opioid usage. Leads were mainly positioned to the top of T5 and T6, and 80% [25] of the patients reported at least 50% of pain relief (pre-trial VAS 8 ± 1.6 to 3.67 ± 2 cm ($p < 0.001$). Last follow-up reported was 1 year and pain scores were maintained at VAS 4.0 ± 2.1 ($p < 0.001$). Opioid usage decreased by two thirds from about 150 mg MSO4 equivalents to about 50 with most of the patients moving from severe functional disability measured by PDI to mild to moderate disability [41].

Other case reports and smaller case series supported above described pain outcomes of the patients with chronic pancreatitis [44–46].

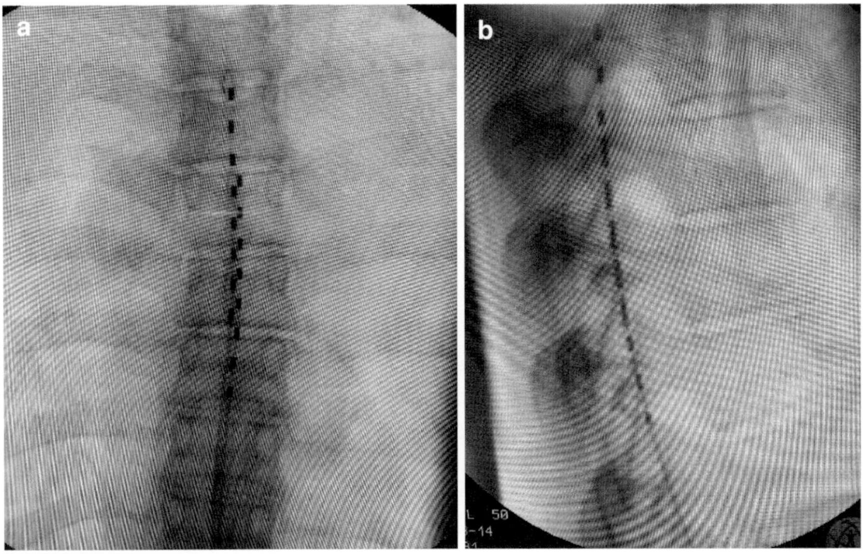

Fig. 4 (**a** and **b**). Lead location for 10 kHz SCS for chronic abdominal pain. Typically, entry point to the epidural space is T9-T10 ligamentum flavum, and leads are uniformly advanced to T4 and T5 levels. Similar approach has been used when novel DTM (TM) SCS is trialed for the same indication. A. Anterior-posterior fluoroscopic view of thoracic spine after the placement of two eight-contact leads. Notice that the tip of one lead is positioned at the top of T4 vertebral body while the other at the top of T5 midline. (**b**). Lateral fluoroscopic view of the same two leads confirming lead placement in the posterior thoracic epidural space

High-frequency SCS therapy (Fig. 4) delivers electrical stimulation at 10 kHz, and lower amplitude (1–5 mA) than conventional SCS is able to reduce pain without any significant paresthesia [47, 48]. 10 kHz SCS was recently approved by the Food and Drug Administration (FDA) following a study reporting equivalent safety and superior relief in back and leg pain compared to conventional SCS [45] with sustained efficacy over 2 years [49]. High-frequency SCS does not require paresthesia mapping during lead implantation which reduces patient discomfort. It has been hypothesized from preclinical studies that afferent pain signal reduction occurs due to inhibition of superficial dorsal horn circuits. Activation of inhibitory interneurons when using a low-intensity 10 kHz SCS might be one of the additional reasons for better outcomes [50]. We recently published a prospective, single-arm study using 10 kHz SCS in 24 patients with CAP of varying etiologies. Epidural leads implanted from the vertebral levels T4 through T8 showed favorable response with high-frequency SCS therapy. 95.8% of the patients had a successful spinal cord stimulator trial and proceeded to a permanent implant. Following 12 months of treatment with 10 kHz SCS, 78.3% of subjects were responders (with pain relief of 50%) and 63.6% were remitters (with sustained <3.0 visual analog scale scores). 10 kHz SCS also greatly improved the quality of life of patients with CAP. Most patients also experienced concurrent reduction or resolution of nausea and vomiting [51].

Complications from SCS placement for chronic abdominal pain and chronic pancreatitis are rare and no different from complications seen with SCS placement for other indications. These include post-dural puncture headache, direct spinal cord or nerve injury, epidural hematoma, epidural abscess, meningitis, epidural fibrosis, lead migration or fracture, IPG failure, IPG seroma, and other infections of SCS implanted hardware [52].

Conclusion

CAP is a complex clinical problem requiring a thorough understanding of the physical and psychosocial features associated with it. Based on preliminary evidence, neuromodulation has proved to be effective for visceral hyperalgesia and chronic abdominal pain, including neuropathic abdominal wall pain and entrapment syndromes [40–46, 51]. Considering widespread availability of new spinal cord stimulation therapeutic options with an established safety profile, along with the poor long-term outcomes using opioids, SCS should be implemented for treatment of chronic abdominal pain. While there is a decent preliminary evidence of the effectivity of SCS for refractory chronic visceral and neuropathic abdominal wall pain, knowledge which waveform/devices would provide the best outcome need to be explored further with well-designed clinical trials.

References

1. Almario CV, Ballal ML, Chey WD, et al. Burden of gastrointestinal symptoms in the United States: results of a nationally representative survey of over 71,000 Americans. Am J Gastroenterol. 2018;113:1701–10.
2. Sandler RS, Stewart WF, Liberman JN, et al. Abdominal pain, bloating, and diarrhea in the United States: prevalence and impact. Dig Dis Sci. 2000;45:1166–71.
3. Greenberger N. Chronic abdominal pain and recurrent abdominal pain. Merck manual: professional version. Kenilworth: Merck & Co., Inc; 2018.
4. Hardt J, Jacobsen C, Goldberg J, et al. Prevalence of chronic pain in a representative sample in the United States. Pain Med. 2008;9:803–12.
5. Klinkman MS. Episodes of care for abdominal pain in a primary care practice. Arch Fam Med. 1996;5:279–85.
6. Veizi IE, Hajek S. Establishing diagnosis of chronic abdominal pain: pain Medicine view. In: Kapural L, editor. Chronic abdominal pain: an evidence-based, comprehensive guide to clinical management. New York: Springer; 2015. p. 33–45.
7. Yadav D, Timmons L, Benson JT, Dierkhising RA, Chari ST. Incidence, prevalence, and survival of chronic pancreatitis: a population-based study. Am J Gastroenterol. 2011;106(12):2192–9. https://doi.org/10.1038/ajg.2011.328.
8. Machicado JD, Dudekula A, Tang G, et al. Period prevalence of chronic pancreatitis diagnosis from 2001-2013 in the commercially insured population of the United States. Pancreatology. 2019;19(6):813–8. https://doi.org/10.1016/j.pan.2019.07.003.

9. Yadav D, Muddana V, O'Connell M. Hospitalizations for chronic pancreatitis in Allegheny County, Pennsylvania. USA Pancreatol. 2011;11(6):546–52. https://doi.org/10.1159/000331498.
10. Wilcox CM, Yadav D, Ye T, et al. Chronic pancreatitis pain pattern and severity are independent of abdominal imaging findings. Clin Gastroenterol Hepatol. 2015;13(3):552–60. https://doi.org/10.1016/j.cgh.2014.10.015.
11. Ammann RW, Muellhaupt B. The natural history of pain in alcoholic chronic pancreatitis. Gastroenterology. 1999;116(5):1132–40. https://doi.org/10.1016/S0016-5085(99)70016-8.
12. Frøkjær JB, Olesen SS, Drewes AM. Fibrosis, atrophy, and ductal pathology in chronic pancreatitis are associated with pancreatic function but independent of symptoms. Pancreas. 2013;42(7):1182–7. https://doi.org/10.1097/MPA.0b013e31829628f4.
13. Bornman PC, Marks IN, Girdwood AH, et al. Is pancreatic duct obstruction or stricture a major-cause of pain in calcific pancreatitis? Br J Surg. 1980;67(6):425–8. https://doi.org/10.1002/bjs.1800670614.
14. Drossman DA. Chronic functional abdominal pain. Am J Gastroenterol. 1996;91:2270–81.
15. Crombie IK, Davies HT, Macrae WA. Cut and thrust: antecedent surgery and trauma among patients attending a chronic pain clinic. Pain. 1998;76:167–71.
16. Muthulingam J, Olesen SS, Hansen TM, et al. Progression of structural brain changes in patients with chronic pancreatitis and its association to chronic pain: a 7-year longitudinal follow-up study. Pancreas. 2018;47(10):1267–76. https://doi.org/10.1097/MPA.0000000000001151.
17. Bouwense SA, Ahmed Ali U, ten Broek RP, et al. Altered central pain processing after pancreatic surgery for chronic pancreatitis. Br J Surg. 2013;100(13):1797–804. https://doi.org/10.1002/bjs.9322.
18. Krames ES, Foreman R. Spinal cord stimulation modulates visceral nociception and hyperalgesia via the spinothalamic tracts and the postsynaptic dorsal column pathways: a literature review and hypothesis. Neuromodulation. 2007;10(3):224–37.
19. North RB, Kidd DH, Piantadosi S. Spinal cord stimulation versus reoperation for failed back surgery syndrome: a prospective, randomized study design. Acta Neurochir Suppl. 1995;64:106–8.
20. Kumar K, Nath RK, Toth C. Spinal cord stimulation is effective in the management of reflex sympathetic dystrophy. Neurosurgery1997;40(3):503–508; discussion 508–9.; 20.
21. Stanton-Hicks M. Complex regional pain syndrome: manifestations and the role of neurostimulation in its management. J Pain Symptom ManagJ Pain Symptom Manage. 2006;31(4 Suppl): S20–4.
22. Jivegard LE, et al. Effects of spinal cord stimulation (SCS) in patients with inoperable severe lower limb ischaemia: a prospective randomised controlled study. Eur J Vasc Endovasc Surg. 1995;9(4):421–5.
23. Reig E, et al. Spinal cord stimulation in peripheral vascular disease: a retrospective analysis of 95 cases. Pain Pract. 2001;1(4):324–31.
24. Linderoth B, Foreman R. Mechanisms of spinal cord stimulation in painful syndromes: role of animal models. Pain Med. 2006;7(Suppl 1):S14–26.
25. Saade NE, et al. Inhibition of nociceptive evoked activity in spinal neurons through a dorsal column-brainstem-spinal loop. Brain Res. 1985;339(1):115–8.
26. Linderoth B, Meyerson BA. Physiology of spinal cord stimulation: mechanism of action. In: Burchiel K, editor. Surgical management of pain. Stuttgart: Thieme Medical Publisher Inc; 2002. p. 505–26.
27. Cui JG, et al. Spinal cord stimulation attenuates augmented dorsal horn release of excitatory amino acids in mononeuropathy via a GABAergic mechanism. Pain. 1997;73(1):87–95.
28. Linderoth B, et al. Gamma-aminobutyric acid is released in the dorsal horn by electrical spinal cord stimulation: an in vivo microdialysis study in the rat. Neurosurgery. 1994;34(3):484–8; discussion 488–9.
29. Campbell JN. Examination of possible mechanisms by which stimulation of the spinal cord in man relieves pain. Appl Neurophysiol. 1981;44(4):181–6.

30. Larson SJ, et al. Neurophysiological effects of dorsal column stimulation in man and monkey. J Neurosurg. 1974;41(2):217–23.
31. Gildenberg PL, Hirshberg RM. Limited myelotomy for the treatment of intractable cancer pain. J Neurol Neurosurg Psychiatry. 1984;47(1):94–6.
32. Becker R, Sure U, Bertalanffy H. Punctate midline myelotomy. A new approach in the management of visceral pain. Acta Neurochir(Wien). 1999;141(8):881–3.
33. Hirshberg RM, et al. Is there a pathway in the posterior funiculus that signals visceral pain? Pain. 1996;67(2–3):291–305.
34. Hwang SL, et al. Punctate midline myelotomy for intractable visceral pain caused by hepatobiliary or pancreatic cancer. J Pain Symptom Manag. 2004;27(1):79–84.
35. Kim YS, Kwon SJ. High thoracic midline dorsal column myelotomy for severe visceral pain due to advanced stomach cancer. Neurosurgery. 2000;46(1):85–90; discussion 90–2.
36. Nauta HJ, et al. Surgical interruption of a midline dorsal column visceral pain pathway. Case report and review of the literature. J Neurosurg. 1997;86(3):538–42.
37. Nauta HJ, et al. Punctate midline myelotomy for the relief of visceral cancer pain. J Neurosurg. 2000;92(2 Suppl):125–30.
38. Kapural L, et al. Spinal cord stimulation is an effective treatment for the chronic intractable visceral pelvic pain. Pain Med. 2006;7(5):440–3.
39. Linderoth B, Fedorcsak I, Meyerson BA. Peripheral vasodilatation after spinal cord stimulation: animal studies of putative effector mechanisms. Neurosurgery. 1991;28(2):187–95.
40. Kapural L, Deer T, Yakovlev A, et al. Technical aspects of spinal cord stimulation for managing chronic visceral abdominal pain: the results from the national survey. Pain Med. 2010;11:685–91.
41. Kapural L, Cywinski JB, Sparks DA. Spinal cord stimulation for visceral pain from chronic pancreatitis. Neuromodulation. 2011;14:423–6; discussion 426–7.
42. Kapural L, Nagem H, Tlucek H, et al. Spinal cord stimulation for chronic visceral abdominal pain. Pain Med. 2010;11:347–55. Narouze S. chronic Abdominal Wall pain: diagnosis and interventional treatment. in L. Kapural (ed.), Chronic abdominal pain: an evidence-based, Comprehensive Guide to Clinical Management, Springer, New York, 2015;189–195.
43. Kapural L, Puyalert M, Walsh M, Sweiss G. Interdisciplinary treatment of the pain from chronic pancreatitis. In: Hayek S, Shah BJ, Desai MJ, Chelimsky TC, editors. Pain medicine, an interdisciplinary case-based approach. New York: Oxford University Press; 2015. p. 289–97.
44. Kapural L, Rakic M. Spinal cord stimulation for chronic visceral pain secondary to chronic non-alcoholic pancreatitis: a case report. Clin Gastroenterol Hepatol. 2008;42(6):750–1.
45. Khan Y, Raza S, Khan E. Application of spinal cord stimulation for the treatment of abdominal visceral pain syndromes: case reports. Neuromodulation. 2005;8:14–27.
46. Kim JK, et al. Spinal cord stimulation for intractable visceral pain due to chronic pancreatitis. J Korean Neurosurg Soc. 2009;46(2):165–7.
47. Kapural L, Yu C, Doust MW, et al. Novel 10-kHz high-frequency therapy (HF10 therapy) is superior to traditional low-frequency spinal cord stimulation for the treatment of chronic back and leg pain: The SENZARCT randomized controlled trial. Anesthesiology. 2015;123:851–60.
48. De Carolis G, Paroli M, Tollapi L, et al. Paresthesia-independence: an assessment of technical factors related to 10 kHz paresthesia-free spinal cord stimulation. Pain Physician. 2017;20:331–41.
49. Kapural L, Yu C, Doust MW, et al. Comparison of 10-kHz high frequency and traditional low-frequency spinal cord stimulation for the treatment of chronic back and leg pain: 24-month results from a multicenter, randomized, controlled pivotal trial. Neurosurgery. 2016;79:667–77.
50. Lee KY, Bae C, Lee DC, Kagan Z, et al. Low-intensity, kilohertz frequency spinal cord stimulation differently affects excitatory and inhibitory neurons in the rodent superficial dorsal horn. Neuroscience. 2020;428:132–9.
51. Kapural L, Mayank G, Richard P, Wyndam S, Vorenkamp Kevin E, Christopher G, Bradford G, Anand R, Jeyakumar S, Rose P-A. Treatment of chronic abdominal pain With 10-kHz spi-

nal cord stimulation: safety and efficacy results from a 12-Month prospective, multicenter, feasibility study, clinical and translational. Gastroenterology. 2020;11(2):e00133. https://doi.org/10.14309/ctg.0000000000000133.

52. Deer TR, Mekhail N, Provenzano D, Pope J, Krames E, Thomson S, et al. Neuromodulation Appropriateness Consensus Committee. The appropriate use of neurostimulation: avoidance and treatment of complications of neurostimulation therapies for the treatment of chronic pain. Neuromodulation Appropriateness Consensus Committee. Neuromodulation. 2014;17:571–97; discussion 597–8

IPG Site Creation, Considerations, and Risk Mitigation

Tory L. McJunkin, Brandon May, Mostafa Maita, and Paul J. Lynch

Introduction and Background

Spinal cord electrical stimulation was first used by neurosurgeon Norman Shealy in 1968. The initial design evolved from external power sources and implanted leads on the spinal cord to internal power sources and dorsal column-stimulating electrodes. The first commercially available systems used external radiofrequency receivers that powered the implanted devices. From here, the field transitioned to using fully implantable systems in 1981 and then fully implantable rechargeable systems in 2004. Subsequently, miniaturized implantable pulse generators (IPGs) and longer-distance maneuverable leads were developed. Currently, the community is focused on advanced miniaturization with enhanced lead target specificity, primary cell (non-rechargeable) IPGs, longer-lasting rechargeable IPGs, a renewed interest in externally powered devices, and even the development of optogenetic modulation therapies [1]. The scope of this chapter will include IPG pocket characteristics, surgical technique, infectious risk reduction, and management strategies related to common complications.

Surgical Technique and Pocket Characteristics

Pulse generator pockets are generally limited to placement at several common locations. The current preferred location of IPG for many physicians has evolved toward the posterolateral flank above the iliac crest and below the last rib (refer to Figs. 1, 2, and 3). This placement is preferred by many because of its stable location close

T. L. McJunkin (✉) · P. J. Lynch
Arizona Pain, Scottsdale, AZ, USA
e-mail: DrMcJunkin@arizonapain.com; DrLynch@arizonapain.com

B. May · M. Maita
UT Health San Antonio, San Antonio, TX, USA

T. d. S. Freitas et al. (eds.), *Neuromodulation Techniques for Pain Treatment*,
https://doi.org/10.1007/978-3-030-84778-4_16

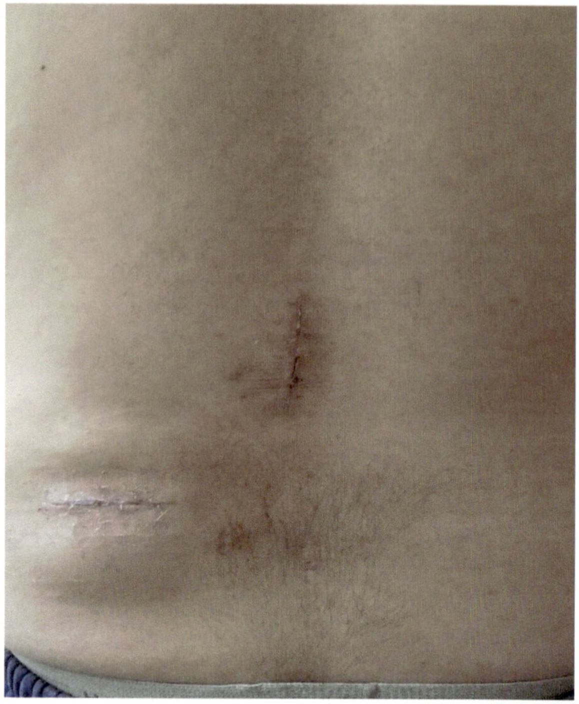

Fig. 1 Well-healed vertical (lead insertion) wound and flank horizontal (IPG site) wound. IPG in close proximity to lead insertion site to reduce risk of lead migration

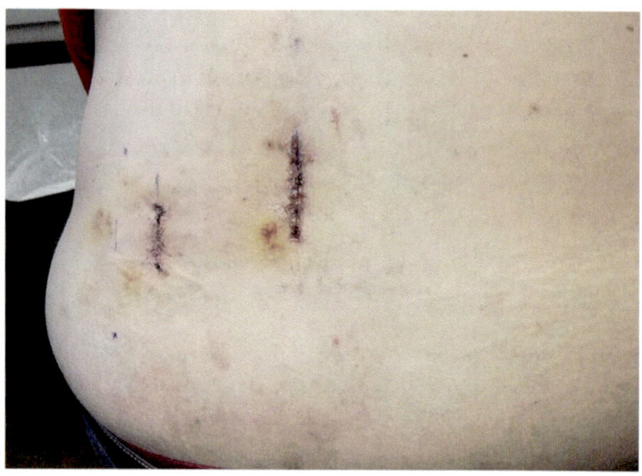

Fig. 2 Well-healed superior vertical (lead insertion) wound and flank vertical (IPG site) wound. IPG in close proximity to lead insertion site to reduce risk of lead migration

to the lead insertion site. Classically, IPGs have been placed in posterolateral buttock pockets below the beltline (refer to Fig. 4). Less commonly, IPGs can be placed in abdominal subcutaneous compartments or in infraclavicular positions, but these implant locations are more typical of intrathecal pumps and VNS/cardiac defibrillators, respectively [2]. As a rule, pocket size should be large enough to accommodate the IPG unit without significant leftover dead space. In practice, clinicians often aim

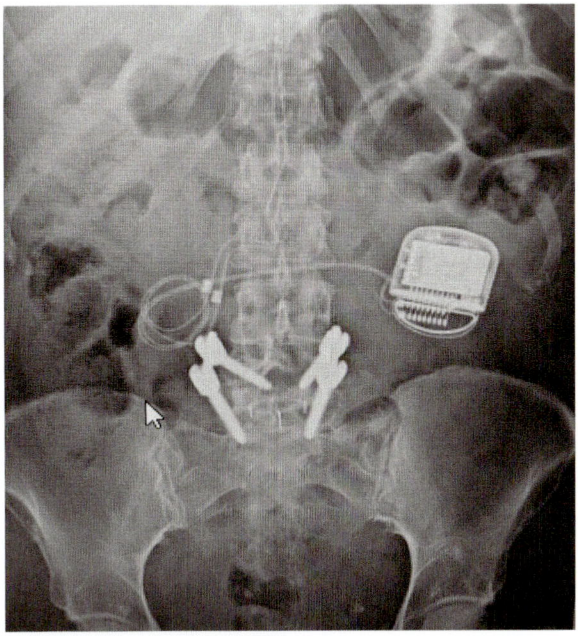

Fig. 3 X-ray of IPG in flank site, above the iliac crest and below the last rib

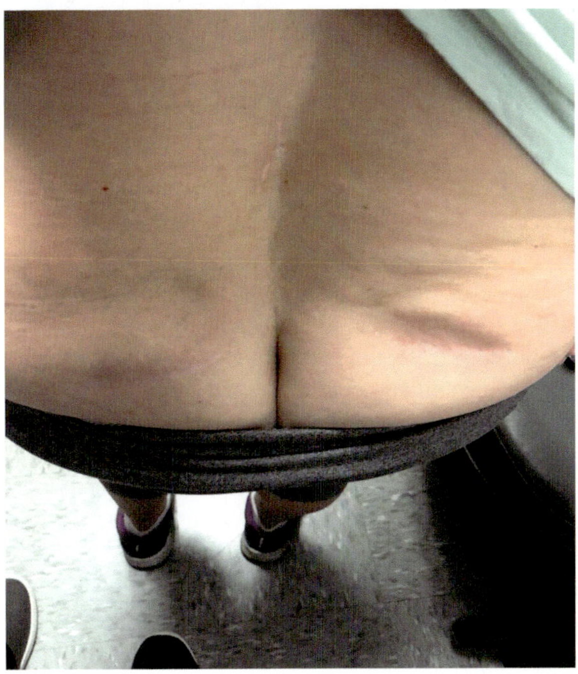

Fig. 4 Patient with two "below-the-belt" buttock SCS IPGs. Right IPG is tilted causing pain in the superior aspect of IPG pocket

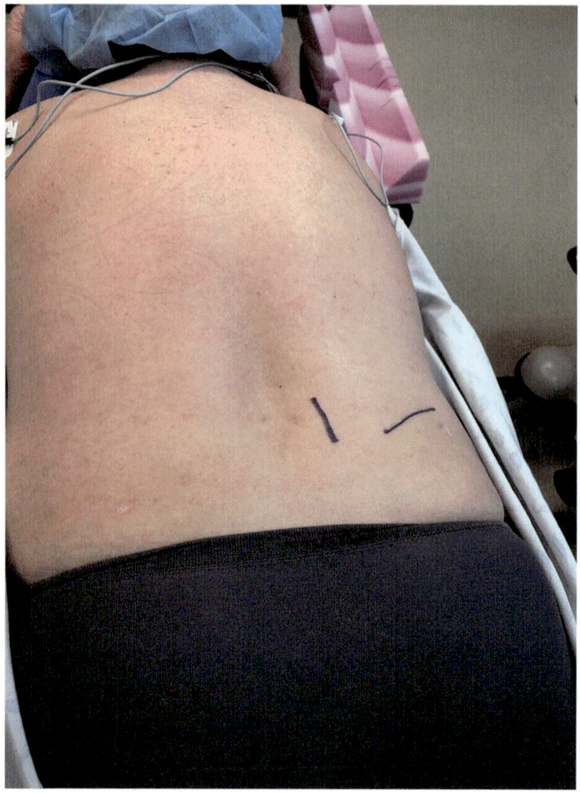

Fig. 5 Preoperative planning, marking of surgical sites and discussion with the patient regarding IPG pocket selection site

to make the pocket 120–130% of the IPG volume and place it at approximately one inch or less in depth below Scarpa's fascia.

The surgical approach generally consists of making two incisions: one for the leads and one for the battery/IPG pocket. Clean-cut incision should be performed with a scalpel in order to create a Class 1 wound with minimal to no desiccation of wound edge (refer to Figs. 5, 6, and 7). Incision length should be as minimal as possible while still allowing for placement of battery and leads. Dead space should be minimized to reduce risk for seroma or hematoma formation. Epinephrine combined with local anesthetic may be used with caution and consideration for the balance between localized peripheral vasoconstriction and reduced blood loss. Vasoconstriction may hinder the healing process and increase risk for infection [3]. Furthermore, electrocautery devices should be used sparingly due to evidence of inferior wound healing, lower threshold for bacterial contamination, increased rates of wound dehiscence, and possibility for thermal tissue damage with excessive use

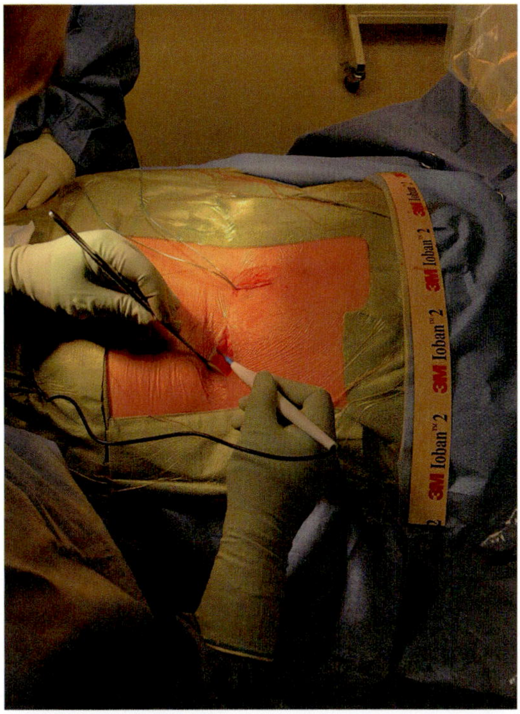

Fig. 6 Surgical approach with two incisions: central vertical incision seen with leads which will be tunneled to lateral horizontal incision at IPG site

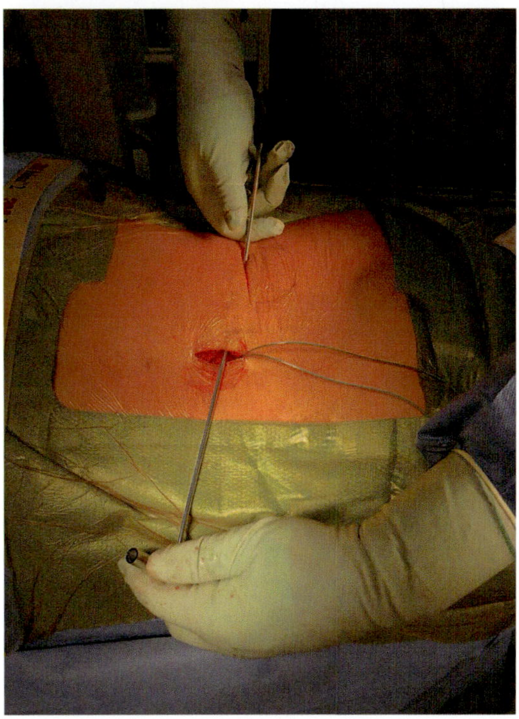

Fig. 7 Tunneling device crating pathway for leads to be tunneled to lateral IPG site

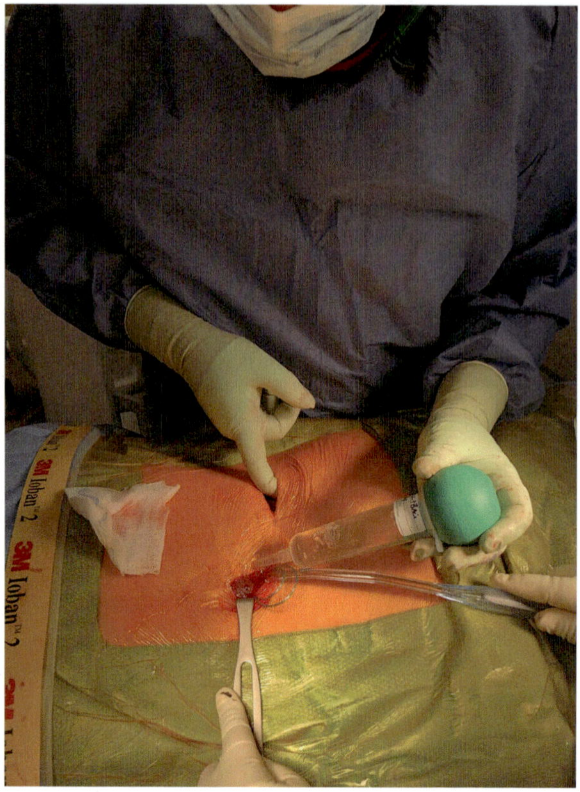

Fig. 8 Tunneling of leads is complete. IPG seen in lateral pocket and coiled redundant leads are seen at central incision. Copious irrigation performed at both incisional sites

[3, 4]. In effect, these devices may be appropriate to optimize hemostasis and reduce operative time, but care must be taken to avoid overzealous use near the surface. Irrigation should be performed with saline via syringe bulb to clean the wound prior to closure [5, 6] (refer to Fig. 7). Superficial skin closure is generally at the discretion of the implanting physician insomuch as neither staples nor suture are clearly superior so long as proper tension is placed on the dead space closure. When using sutures to close deeper layers, simple interrupted sutures are optimal, while running locked sutures should generally be avoided; smaller stitches and knots with minimal tension are preferred [3, 7] (refer to Figs. 8, 9, 10, and 11).

Reducing Infectious Risk

Surgical site infection (SSI) rates of implanted spinal cord stimulators (SCS) have ranged between one and ten percent with two large studies reporting rates of 3.4% to 4.6% [8, 9]. More recent data from retrospective multicenter studies suggest

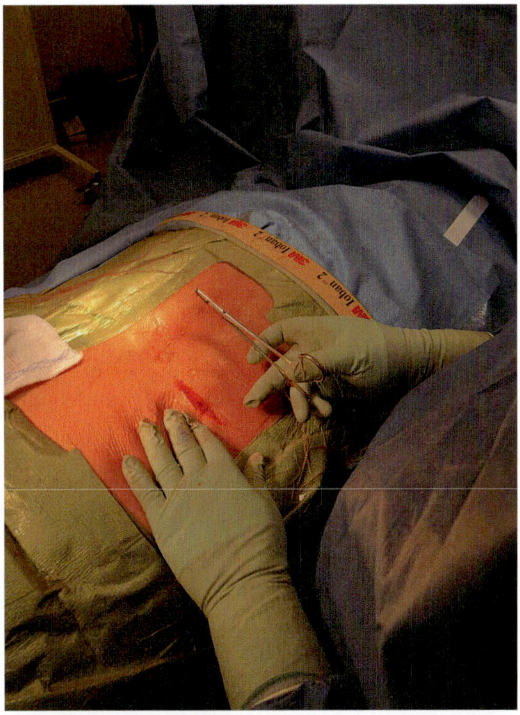

Fig. 9 Closure of both incisional sites with deep and superficial layers with 2.0 Vicryl

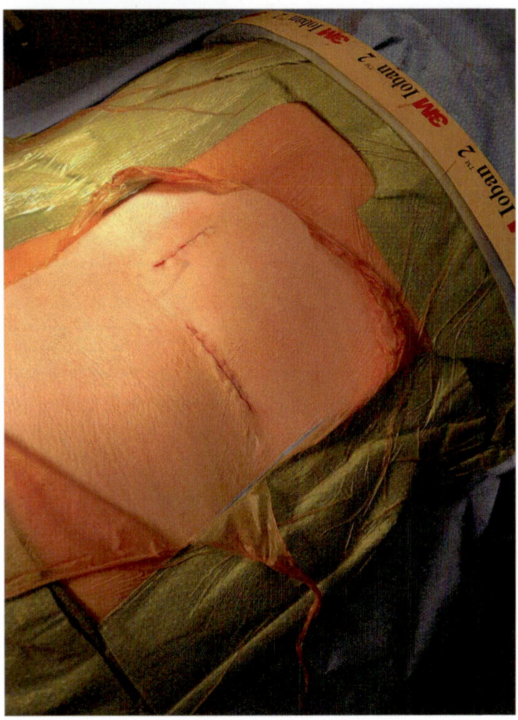

Fig. 10 Closure of both wounds is complete

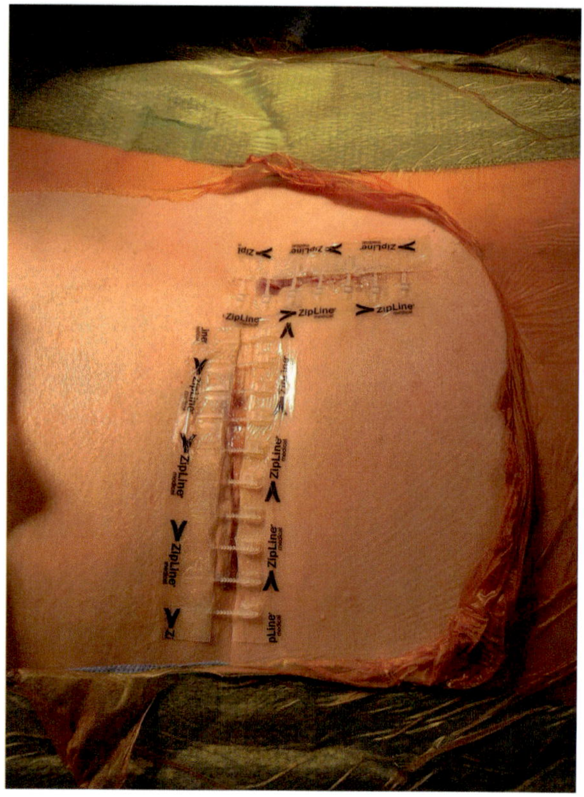

Fig. 11 Zipline™ noninvasive skin closure device used and removed after 14 days

lower SSI incidence of 2.45% [10]. The Neurostimulation Appropriateness Consensus Committee (NACC) has created recommendations for infection prevention and management as follows.

Preoperative

Preop workup is the first step in reducing SSI risk. Physicians must take a comprehensive history and perform pertinent physical exam maneuvers to assess potential implantation candidates for underlying comorbid medical conditions that predispose to SSI. Notably, uncontrolled diabetes, obesity, hyperglycemia, recent smoking, chronic preoperative corticosteroid use, HIV seropositivity, active chemotherapy, malnourishment, and high-dose opioid therapy are associated with increased occurrence of SSI and are relative contraindications to surgery depending on severity [11]. In this regard, the NACC recommends HbA1C optimization, 4 weeks of preoperative smoking cessation, limitation of corticosteroids, nutritional status optimization, infectious disease consultation with HIV viral load, and oncology consultation to assess implantation risk versus benefit [12]. Physical exam findings of concern include inspection of surgical site area skin and monitoring of vital signs to evaluate for ongoing local or systemic infectious process or disruption of skin integrity. Communication with prescribing physician of anticoagulation medication should occur to ensure appropriate preoperative anticoagulation [13]. There is no specific set of preoperative labs to order for IPG implantation surgery; however it may be prudent to consider ordering ESR, CRP, CBC, and any labs deemed pertinent for monitoring of medical comorbidities [14, 15]. Preoperative screening for MRSA and MSSA is recommended in all IPG candidates because *S. aureus* is responsible for 50–60% of SSIs in orthopedic and neurological procedures and 30% of SSIs overall; carrier individuals are two to nine times higher risk of developing SSIs, and decolonization protocols are effective in SSI risk reduction (3.4% SSI rate in decolonization group compared to 7.7% in placebo group) [16–19]. Decolonization treatment primarily consists of a 5-day preoperative course of intranasal mupirocin and daily chlorhexidine baths [16]. Furthermore, since hair removal by clipping or shaving 24 hours or more before surgery increases SSI risk, the NACC recommends hair removal to be done immediately preop using electrical clippers if necessary [20].

Appropriate antibiotic prophylaxis has resulted in approximately 50% SSI reduction in clinical studies [21]. *S. epidermidis* and *S. aureus* are the two most commonly implicated pathogens in neuromodulation implant SSIs. In most cases, a single dose of a cephalosporin such as cefazolin is appropriate with clindamycin or vancomycin as options for patients with a beta-lactam allergy. Local and community patterns of antibiotic resistance/susceptibility may warrant alternative antibiotic choice. Otherwise, vancomycin should be used in MRSA carriers and patients at high risk for colonization by MRSA [22]. Furthermore, weight-based dosing reduces SSI rates. SSI risk reduction was achieved when morbidly obese patients were given 2 g dosing of cefazolin to achieve minimum inhibitory concentration rather than the standard single 1 g dose [23, 24]. In addition, dose timing is important in SSI risk reduction. Cefazolin and clindamycin should be dosed 30–60 minutes prior to incision, while vancomycin should be dosed within 120 minutes prior to incision [25, 26].

Ideal surgical scrub technique should include 2–5 minutes of hand washing, removal of upper extremity jewelry, nails to be kept short [27–29]. Chlorhexidine use is supported over povidone-iodine due to superior effect in reducing hand bacterial colony-forming unit counts [30, 31].

Intraoperative

For intraoperative infectious risk reduction, the NACC recommends using combination chlorhexidine-isopropyl alcohol products for preparation of the skin prior to first incision [32]. Furthermore, sterile barrier precautions and double gloving are preferred for implanting neuromodulation devices. Traffic through the operating room should be kept to a minimum, and draping should be performed with sterile C-arm drapes. If adhesive drapes are used, they should be iodophor-impregnated due to potential for improved bacterial penetration of wet traditional cloth drapes [33].

As a standard for surgical training, neuromodulation-credentialed physicians should be trained on at least ten supervised IPG cases as the primary implanter prior to independent practice, especially if these physicians come from non-ACGME programs [12]. The supervisor for these initial cases should have prior credentialing from a Joint Commission-approved facility.

Several different trial and implant pathways exist. The two most common are initial trial followed by separate complete implant versus staged trial with completion implant integrated. If all of the aforementioned risk reduction methods are properly employed, current evidence suggests that the staged variant does not significantly increase infection rate [34]. Importantly, increased rates of SSI are observed with increased duration of trial [35].

Surgical techniques to limit infection are indicated as described in the Surgical Technique and Pocket Characteristics section. In addition to surgical technique, intraoperative SSI reduction efforts also include various antimicrobial strategies. Most notably, chlorhexidine-impregnated dressings are recommended in patients with high-risk comorbidities to reduce exit-site colonization and related infection [36]. Furthermore, intrasite vancomycin powder shows promise but is awaiting further study for neuromodulation patients with promising existing results for spine surgery patients [37, 38]. Bioabsorbable antimicrobial mesh envelopes are approved for ICD implants and have likely benefit in SCS implant patients such that high-risk SCS implant patients may benefit from use, despite a lack of SCS-specific data at current time [39].

Postoperative

Several large multicenter retrospective reviews have been done with focus on post-implantation infection incidence and associated risk factors. Their findings demonstrate reduced SSI rates with use of occlusive dressings, continuation of antibiotics beyond 24 postoperative hours, and limiting SCS trials to 5 days or less in length if possible [10, 40]. Notably, cephalexin and clindamycin were the most used postoperative antibiotics, and no statistical difference in SSI rates were found between paddle leads versus cylindrical leads. SSIs may occur more than 1 year after implantation, but the median time to onset in the studied population was 27 days [40]. Lastly, education of the patient and family to recognize signs of site infection helps with earlier detection in the small percentage that do develop SSI. In such patients it is good practice to consult with an infectious disease specialist if the device is to be removed to determine appropriate antimicrobial treatment and to discuss timing of reimplantation. Neuraxial imaging (CT or MRI often with and without contrast) is warranted in scenarios involving suspicion for epidural involvement or deep infection [41].

Management of Common Complications

Overall implant complication rates range from 30% to 40% and include both hardware-related and biologic complications. The leading biologic complications are superficial surgical site infections, while the leading mechanical or hardware-related complications are lead migration and implant site pain. In Senza's 24-month multicenter randomized control trial comparing 10 kHz high-frequency (HF10) and traditional low-frequency SCS, implant site pain was most common (observed in 12.9% of HF10 versus 13.4% of traditional SCS patients, $P = 0.91$) [42]. Of the various hardware issues, lead migration and lead fracture are the most common [43], with lead migration being observed in 13% of implantation cases [44]. Mechanical implant site pain can result from the IPG tilting, rotating within the pocket or simply extruding which usually occurs on thinner patients.

Lead fracture or connection loss from the IPG can be diagnosed grossly by radiography and directly by impedance testing. It is managed by surgical replacement, programming around the break, or cessation of use. This complication may be reduced by incorporating strain relief loops, adequate anchoring techniques, avoiding placement in areas with large ranges of motion, implanting the pulse generator close to the lead termination site, and limiting patient movement during the postoperative interval [45–47]. When lead migration is visualized on X-ray, lead replacement or paddle lead placement may be considered.

Battery or IPG failure has been observed to occur but may be limited by proper testing of the lead connection. Unexpected battery failure prior to the specified battery lifetime occurs more frequently with non-rechargeable IPG systems [48]. These complications may necessitate device replacement, and it is advisable to contact the manufacturer to rule out known device defects. Lastly, MRI incompatibility may serve as another cause for battery removal or for initial IPG refusal depending on the predicted imaging needs warranted by the patient health profile. This is because MRI exposure can cause magnetic field-induced rotation, translation, and acceleration of the IPG device and the accumulated RF exposure can lead to device heating and subsequent burn injury to the patient. Here lies a focus of clinical reasoning insomuch as 82–84% of SCS-implanted patients in a studied population were evaluated to have a likely need for one or more MR imaging appointments within 5 years of SCS implantation [49]. Having said this, most current-generation IPGs are MRI compatible.

The most common biologic complication is infection and may be evidenced by wound dehiscence (refer to Fig. 12), purulent IPG site drainage (refer to Fig. 13), or systemic signs of infection in disseminated cases. Most surgical site infections originate from endogenous bacteria that are introduced due to surgical trauma [50–52]. Clinical suspicion should make the physician consider computed tomography scanning with contrast, serum cultures, wound culture, CBC, CRP, ESR, and infectious disease specialist care if clinical picture is more concerning. Management typically includes reopening the IPG pocket with subsequent device removal and culture of surrounding tissue with fluid or purulent drainage sent to pathology [53].

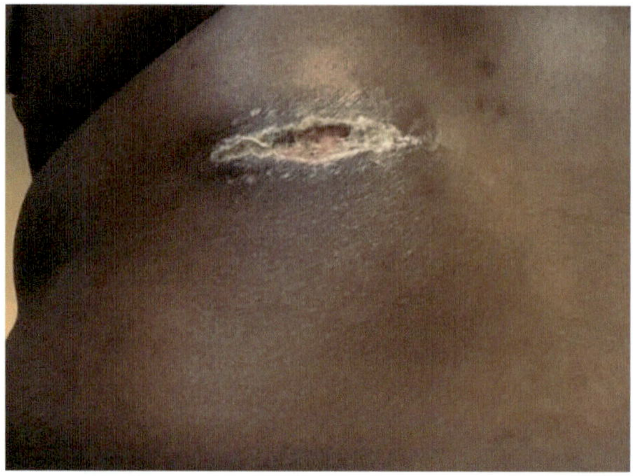

Fig. 12 Wound dehiscence and early signs of infection

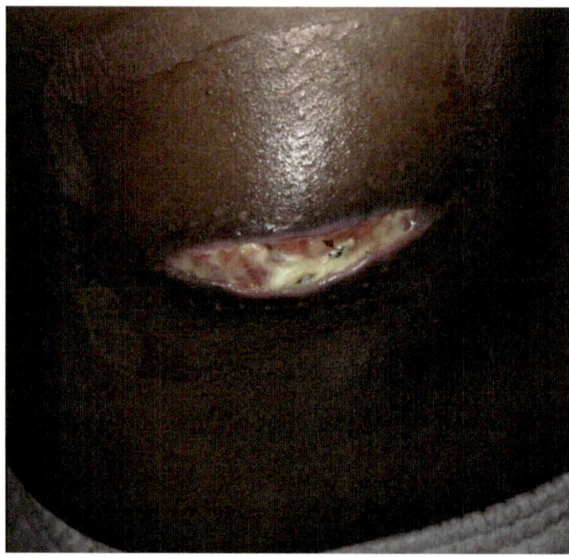

Fig. 13 Granulation tissue, purulent drainage, and swelling at IPG site

Contrastingly, infection limited to the superficial skin area around the IPG site may be managed with oral antibiotics and early follow-up so long as it does not involve the neuraxial entry point. Antibiotic treatment should be directed based on pathology profile of cultured microbes [54].

Allergic reactions may occur based on case reports and include symptoms of malaise, itching, and pain. The diagnosis may be sought out via skin patch testing and serum panels to rule out infectious etiology. Severe allergic reactions may warrant explant. Physicians may prevent or reduce likelihood of allergic reaction by suggesting skin patch testing in individuals with high-risk history of atopy [43]. Care should be taken to rule out other common allergen sources such as latex or adhesive.

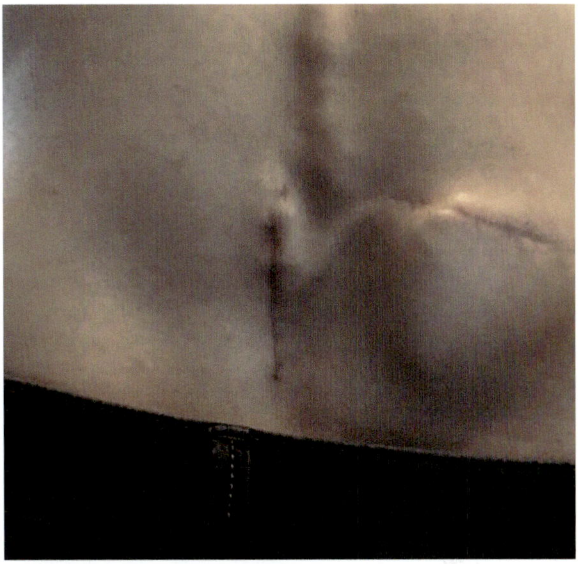

Fig. 14 Fluid and swelling at IPG site with tracking along leads to lead insertion incision site

IPG seromas are also quite common and usually manifest as swelling, pain, and redness at battery implant site (refer to Fig. 14). They can occur spontaneously or as a result of swelling from IPG site trauma. CT with contrast may identify the seroma and serum panel may be ordered for infectious rule out. Seromas may be managed conservatively with sterile drainage and abdominal binder placement. Drained fluid may be sent to pathology if infectious cause is suspected. Risk is reduced by limiting blunt dissection, avoiding overuse of electrocautery, using minimal pocket size with layered closure, and appropriate hemostasis. Abdominal binders may be used prophylactically for the initial 2 postoperative months [55]. Usually IPG seromas can be conservatively treated and do not require explant, but some may require revision or removal of implant.

Erosion of lead or IPG site are rare complications but can occur (see Fig. 15). They can occur due to inflammation and infectious and likely allergic causes. They are more commonly seen in superficial locations like supraorbital PNS stimulation but can occur anywhere. Generally, they require removal of the leads and/or IPG.

Epidural hematomas typically present as new-onset neurologic findings including worsening of pain, or shifting of pain to a new area, numbness, weakness, and bowel and/or bladder changes. Epidural hematomas are notably most prevalent in the male population and in those in their fifth or sixth decade [56]. Diagnosis is reached by clinical picture and with emergent CT or MRI with or without contrast and subsequent surgical consultation [57]. Epidural hematomas should be evacuated, and often at the same time device should be removed within 8 hours of neurological symptom onset. Careful attention should be paid to patients on chronic anticoagulation [58].

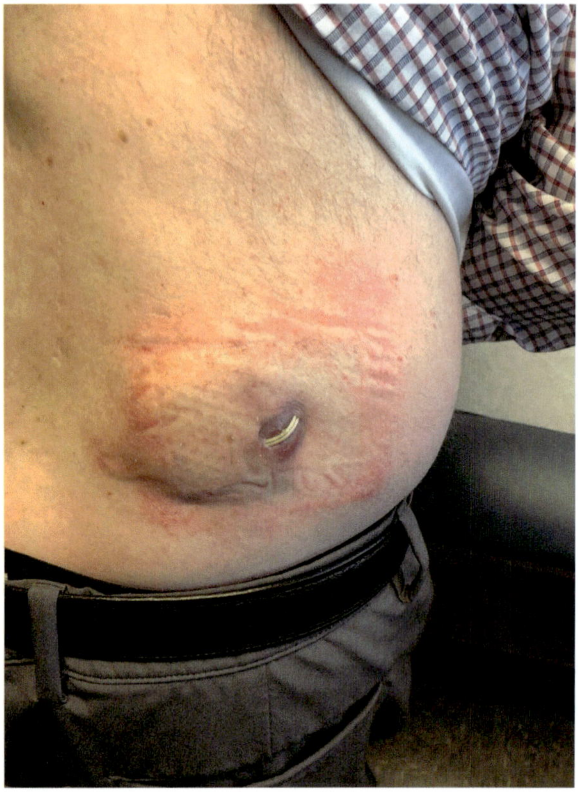

Fig. 15 Skin erosion of coiled leads at IPG site in a patient 5 years after implant

Epidural fibrosis has been reported in case reports and may be evidenced by change in stimulation pattern due to scarring around leads [34]. Reprogramming may result in regain of efficacy.

Dural puncture is another less common complication. Patients classically experience a positional postoperative headache in the context of surgeon observing spinal fluid in the surgical field or spinal fluid leakage from incision site after closure [59]. IV fluids, supine positioning, and caffeine are the conservative treatment options. Some physicians will abort the procedure upon noticing a tear, while others will move vertically to a different spinal level. Blood patches are a treatment for dural puncture, but their recommendation is controversial due to the patch providing a source for infection. This complication should be considered especially in patients with spinal stenosis, with calcification of ligamentum flavum, or with history of previous surgery at the site [53].

Compressive neurologic pathology and nerve or cord injury are listed in case reports. They present with new-onset neurologic deficits and warrant evaluation with emergent CT with contrast. Neurosurgery should be consulted. Cord and nerve damage is more common when the implanter makes multiple needle placement attempts, multiple attempts passing electrodes, or multiple attempts passing paddles. Many physicians are using real-time neuromonitoring for additional safety while performing implant procedures. Compressive pathology may require mechanical decompression procedures such as lead removal and/or laminectomy [60]. This risk can be limited by taking adequate time to review preoperative imaging and to take particular care with spinal stenosis patients.

IPG Site Reimplantation or Revision

After complications result in explant, reimplantation should be considered. However, there are no clearly established protocols for timeline, site change, and preoperative preparation. Existing protocols are largely anecdotal, and as such, physician practice varies considerably. If reimplantation is chosen, preoperative planning should be considered to lower the rates of early complication and need for replacement. For instance, if an IPG was removed secondary to infection, many would recommend consultation with an infectious disease physician for additional guidance to prevent another site infection.

IPG positional problems can occur for many reasons including weight loss, trauma to the site, change in body habitus, additional surgery, and internal pocket problems like a seroma. IPG positional problems often result in tilting, rotation, or even flipping of the IPG in the pocket. If revision of IPG site is considered which is usually due to patient discomfort, careful discussion of site change and preoperative planning is also recommended to prevent further surgery if possible.

References

1. Fishman MA, Antony A, Esposito M, Deer T, Levy R. The evolution of neuromodulation in the treatment of chronic pain: forward-looking perspectives. Pain Med. 2019;20(Supplement_1):S58–68. https://doi.org/10.1093/pm/pnz074.
2. Deer TR, et al. The neuromodulation appropriateness consensus committee on best practices for dorsal root ganglion stimulation. Neuromodulation. 2019;22(1):1–35. https://doi.org/10.1111/ner.12845.
3. Gabriella Gutman JZ. A review of surgical techniques in spinal cord stimulator implantation to decrease the post-operative infection rate. J Spine. 2015;04(01):1–12. https://doi.org/10.4172/2165-7939.1000202.
4. Soballe PW, Nimbkar NV, Hayward I, Nielsen TB, Drucker WR. Electric cautery lowers the contamination threshold for infection of laparotomies 11This work was supported by the Naval Medical Research and Development Command, work unit 61153N MR04120.001-1002.22The first two authors contributed equally to this work. Am J Surg. 1998;175(4):263–6. https://doi.org/10.1016/S0002-9610(98)00020-8.
5. Anglen JO. Wound irrigation in musculoskeletal injury. J Am Acad Orthop Surg. 9(4):219–26. s10.5435/00124635-200107000-00001.
6. Barnes S, Spencer M, Graham D, Johnson HB. Surgical wound irrigation: a call for evidence-based standardization of practice. Am J Infect Control. 2014;42(5):525–9. https://doi.org/10.1016/j.ajic.2014.01.012.

7. Smith TO, Sexton D, Mann C, Donell S. Sutures versus staples for skin closure in orthopaedic surgery: meta-analysis. BMJ. 2010;340(mar16 1):c1199. https://doi.org/10.1136/bmj.c1199.
8. Waszak PM, et al. Spinal cord stimulation in failed back surgery syndrome: review of clinical use, quality of life and cost-effectiveness. Asian Spine J. 2016;10(6):1195. https://doi.org/10.4184/asj.2016.10.6.1195.
9. Jeon YH. Spinal Cord Stimulation in Pain Management: A Review. Korean J. Pain. 2012;25(3):143. https://doi.org/10.3344/kjp.2012.25.3.143.
10. Hoelzer BC, et al. Spinal cord stimulator implant infection rates and risk factors: a multicenter retrospective study. Neuromodulation. 2017;20(6):558–62. https://doi.org/10.1111/ner.12609.
11. Pull ter Gunne AF, Cohen DB. Incidence, prevalence, and analysis of risk factors for surgical site infection following adult spinal surgery. Spine (Phila Pa 1976). Jun. 2009;34(13):1422–8. https://doi.org/10.1097/BRS.0b013e3181a03013.
12. Deer TR, et al. The Neurostimulation appropriateness consensus committee (NACC) recommendations for infection prevention and management. Neuromodulation. 2017;20(1):31–50. https://doi.org/10.1111/ner.12565.
13. Narouze S, et al. Interventional spine and pain procedures in patients on antiplatelet and anticoagulant medications (Second Edition). Reg Anesth Pain Med. 2017:1. https://doi.org/10.1097/AAP.0000000000000700.
14. Spangehl MJ, Masri BA, O'connell JX, Duncan CP. Prospective analysis of preoperative and intraoperative investigations for the diagnosis of infection at the sites of two hundred and two revision Total hip arthroplasties*. J Bone Jt Surg. 1999;81(5):672–83. https://doi.org/10.2106/00004623-199905000-00008.
15. King MS. Preoperative evaluation. Am Fam Physician. 2000;62(2):387–96, [Online]. Available: http://www.ncbi.nlm.nih.gov/pubmed/10929701.
16. Perl TM, et al. Intranasal mupirocin to prevent postoperative Staphylococcus aureus infections. N Engl J Med. Jun. 2002;346(24):1871–7. https://doi.org/10.1056/NEJMoa003069.
17. Parvizi J, Matar WY, Saleh KJ, Schmalzried TP, Mihalko WM. Decolonization of drug-resistant organisms before total joint arthroplasty. Instr Course Lect. 2010;59:131–7.
18. Wenzel RP, Perl TM. The significance of nasal carriage of Staphylococcus aureus and the incidence of postoperative wound infection. J Hosp Infect. 1995;31(1):13–24. https://doi.org/10.1016/0195-6701(95)90079-9.
19. Kluytmans J, van Belkum A, Verbrugh H. Nasal carriage of Staphylococcus aureus: epidemiology, underlying mechanisms, and associated risks. Clin Microbiol Rev. 1997;10(3):505–20, [Online]. Available: http://www.ncbi.nlm.nih.gov/pubmed/9227864
20. Seropian R, Reynolds BM. Wound infections after preoperative depilatory versus razor preparation. Am J Surg. 1971;121(3):251–4. https://doi.org/10.1016/0002-9610(71)90199-1.
21. Bowater RJ, Stirling SA, Lilford RJ. Is antibiotic prophylaxis in surgery a generally effective intervention? Ann Surg. 2009;249(4):551–6. https://doi.org/10.1097/SLA.0b013e318199f202.
22. Matar WY, Jafari SM, Restrepo C, Austin M, Purtill JJ, Parvizi J. Preventing infection in total joint arthroplasty. J Bone Jt Surg - Ser A. 2010;92(SUPPL. 2):36–46. https://doi.org/10.2106/JBJS.J.01046.
23. Alexander JW, Solomkin JS, Edwards MJ. Updated recommendations for control of surgical site infections. Ann Surg. 2011;253(6):1082–93. https://doi.org/10.1097/SLA.0b013e31821175f8.
24. Hranjec T, Swenson BR, Sawyer RG. Surgical site infection prevention: how we do it. Surg Infect. 2010;11(3):289–94. https://doi.org/10.1089/sur.2010.021.
25. Olsen MA, et al. Risk factors for surgical site infection following Orthopaedic spinal operations. J Bone Jt Surg Am. 2008;90(1):62–9. https://doi.org/10.2106/JBJS.F.01515.
26. Bratzler DW. Use of antimicrobial prophylaxis for major surgery. Arch Surg. 2005;140(2):174. https://doi.org/10.1001/archsurg.140.2.174.
27. Kappstein I, Schulgen G, Waninger J, Daschner F. Microbiological and economic studies of abbreviated procedures for surgical hand disinfection. Chirurg. 1993;64(5):400–5, [Online]. Available: http://www.ncbi.nlm.nih.gov/pubmed/8330498

28. Wheelock SM, Lookinland S. Effect of surgical hand scrub time on subsequent bacterial growth. AORN J. 1997;65(6):1087–98. https://doi.org/10.1016/S0001-2092(06)62949-9.
29. Pereira LJ, Lee GM, Wade KJ. An evaluation of five protocols for surgical handwashing in relation to skin condition and microbial counts. J Hosp Infect. 1997;36(1):49–65. https://doi.org/10.1016/S0195-6701(97)90090-6.
30. Furukawa K, Tajiri T, Suzuki H, Norose Y. Are sterile water and brushes necessary for hand washing before surgery in Japan? J Nippon Med Sch. 2005;72(3):149–54. https://doi.org/10.1272/jnms.72.149.
31. Pereira LJ, Lee GM, Wade KJ. The effect of surgical handwash routines on the microbial counts operating room nurses. Am J Infect Control. 1990;18(6):354–64. https://doi.org/10.1016/0196-6553(90)90249-R.
32. Lee I, Agarwal RK, Lee BY, Fishman NO, Umscheid CA. Systematic review and cost analysis comparing use of chlorhexidine with use of iodine for preoperative skin antisepsis to prevent surgical site infection. Infect Control Hosp Epidemiol. 2010;31(12):1219–29. https://doi.org/10.1086/657134.
33. J. Webster and A. Alghamdi. Use of plastic adhesive drapes during surgery for preventing surgical site infection. Cochrane Database Syst Rev. 2015. https://doi.org/10.1002/14651858.CD006353.pub4.
34. Kumar K, et al. Spinal cord stimulation versus conventional medical management for neuropathic pain: a multicentre randomised controlled trial in patients with failed back surgery syndrome. Pain. 2007;132(1–2):179–88. https://doi.org/10.1016/j.pain.2007.07.028.
35. North R, et al. Postoperative infections associated with prolonged spinal cord stimulation trial duration (PROMISE RCT). Neuromodulation. 2020;23(5):620–5. https://doi.org/10.1111/ner.13141.
36. Ho KM. Use of chlorhexidine-impregnated dressing to prevent vascular and epidural catheter colonization and infection: a meta-analysis. J Antimicrob Chemother. 2006;58(2):281–7. https://doi.org/10.1093/jac/dkl234.
37. Aleem IS, Tan LA, Nassr A, Riew KD. Surgical site infection prevention following spine surgery. Glob Spine J. 2020;10(1_suppl):92S–8S. https://doi.org/10.1177/2192568219844228.
38. Amrani J. Intraoperative powdered vancomycin use with paddle lead placement. Neuromodulation. 2015;18(3):177–81. https://doi.org/10.1111/ner.12216.
39. Pranata R, Tondas AE, Vania R, Yuniadi Y. Antibiotic envelope is associated with reduction in cardiac implantable electronic devices infections especially for high-power device—systematic review and meta-analysis. J Arrhythmia. 2020;36(1):166–73. https://doi.org/10.1002/joa3.12270.
40. Bendel MA, et al. Spinal cord stimulator related infections: findings from a multicenter retrospective analysis of 2737 implants. Neuromodulation. 2017;20(6):553–7. https://doi.org/10.1111/ner.12636.
41. Horn JA, Cole PJ. Severe neurological damage following epidural analgesia. Acute Pain. 2003;5(2):69–72. https://doi.org/10.1016/j.acpain.2003.08.003.
42. Kapural L, et al. Comparison of 10-kHz high-frequency and traditional low-frequency spinal cord stimulation for the treatment of chronic back and leg pain. Neurosurgery. 2016;79(5):667–77. https://doi.org/10.1227/NEU.0000000000001418.
43. Deer TR, et al. The appropriate use of neurostimulation: avoidance and treatment of complications of neurostimulation therapies for the treatment of chronic pain. Neuromodulation. 2014;17(6):571–98. https://doi.org/10.1111/ner.12206.
44. Abejón D, Arango S, Riquelme I, Del Saz J. Neuromodulation techniques, complications, and troubleshooting. Tech Reg Anesth Pain Manag. Jan. 2014;18(1–2):49–57. https://doi.org/10.1053/j.trap.2015.01.008.
45. Cameron T. Safety and efficacy of spinal cord stimulation for the treatment of chronic pain: a 20-year literature review. J Neurosurg Spine. 2004;100(3):254–67. https://doi.org/10.3171/spi.2004.100.3.0254.

46. Kumar K, Buchser E, Linderoth B, Meglio M, Van Buyten J-P. Avoiding complications from spinal cord stimulation: practical recommendations from an international panel of experts. Neuromodulation. 2007;10(1):24–33. https://doi.org/10.1111/j.1525-1403.2007.00084.x.
47. Henderson JM, Schade CM, Sasaki J, Caraway DL, Oakley JC. Prevention of mechanical failures in implanted spinal cord stimulation systems. Neuromodulation. 2006;9(3):183–91. https://doi.org/10.1111/j.1525-1403.2006.00059.x.
48. Abejón D, Reig E, del Pozo C, Contreras R, Insausti J. Dual spinal cord stimulation for complex pain: preliminary study. Neuromodulation. 2005;8(2):105–11. https://doi.org/10.1111/j.1525-1403.2005.00226.x.
49. Desai MJ, et al. The rate of magnetic resonance imaging in patients with spinal cord stimulation. Spine (Phila Pa 1976). 2015;40(9):E531–7. https://doi.org/10.1097/BRS.0000000000000805.
50. Bedder MD, Bedder HF. Spinal cord stimulation surgical technique for the nonsurgically trained. Neuromodulation. 2009;12:1–19. https://doi.org/10.1111/j.1525-1403.2009.00194.x.
51. Moucha CS, Clyburn T, Evans RP, Prokuski L. Modifiable risk factors for surgical site infection. J Bone Joint Surg Am. 2011;93(4):398–404, [Online]. Available: http://www.ncbi.nlm.nih.gov/pubmed/21325594.
52. Bode LGM, et al. Preventing surgical-site infections in nasal carriers of Staphylococcus aureus. N Engl J Med. 2010;362(1):9–17. https://doi.org/10.1056/NEJMoa0808939.
53. Deer TR, Stewart CD. Complications of spinal cord stimulation: identification, treatment, and prevention. Pain Med. 2008;9(suppl 1):S93–S101. https://doi.org/10.1111/j.1526-4637.2008.00444.x.
54. Deer TR, Pope JE. Complications of spinal cord stimulation. In: Atlas of implantable therapies for pain management. New York: Springer New York; 2016. p. 93–103.
55. Beer GM, Wallner H. Prevention of seroma after abdominoplasty. Aesthetic Surg J. 2010;30(3):414–7. https://doi.org/10.1177/1090820X10374116.
56. Kloss BT, Sullivan AM, Rodriguez E. Epidural hematoma following spinal cord stimulator implant. Int J Emerg Med. 2010;3(4):483–4. https://doi.org/10.1007/s12245-010-0174-z.
57. Vandermeulen EP, Van Aken H, Vermylen J. Anticoagulants and spinal-epidural anesthesia. Anesth Analg. 1994;79(6):1165–77. https://doi.org/10.1213/00000539-199412000-00024.
58. Horlocker TT, et al. Regional anesthesia in the patient receiving antithrombotic or thrombolytic therapy; American Society of Regional Anesthesia and Pain Medicine evidence-based guidelines (Third Edition). Reg Anesth Pain Med. 2010;35(1):64–101. https://doi.org/10.1097/AAP.0b013e3181c15c70.
59. Franzini A, Ferroli P, Marras C, Broggi G. Huge epidural hematoma after surgery for spinal cord stimulation. Acta Neurochir. 2005;147(5):565–7. https://doi.org/10.1007/s00701-004-0470-6.
60. Lennarson PJ, Guillen FT. Spinal cord compression from a foreign body reaction to spinal cord stimulation: A previously unreported complication. Spine (Phila. Pa. 1976). 2010;35(25):E1516. https://doi.org/10.1097/BRS.0b013e3181ecc965.

Intrathecal Drug Delivery System: Surgical Technique

Antônio Jorge Barbosa de Oliveira, Plinio Duarte Mendes, Gilberto de Almeida Fonseca Filho, and Fabian C. Piedimonte

History and General Indications

From a historic point of view, the first report on the use of an analgesic substance in the subarachnoid space dates back to 1898, when August Bier, a famous German surgeon, described the analgesic effects of a solution containing cocaine, which he injected in himself and in his assistant [1]. The discovery of opioid receptors in the nervous system was reported by Pert and Snyder in 1973 [2]. Ten years later, Coombs and colleagues published the first study on the use of an implanted system of continuous intrathecal administration in ten patients, demonstrating satisfactory pain control [3]. The aim of the present chapter is to describe the main aspects related to patient selection, surgical technique, the refill technique for the implanted device, and the main complications in intrathecal drug delivery system (IDDS).

Implantable intrathecal opioid administration systems constitute well-established treatment for oncological pain and select cases of noncancer chronic pain [4]. With this method of analgesia, the medication is administered directly into the intrathecal space, reaching the dorsal horn of the spinal cord, which houses a high

A. J. Barbosa de Oliveira (✉)
Functional Neurosurgery / Pain treatment; Brasilia Pain Institute (INDOR), Brasilia, Brazil

Functional Neurosurgery Department, Hospital Sirio Libanes, Brasilia, Brazil

Neurosurgery Department, Associação de Assistência à Criança Deficiente – AACD, Sao Paulo, Brazil

P. Duarte Mendes · G. de Almeida Fonseca Filho
Functional Neurosurgery Department, Madre Teresa Hospital, Belo Horizonte, Brazil

Functional Neurosurgery Department, Biocor Institute, Nova Lima, Brazil

F. C. Piedimonte
Functional Neurosurgery, Fellow of Interventional Pain Procedures (FIPP/WIP), Buenos Aires, Argentina

T. d. S. Freitas et al. (eds.), *Neuromodulation Techniques for Pain Treatment*,
https://doi.org/10.1007/978-3-030-84778-4_17

concentration of receptors responsible for processing pain. This particularity minimizes systemic exposure to metabolites of the administered drug and enables pain relief with lower doses in comparison to oral or venous administration, thereby exerting fewer side effects [4].

Patient selection is the most important initial factor for therapeutic success. Thus, a comprehensive multidisciplinary assessment should be a prerequisite for decision-making, including all cases of neuropsychological and/or psychiatric evaluation. Patients with pain that is refractory to clinical treatment or those with satisfactory analgesia but intolerable side effects related to the proposed therapeutic regimen can be considered candidates for intrathecal therapy [4]. In patients with a weak response to systemic opioids, however, it is unlikely that satisfactory analgesia will result from the subarachnoid route [5]. In such cases, ziconotide may be an option. The IDDS is recommended for oncological patients whose life expectancy is longer than 3 months [4]. For those with a shorter life expectancy, the option is to use an epidural or subarachnoid catheter for analgesia.

According to the most recent Polyanalgesic Consensus Conference (PACC) held in 2017, the treatment of oncological and noncancer pain using an IDDS with morphine or ziconotide has level 1A evidence and recommendation. In cases of non-oncological pain, the preference is to initially use neurostimulation techniques (evidence level 3C) [4]. At present, IDDS is utilized for severe refractory pain and spasticity that has any other possibility to be treated with more conservative managements. There are other many clinical conditions under investigational trials with intrathecal therapy drugs such as epilepsy, psychiatric disorders, movement disorders, Alzheimer's disease, multiple sclerosis, and malignant hypertension.

Among exclusion criteria for therapy, we have [1] patients with a life expectancy less than 3 months, [2] skin infection near the implant site, [3] systemic infection, [4] coagulopathy (platelet count <7000/μL), [5] sparse drainage of cerebrospinal fluid (CSF) after the lumbar puncture, [6] a large spinal injury that impedes the free distribution of CSF, and [7] intolerance to the effect of the pre-implant test [6].

Trialing Techniques

After adequate patient selection, the next step is the pre-implant trial through epidural or intrathecal administration of the drugs to be tested (Table 1). It is important to perform this test in the hospital setting due to the possible emergence of the typical side effects of opioid use (nausea, vomiting, urinary retention, pruritus, sedation, and respiratory depression).

The test is considered positive when there is at least a 50% reduction in the numeric pain rating score. An improvement in functional performance and a reduction in the side effects of systemic medications are other indicators of success. The therapeutic effect of the bolus of morphine in the subarachnoid space begins about 30 minutes after administration and lasts 6 to 24 h [6, 7]. When ziconotide is

Table 1 Dose ranges for IT bolus trialing recommended [5]

Medications	Dose
Morphine	0.1–0.5 mg
Hydromorphone	0.025–0.1 mg
Ziconotide	1–5 mcg
Fentanyl	15–75 mcg
Bupivacaine	0.5–2.5 mg
Clonidine Sufentanil	5–20 mcg 5–20 mcg

chosen, the test should only be performed intrathecally; epidural administration of this drug is not permitted [8]. There is also the possibility of performing the test with an external pump connected to a catheter for the administration of the medication [5].

The pre-implant test has two purposes: [1] to define whether pain control is effective through the intrathecal route and [2] to guide the initial dose of the medication after the implant. There is no consensus on the administration method; it may be a single, multiple, or continuous [9]. The single administration option is considered a safe strategy (evidence level 2B) [10]. For patients with pain associated with cancer, it is necessary to assess the treatment options quickly and efficiently. In such cases, the PACC states that the test can be waived [5].

Surgical Technique

Preoperative Practices

The step-by-step process of the intraoperative procedure will be explained in the images below. The following practices are important to adopt prior to the surgical procedure: optimization of glycemic control, cessation of smoking (2 months before, if possible), screening for *Staphylococcus* colonization, and suspension of anticoagulant and antiplatelet agents (warfarin 5–7 days before and INR < 1.5; therapeutic heparin 24 h before; antiplatelet 7 days before; nonsteroidal anti-inflammatory 7 days before [no need to suspend selective COX-2 inhibitors]; consumption of ginseng, ginkgo biloba, and garlic 7 days before; new anticoagulants 3–5 days before). Anticoagulant and antiplatelet agents can be used again 24 h after the end of the procedure. A chlorhexidine wash 24 h prior to the surgery is also recommended [10].

A prophylactic antimicrobial should be administered 30 minutes prior to the skin incision. The options typically include cefuroxime IV or, if the patient is allergic to beta-lactam, clindamycin IV. These orientations may have variations in specific cases or depending on the infection control service of each hospital. Two sterile gloves shall be worn habitually during the procedure.

Marking

The definition of the flank in which the device will be implanted is performed with the patient awake and in dorsal decubitus to avoid errors due to the deviation of the abdominal wall when in lateral decubitus. Assess the patient decubitus preference to reduce the possibility of routinely lying atop the device; ensure intact skin with no scars from previous procedures; and, in cases of colostomy or gastrostomy, implant the device on the contralateral side as far away as possible. Consider an appropriate site so that the device does not rub against the iliac crest below or the costal arches above. The location of the pump on the abdominal wall should be planned in advance and based on the possible need for future surgical interventions related to the baseline disease. If the patient has no preference for either of the sides and there is no special circumstance that justifies a specific location, opt for the left side due the lower frequency of diseases requiring surgery in this region; for example, appendicitis and cholecystitis are conditions that affect the right side of the abdomen. All such planning should occur previously during office visits, reserving the day of the procedure only for the marking of the skin.

Positioning

Under general anesthesia, the patient should be carefully positioned in lateral decubitus, comfortably supporting the upper and lower limbs. Tethers should be used to secure the thoracic region, pelvic region, and lower limbs to avoid accidents in case there is a need to move the surgical table (Fig. 1a). Place cushions under the flank and axilla for protection (Fig. 1b). Prior to antisepsis of the skin, the C-arm of the X-ray machine should be positioned freely to be moved to enable the anteroposterior view and profile, facilitating the lumbar puncture, the visualization of the passage of the catheter, and the appropriate localization of the tip in the desired target. Although some guidelines suggest performing the procedure only under sedation and local anesthesia so that the patient can report any possible neurological effects due to the progression of the catheter, we routinely perform it under general anesthesia, considering the surgical procedure and steps following the lumbar puncture.

Skin Preparation and Draping

The patient is submitted to epilation, followed by rigorous antisepsis of the lumbar region, flank, and abdomen (Fig. 2a and b). Sterile adhesive and surgical fields are draped with adequate exposure for the procedure. The C-arm also needs to be draped with sterile fields (Fig. 2c).

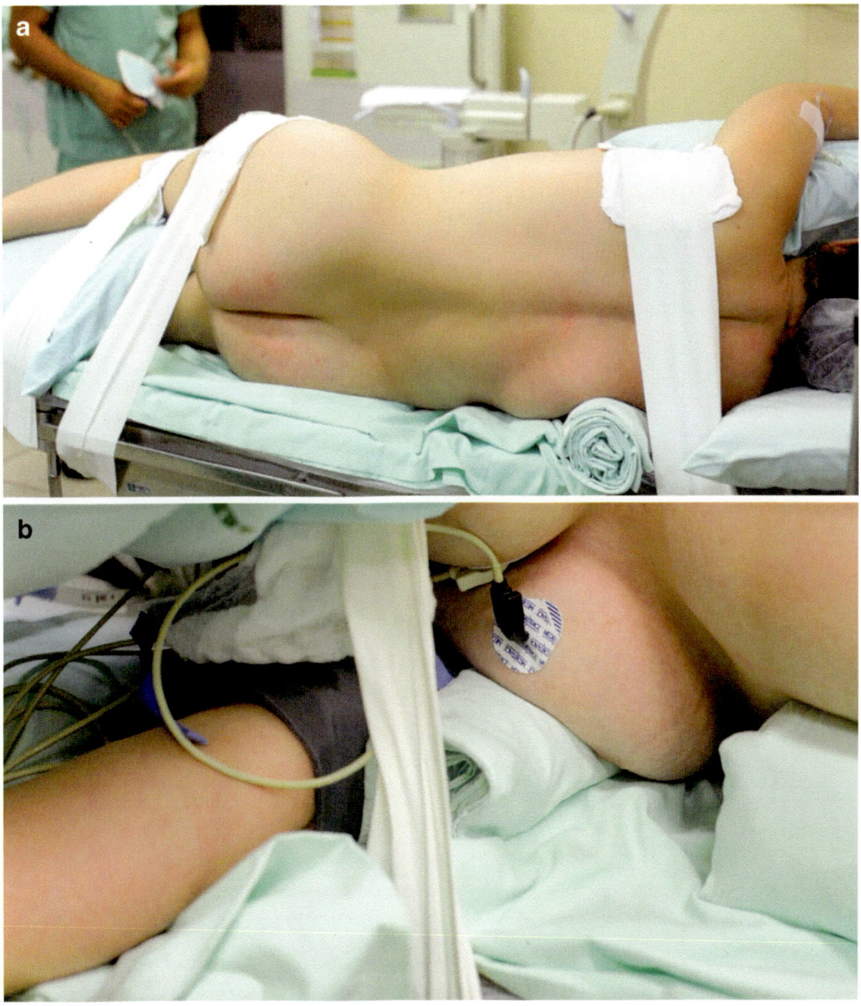

Fig. 1 (**a**) Positioning. Tethers to secure the thoracic region, pelvic region, and lower limbs. (**b**) Cushions under the flank and axilla for protection

Preparation of Pump

At the onset of the operation, the pump should be taken out of the sterile package and be prepared in accordance with the manufacturer's instructions simultaneously to the progression of the surgery in order to be ready for use at the proper time. Fill it carefully after verifying the chosen medication and concentration (Fig. 3).

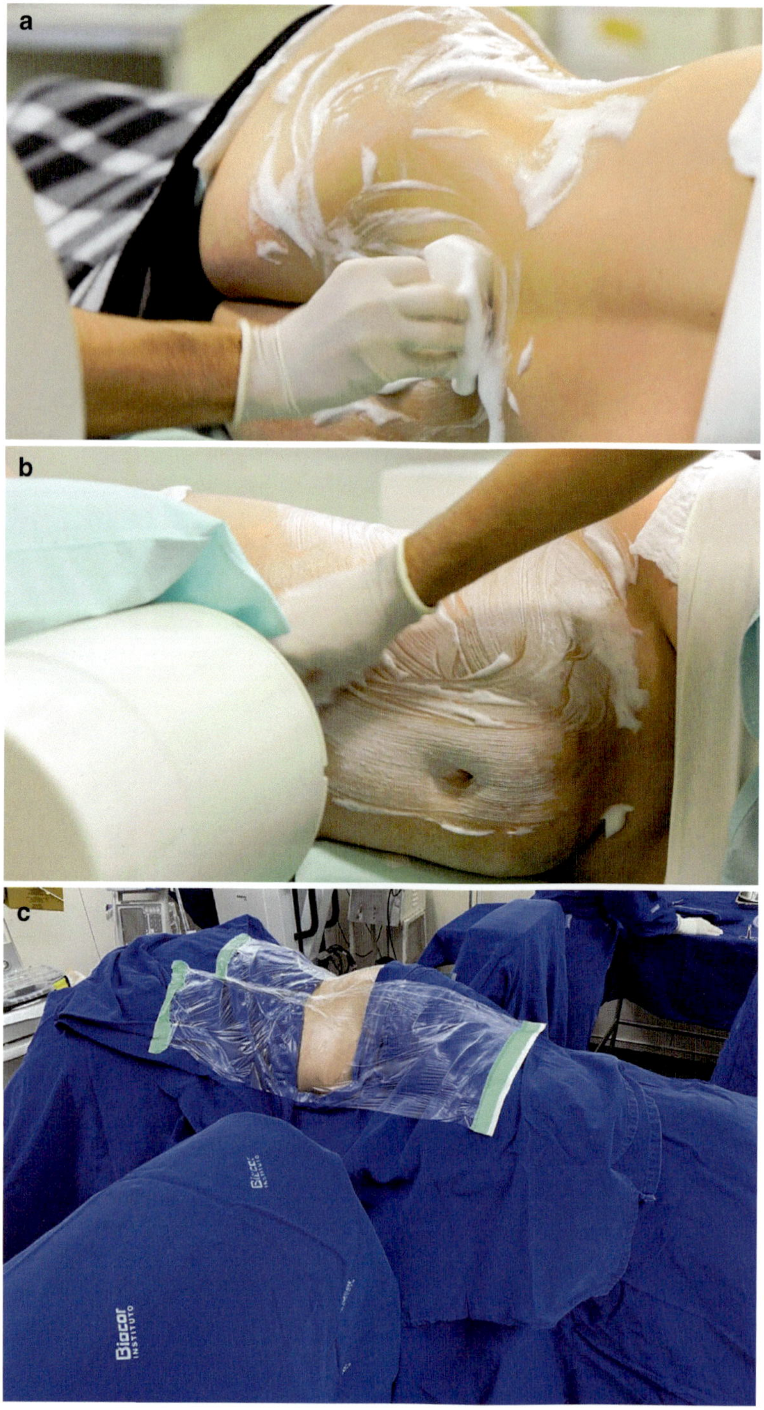

Fig. 2 (**a**) Skin preparation. (**b**) Skin preparation. (**c**) Fluoroscopy positioning, sterile fields, and draping

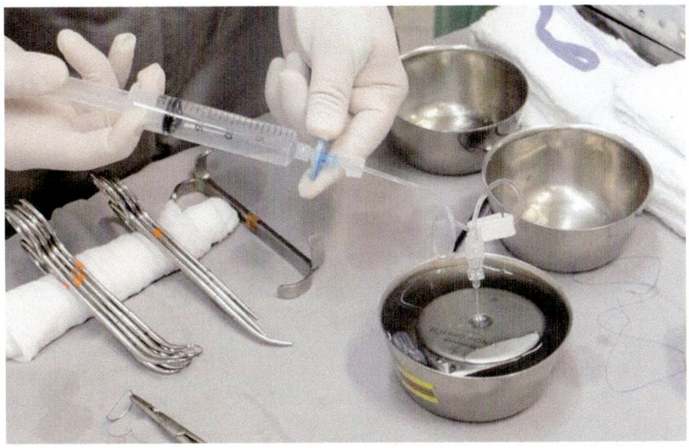

Fig. 3 Preparing the pump

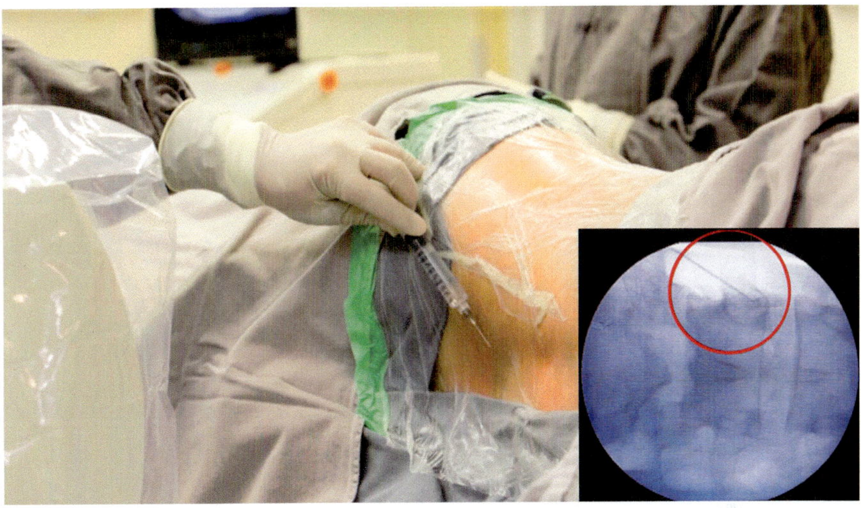

Fig. 4 Anesthesia of the paramedian puncture site and needle path

Intrathecal Access and Catheter Placement

The first step of the operation is the administration of the anesthesia of the puncture site and needle path (Figs. 4 and 5a). Next, guided by the X-ray machine, a paramedian lumbar puncture is performed at an angle of approximately 30–45 degrees, ideally on the same side on which the tunneling will be performed to the subarachnoid space (Fig. 5b). The entry point on the skin should be 1–2 levels below the entry site in the dura mater (L2–L4) and should ensure abundant drainage of the CSF through the catheter after the puncture (Fig. 5c). With regard to the final positioning of the tip of the spinal catheter, although we are aware that morphine, which is water soluble, diffuses to higher levels of the spinal cord, we prefer to position the catheter closer in accordance with the pain site (Figs. 6 and 7). Whenever possible, leave the tip of the catheter posterior to

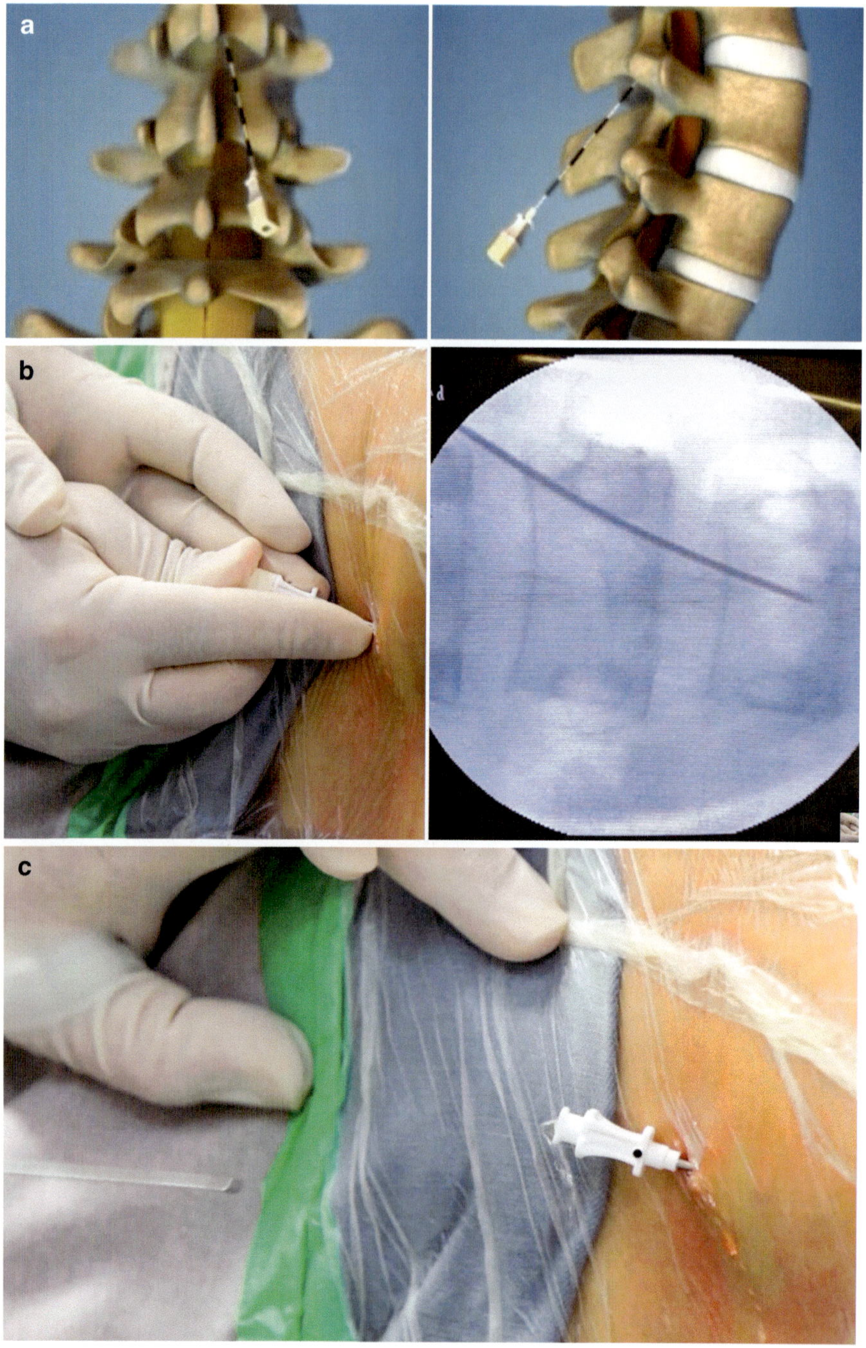

Fig. 5 (**a**) Puncture planning (authorized by Medtronic). (**b**) Paramedian lumbar puncture. Fluoroscopic view of the needle being advanced toward the interlaminar space. (**c**) Abundant CSF drainage

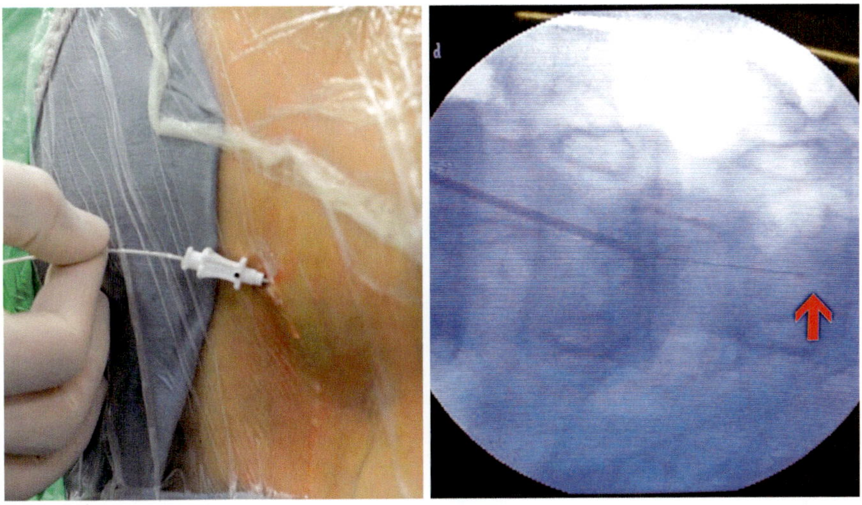

Fig. 6 The catheter has been placed through the needle and into the intrathecal space

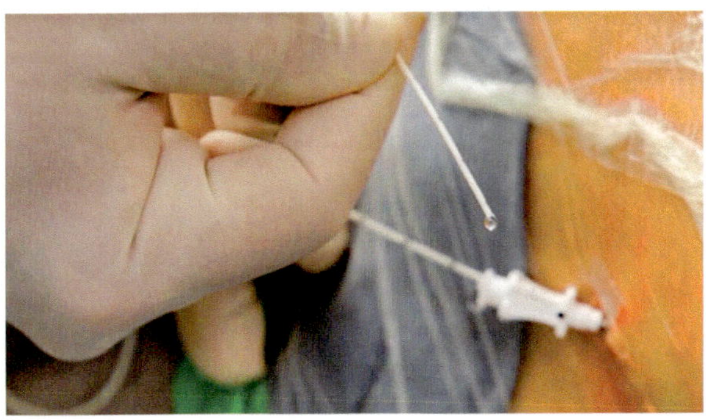

Fig. 7 CSF drainage

the spinal cord. The progression of the spinal catheter should be performed carefully and accompanied by the X-ray machine (Fig. 8), so that, in the occurrence of resistance, the mandrel can be removed to enable proceeding with the desired positioning. The habitual location is between T2 and T8 for cases of thoracic pain, between T4 and T12 for pain in the upper floor of the abdomen, between T10 and L3 for cases of pain in the lower floor of the abdomen, between C4 and C7 for pain in the upper limbs, and between T12 and L3 for pain in the lower limbs. In cases of craniofacial pain, we place the catheter at the C2 or intraventricular level [7]. Better results are expected when there is adequate correlation of dermatomes and the level corresponding to the pain (evidence level 2B) [4].

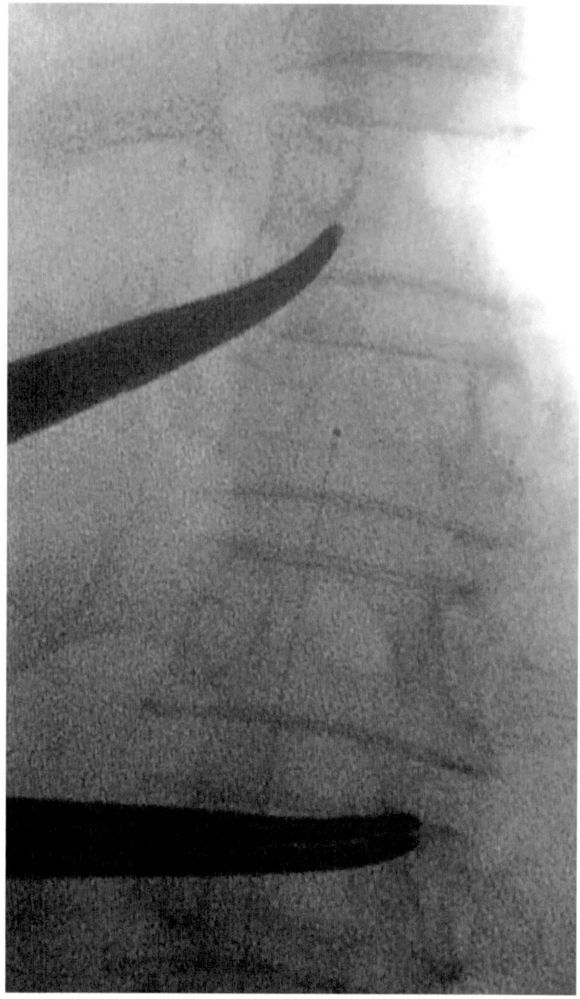

Fig. 8 Catheter tip X-ray view

Lumbar Incision, Dissection, and Catheter Anchoring

The next step is to make an incision approximately 3–5 cm along the needle through the subcutaneous and adipose tissue until the exposure of its entry in the muscle fascia (Fig. 9). Before removing the needle, position the nonabsorbable threads that will affix the anchor of the catheter to maintain the catheter protected. The needle should then be carefully removed, maintaining the position of the catheter stable by securing it with the fingers as soon it appears after the exiting of the needle from the fascia (Fig. 10). Finalize the removal of the rest of the needle and mandrel of the catheter if it had not previously been removed. At this point, check the positioning of the X-ray machine and the presence of CSF. Using a device furnished by the

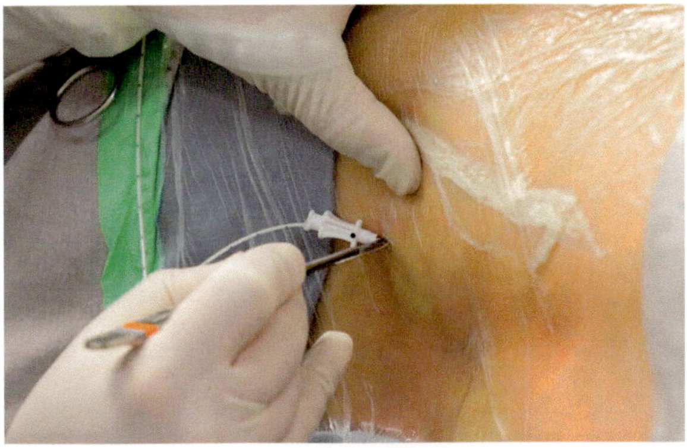

Fig. 9 Incision along the needle

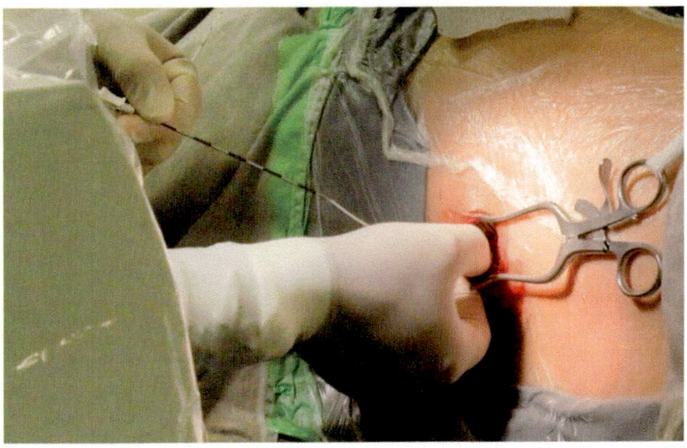

Fig. 10 Needle removal

manufacturer, affix the catheter after verifying its final position and perform suturing so that the anchor is preferable lying to the side to be tunneled (Figs. 11a, b and 12).

Pump Pocket Creation and Anchoring Suture Placement

Make a rectilinear incision in the abdomen parallel to and approximately 5 cm from the costal arch, dissecting to the fascia of the rectus abdominis/external oblique muscle and creating a pouch where the pump will be housed (Fig. 13). Avoid electrocauterization due to the risk of skin injuries and infection. The pouch should be wide enough so that the pump does not place pressure on the subcutaneous tissue, which could lead to its exposure to the external environment. The size of the pouch should not surpass the dimensions of the device excessively, as this could lead to the accumulation of seroma and the displacement of the device (Fig. 14). The anchoring sutures are then minimally placed at two points to avoid movements (Fig. 15).

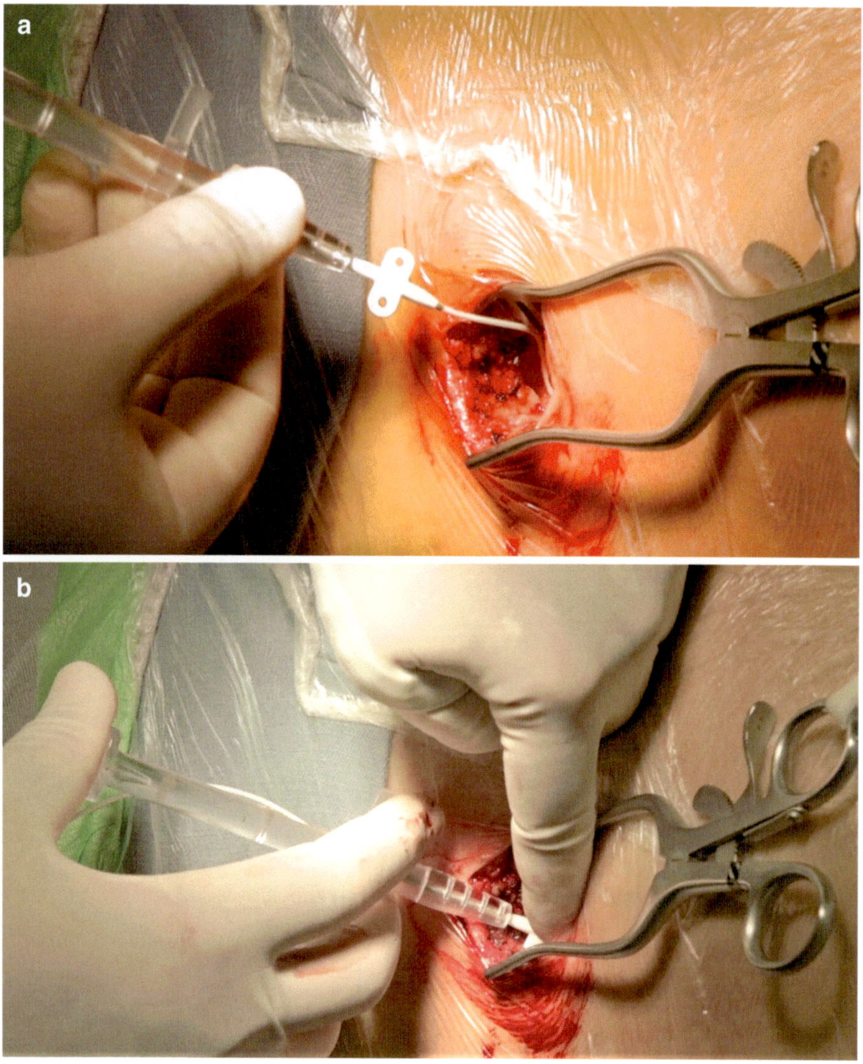

Fig. 11 (**a**) Positioning of anchor, (**b**) Positioning of anchor

Tunneling

Tunneling of the catheter is performed from the lumbar region to the pouch where the pump will be implanted on the anterior face of the abdomen between the iliac crest and costal margin (Fig. 16a, b, and c). We recommend the administration of local anesthetic with a vasoconstrictor for better postoperative analgesia and less

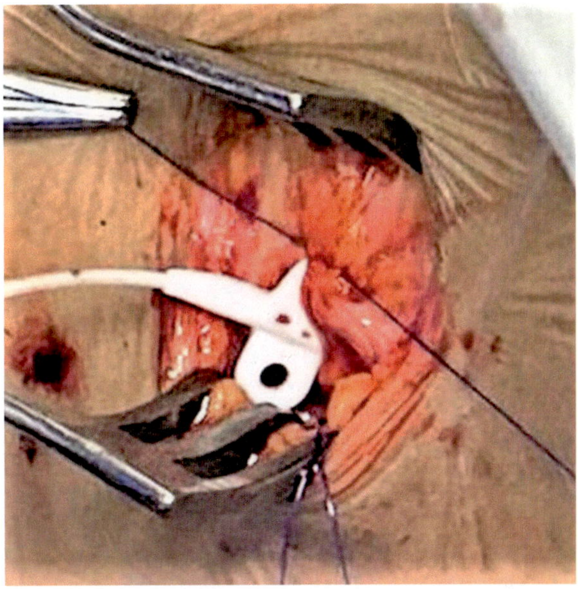

Fig. 12 Catheter anchoring

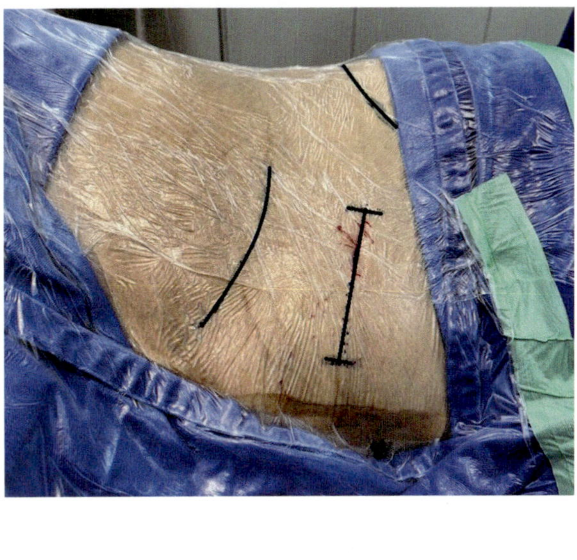

Fig. 13 The rectilinear abdominal incision. Far away from costal arches above and the iliac crest

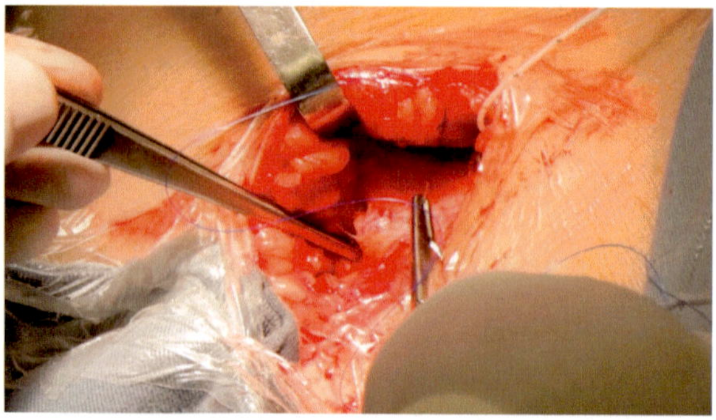

Fig. 14 Dissection down to the rectus fascia. Placement of anchoring sutures

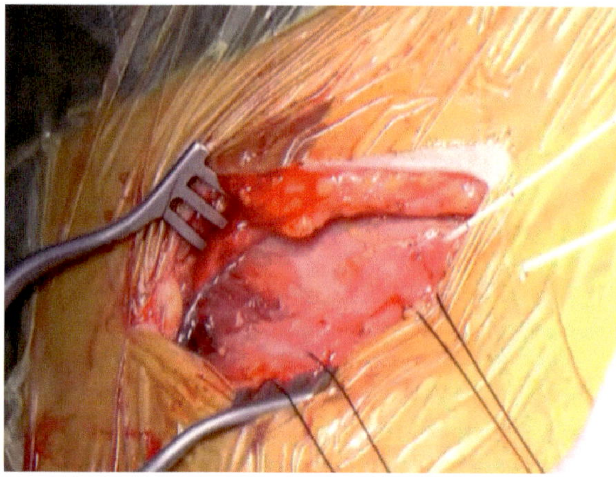

Fig. 15 2 points anchoring suture

likelihood of hematomas along the catheter path. Connect the catheter to the pump (Fig. 17). A small part of the catheter should be maintained adjacent to the lumbar fixation point to avoid traction and possible migration. For obese patients, it may be necessary to perform the tunneling in two steps, making a small incision in the skin in order to externalize the tunneling tool and make a new passageway. Whenever possible, give preference to maintaining the catheter in its original size without sectioning it.

Pump Insertion and Skin Closure

The pump is inserted and positioned in the pouch, followed by the closing of the incision, beginning with the deepest layer, followed by the subcutaneous layer and skin. The catheter excess should be folded together and positioned posterior to the pump to avoid accidents during the refill punctures. The device should be placed such that the access port to the catheter is positioned caudally to avoid pressure on

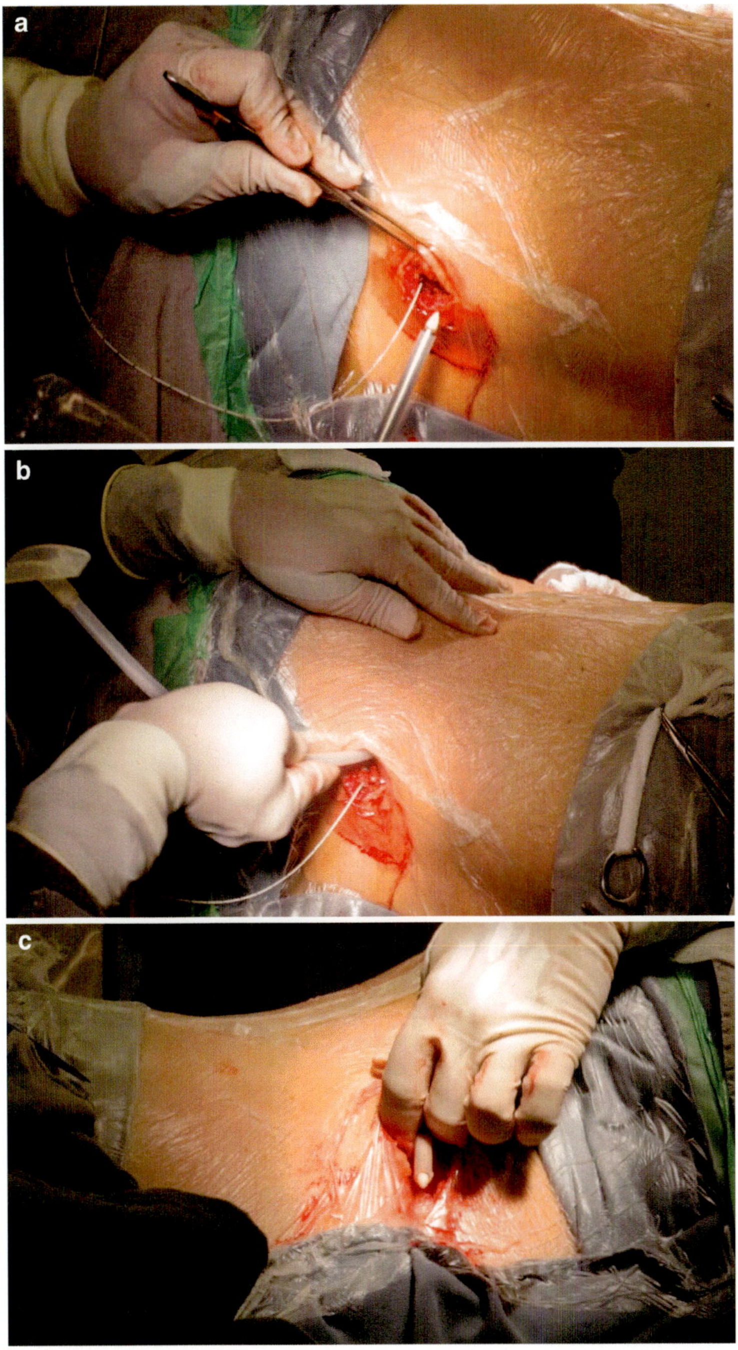

Fig. 16 (**a**) Tunneling from the lumbar incision to the pump pocket. (**b**) Tunneling from the lumbar incision to the pump pocket. (**c**) Tunneling from the lumbar incision to the pump pocket

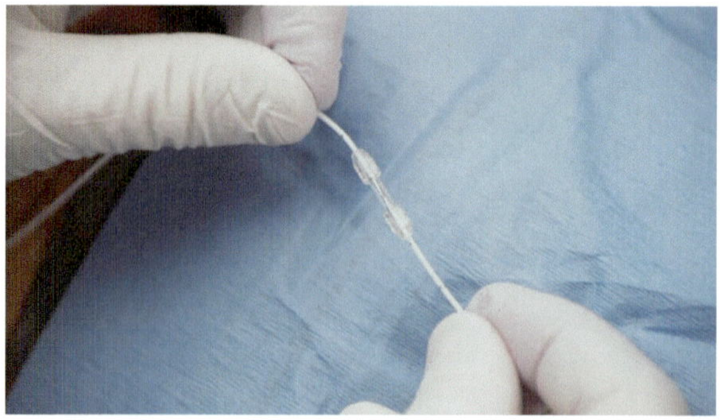

Fig. 17 Attaching the intrathecal segment to the pump segment and the catheter to the pump

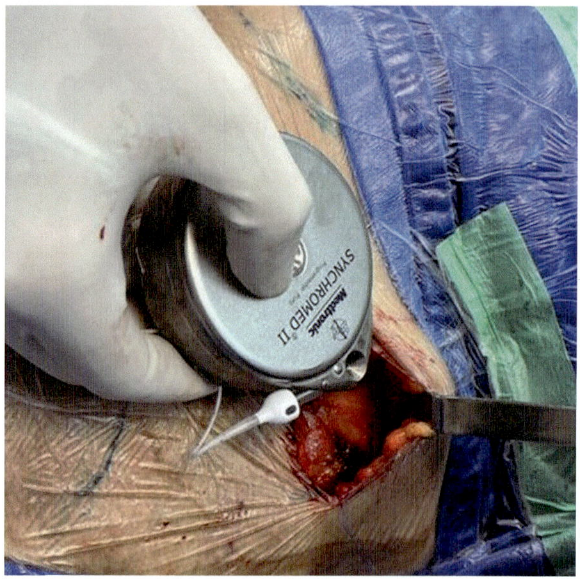

Fig. 18 Pump being inserted into the pocket

the wound (Figs. 18, 19, 20, 21a and b). We suggest occlusive dressing for 24–48 h and antibiotic prophylaxis for only 24 h, with no use of topical antibiotics (evidence level 1A–B) [10].

Pump Refills

The pump should be refilled a maximum of every 6 months, even when it is not completely empty, due to possible changes in the stability of the medication over a long period [11]. The refill frequency commonly ranges from several weeks to

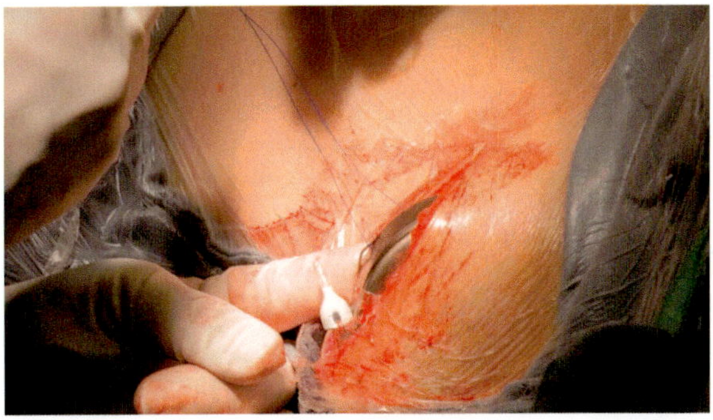

Fig. 19 Anchoring suture placement

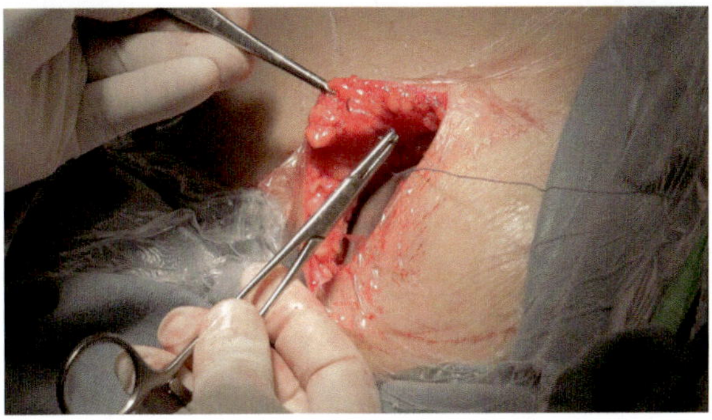

Fig. 20 Skin closure. Beginning with the deepest layer

6 months depending on the infusion speed, which is fixed in continuous flow pumps and predetermined or individualized in programmable electronic pumps.

We strongly recommend the use of the kit provided by the manufacturer with the material to be used during the refill procedure (Fig. 22a). Adequate antisepsis is first performed of the skin over the pump, followed by the draping of a sterile field. Next, a puncture is performed of the septum made of self-sealing silicone, which is located in the central portion of the device (Fig. 22b and c). In some cases, the identification of the pump septum is hindered due to scar tissue or excess adipose tissue, which may require the use of ultrasound or C-arm imaging for the proper localization. After the insertion of the needle through the septum, the residual medication solution is removed prior to refilling, with care taken to avoid the entrance of air during the process. The new medication is then injected into the reservoir and the refilling is concluded (Fig. 22d). With a programmable electronic pump, the reading should then be made, followed by reprogramming with the new medication volume and new concentration, if necessary [11]. With a gas pump, care must be taken to previously calculate the concentration of the medication to be administered.

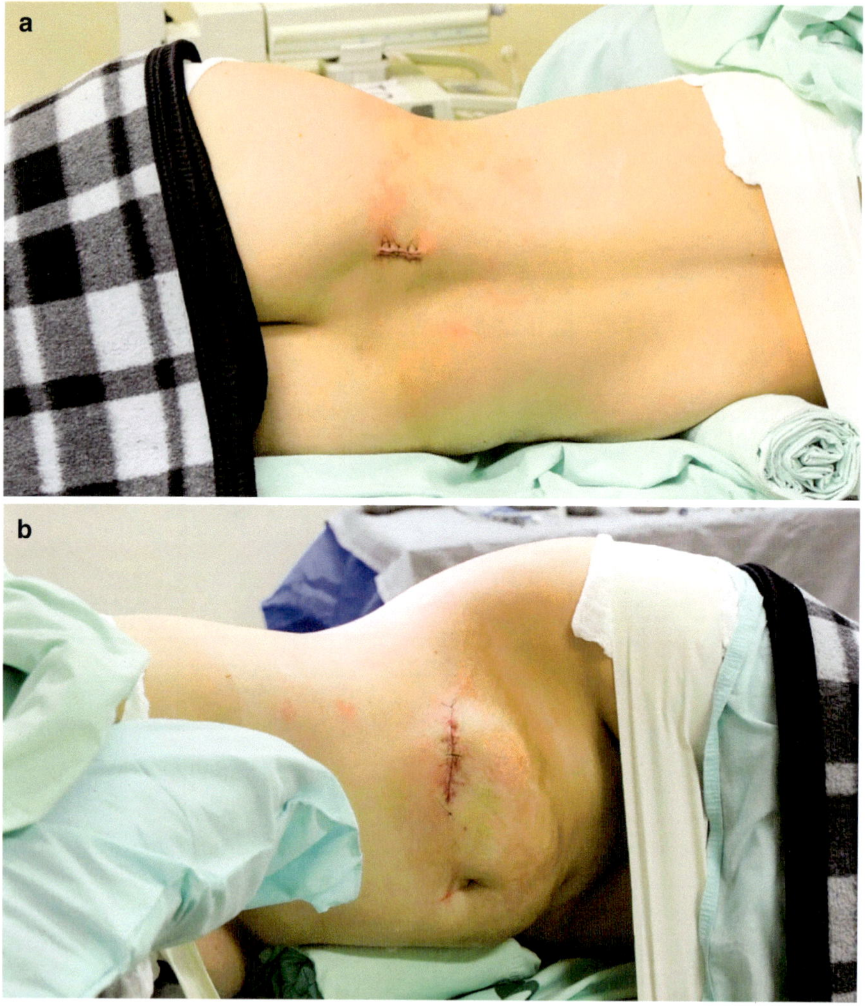

Fig. 21 (a) Final aspect of lumbar skin closure. (b) Final aspect of abdominal skin closure

Types of Infusion Pumps

Mechanically Driven

This is operated by the patient himself or a family member. It comprises a drug reservoir that is connected to a one-direction valve system, which in turn is connected to a catheter that takes the medication flow into the subarachnoid space. Access to the reservoir is done through a space designed for refilling. Digital pressing of the buttons on the device activate bolus release of the drug (Fig. 23).

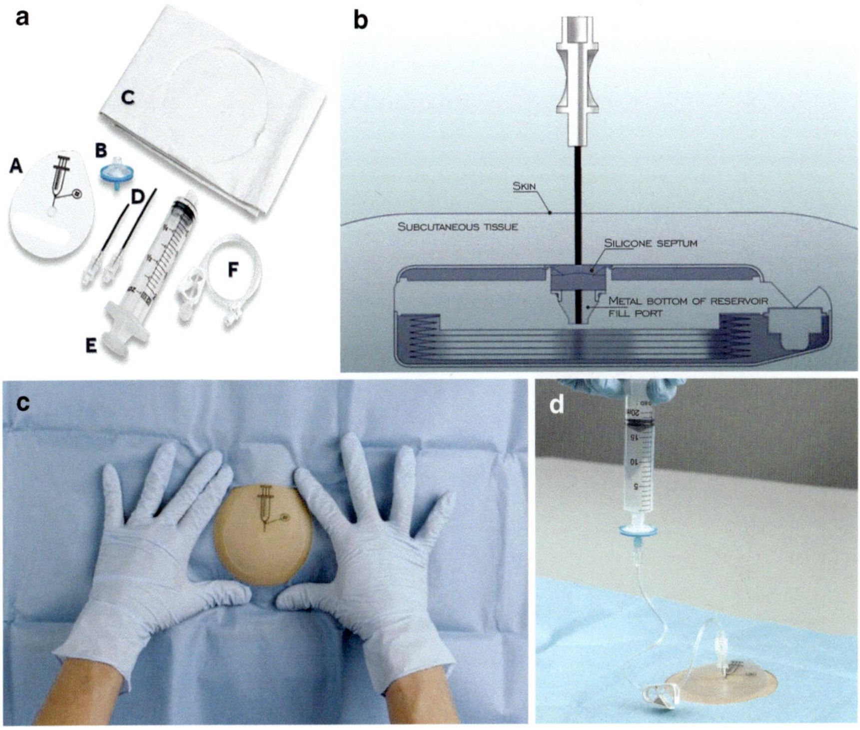

Fig. 22 (**a**) Refill kit (authorized by Medtronic). (**b**) Puncture pump central septum. (**c**) Skin prepare (authorized by Medtronic). (**d**) Pump refill (authorized by Medtronic)

The disadvantages of this device include only bolus dosing, need for self-administration, and risk of intoxication, although it contains safety mechanisms that prevent subsequent doses. In addition, the assessment during days following implantation can be challenging, due the postoperative edema and serosal collection.

Gas Propulsion

These systems enable continuous infusion into the intrathecal space by gas propulsion mechanism. They have two compartments: a reservoir, which can be accessed through a silicone septum for regular refilling and other containing an inert gas (Freon, butane, or R114) performing constant pressure on the first providing outflow to intrathecal space. Most of these devices are fitted with a lateral septum that provides access to the spinal catheter and allows for withdrawing cerebrospinal fluid (CSF) for examination, injection of contrast dye, or even for medication injection. There is a constant flow preset by

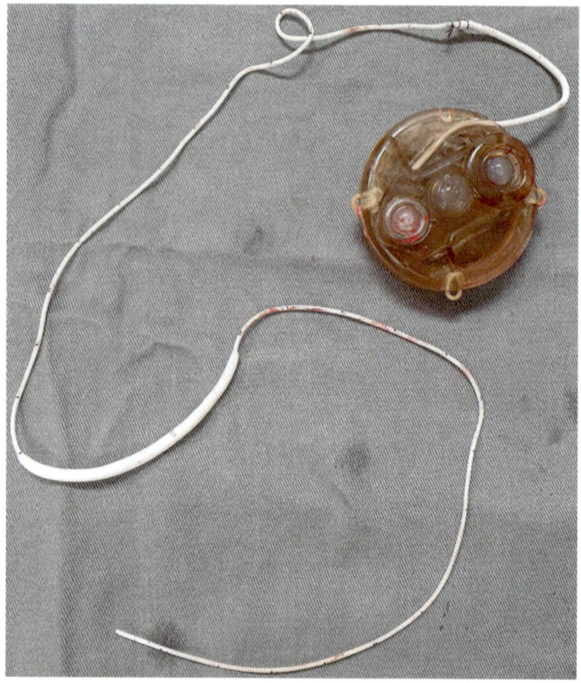

Fig. 23 Mechanical pump

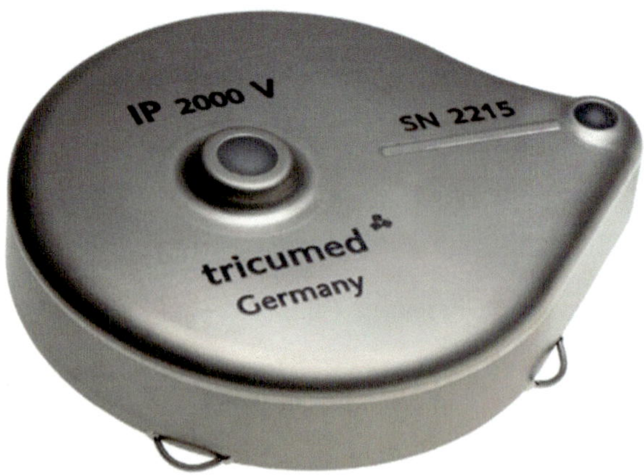

Fig. 24 Gas-flow pump IP 2000 V (authorized by Tricumed Medizintechnik GmbH)

the manufacturer and varies between 0.3 and 4.0 ml/day and its volume capacity about 20–60 ml (Fig. 24). It's necessary changing concentrations to shift medication dosage. The shelf-life depends mainly of the puncture frequency, up to 1000 recharges with correct refill kit. It can be advantageous cause is usually cheaper than other devices and cases with difficulty in regular medical access.

Programmable Infusion Pump

The most used nowadays comprises a drug reservoir, which is accessible through a silicon septum for regular replacement of the drug: a different compartment containing gas that forces the content into a rotor driven on a battery engine that collapses at each tube revolution of the roulette pump and a microprocessor that allows flexible programming, for example, bolus, continuous, or variable (Figs. 25 and 26). There are also auto-checking software and alarms to verify volume, battery, and other functions. The major volume capacities are between 10 and 40 ml. Still, the patient can control the therapy by itself with an external device (Fig. 27), if allowed by the attending physician. On the other hand, it is necessary to have regular battery changes.

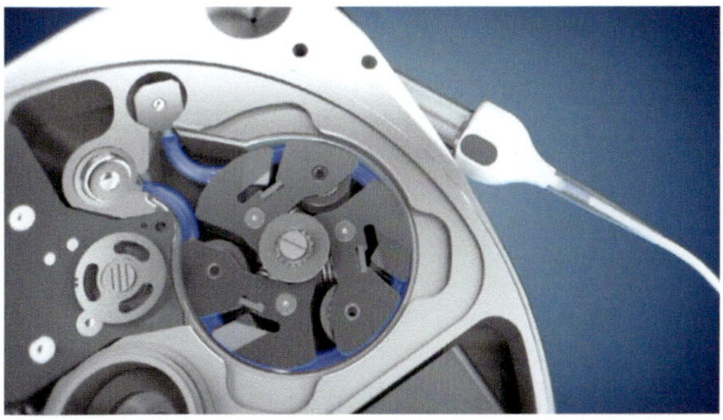

Fig. 25 Roulette programmable pump (authorized by Medtronic)

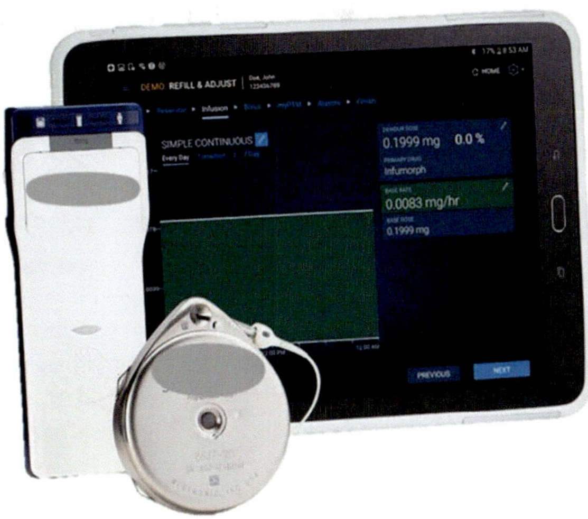

Fig. 26 Programmable pump (authorized by Medtronic)

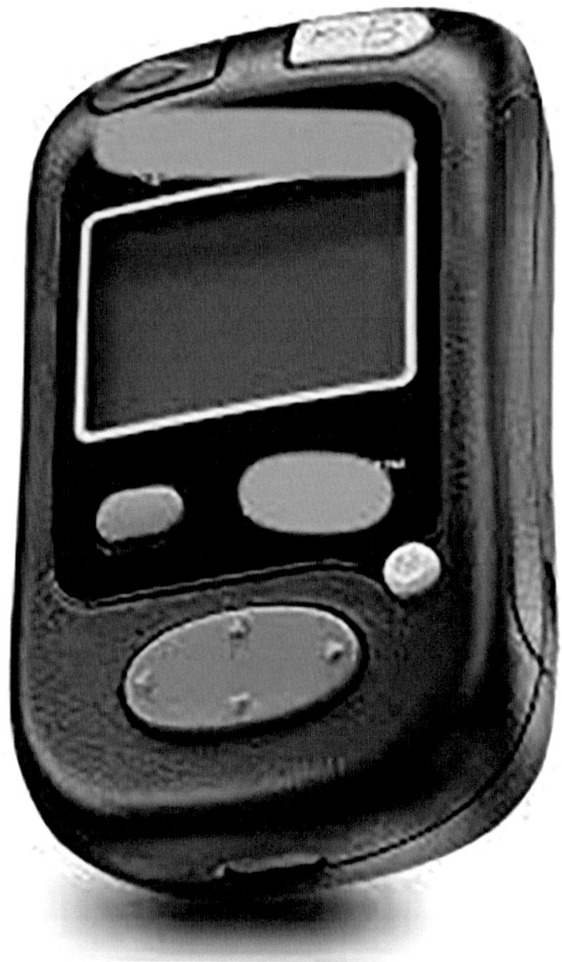

Fig. 27 Patient control (authorized by Medtronic)

Complications

There are various complications that may occur during the use of the IDDS related to the indication, effects of the medication in use, the surgical procedure, the implanted device, the refill, and the telemetric programming of the device. The main complications are listed in Table 2 [8]. The most frequent is post-puncture headache (15.5%), followed by infection (3.5–4.5%) and seroma (2.5%) [9].

Although rare, the formation of catheter-tip granuloma is a feared and potentially serious complication. The reported prevalence is up to 8%, with symptoms in 0.5 to 3% of cases. This condition results from the growth of macrophages, neutrophils, and monocytes that adhere to the dura mater and, at times, the spinal cord [12]. The

Table 2 Complications during the use of the IDDS [9]

Medication
Pruritus
Nausea and vomiting
Urinary retention
Constipation
Fluid retention
Respiratory depression
Sedation
Intraoperative
Bleeding
Neurological deficits related to tissue damage
Cerebrospinal fluid leaks
Infections
Skin ulcers
Catheter
Breaking
Kinking
Disconnections
Catheter-tip granuloma
Migration
Pump
Overfilling
Battery failure
Pump torsion
Wrong refill
Programming errors

formation of catheter-tip granuloma seems to be linked to the greater concentration of the infused drug in a small area, with little CSF flow and for a long period. There are reports of this occurrence with all drugs, except ziconotide. Any new focal neurological condition should be actively investigated with imaging exams, such as magnetic resonance with gadolinium or myelotomography. The most common presentations are the loss of effective pain relief, the frequent need for adjusting the dose, residual volume greater than the predicted volume during the refilling of the pump, altered proprioception and sensitivity, and, in more advanced cases, motor, bladder, and intestinal impairment [13]. The use of flexible systems with a bolus during therapy seems to diminish the incidence (evidence level 3C) [10].

Surgical site infection corresponds to 3.5–4.5% [14]. Inherent of any surgery, it has similar patterns as neurostimulation. The PACC/CDC consensus has specific recommendations at each stage to mitigate such situations (Fig. 28a, b, c, and d).

In addition, other complication is hematoma, difficult to assess, with variable incidence around 0.3–0.7% [4, 14], the same as other interventional pain procedures in neuroaxis and must follow standard precautions. In general, it is classified as an intermediate risk. Although rare, the most cited is epidural, subdural, and pocket hematoma, which must be highly suspicious and treated early due to the risk of serious sequelae (Fig. 29a and b).

The following are some more images about illustrative case complications (Fig. 30a–e).

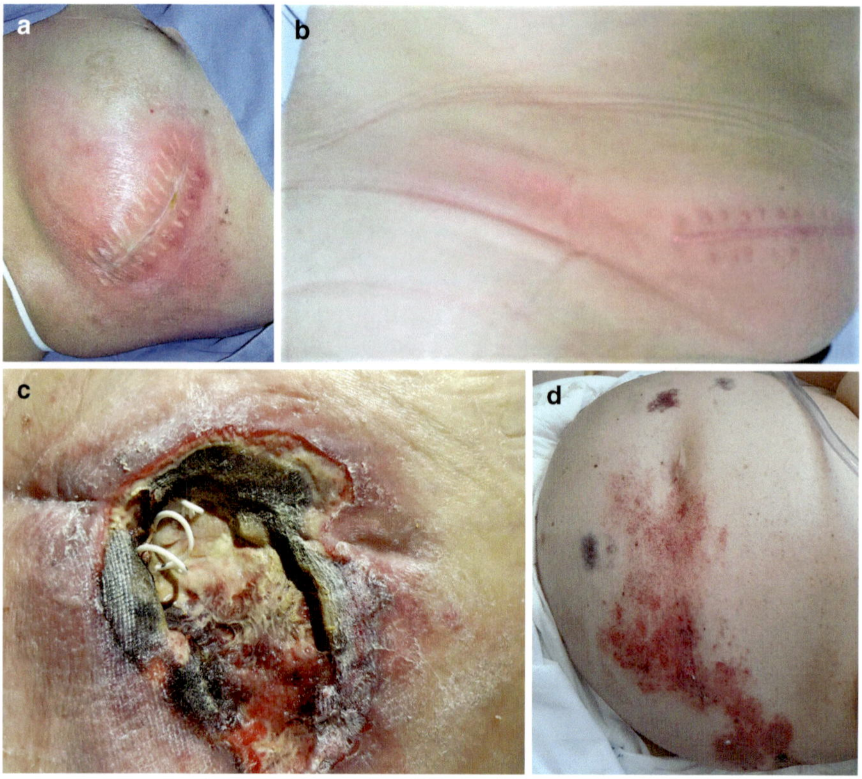

Fig. 28 (**a**) Pump infection. (**b**) Pump and catheter infection. (**c**): Intrathecal catheter exposed. (**d**) Herpes zoster infection on IDDS trajectory (oncology patient)

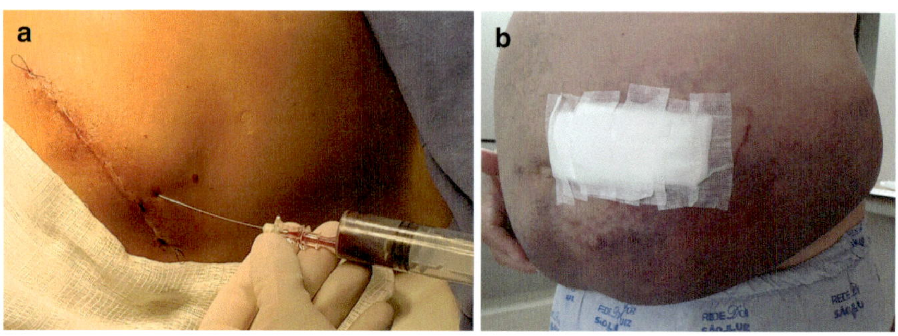

Fig. 29 (**a**) Hematoma. (**b**) Trajectory hematoma

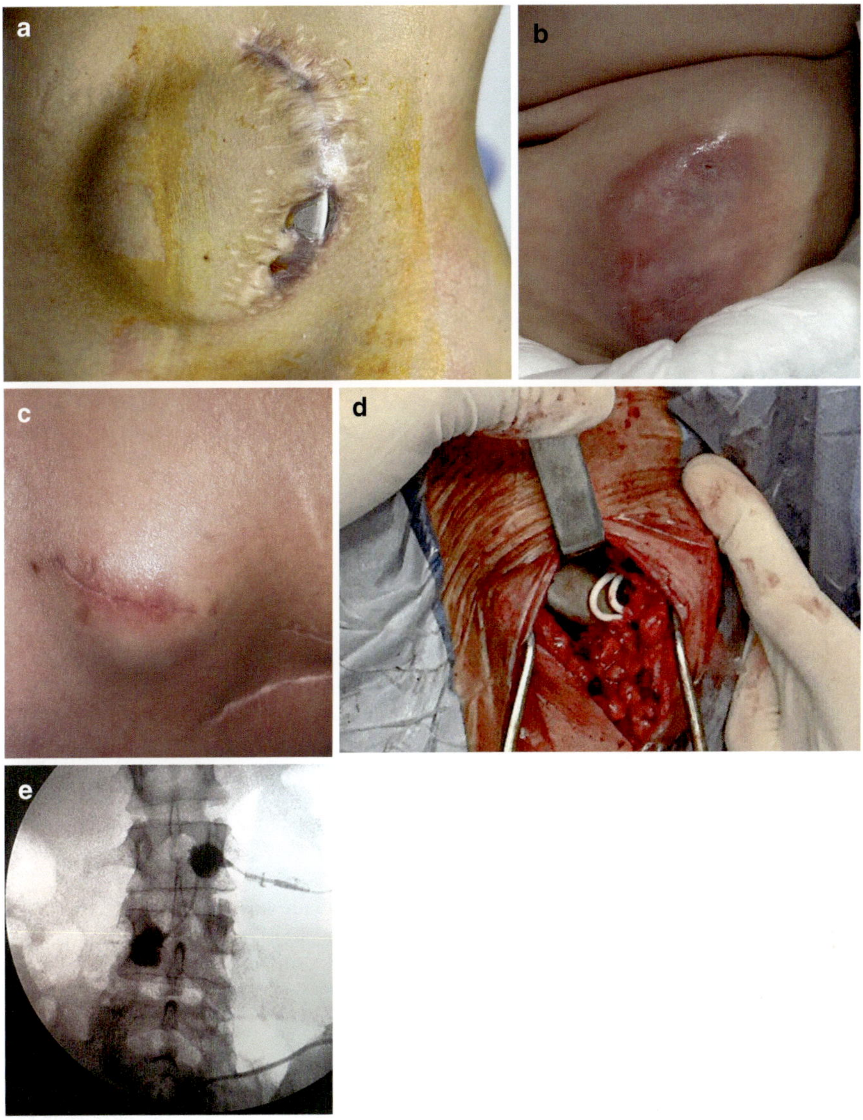

Fig. 30 (**a**) Skin ulcer. (**b**) Skin ulcer 2. (**c**) Pseudomeningocele (hygroma). (**d**) Mispositioned multi-perforated catheter. (**e**) Contrast dye study with system leakage

Medications

Although there are studies with several drugs, below a brief summary with the main ones used for knowledge of the main aspects will be highlighted. According to the last PACC consensus, only morphine and ziconotide have 1A level of evidence for intrathecal use [4].

Morphine

Morphine is the most widely used, with proven efficacy both in cancer patients and those with benign diseases. With IDDS, there is a downward trend of opioids by other routes. Different studies show more than 70% improvement in pain levels in more than a half of patients [15]. The most serious side effect is respiratory depression [16], especially at the beginning of therapy or when concomitant use of central nervous system depressants, such as benzodiazepines, besides the other classical ones that may occur with opioid users. In the long term, it can also result in suppression of the pituitary and gonadal axis [4].

Ziconotide

Considered the first line of treatment for both neuropathic and nociceptive pain by Food and Drug Administration (FDA), it can be useful in patients with trial failure with opioids, although it needs special care due to the proximity of the therapeutic dose and the toxic one [4]. It acts by blocking presynaptic N-type calcium channels in the dorsal horn of the spinal cord. This targeting is distinctly different from mu agonism and allows ziconotide to be helpful in the opioid-tolerant patient [17]. There isn't evidence of any spinal toxicity, however contraindicated in case of suspected psychosis, when must be stopped immediately [18].

References

1. Brill S, Gurman GM, Fisher A. A history of neuraxial administration of local analgesics and opioids. Eur J Anaesthesiol. 2003;20:682–9.
2. Pert CB, Snyder SH. Opiate receptor: demonstration in nervous tissue. Science. 1973;179:1011–4.
3. Coombs DW, Saunders RL, Gaylor MS, Block AR, Colton T, Harbaugh R, et al. Relief of continuous chronic pain by intraspinal narcotics infusion via an implanted reservoir. JAMA. 1983;250:2336–9.
4. Deer TR, Pope JE, Hayek SM, Bux A, Buchser E, Eldabe S, et al. The Polyanalgesic Consensus Conference (PACC): recommendation on intrathecal drug infusion systems best practices and guidelines. Neuromodulation. 2017;20(2):96–132.
5. Deer TR, Hayek SM, Pope JE, Lamer TJ, Hamza M, Grider JS, et al. The Polyanalgesic Consensus Conference (PACC): recommendations for trialing of intrathecal drug delivery infusion therapy. Neuromodulation. 2017;20(2):133–54.
6. Wallace M, Yaksh TL. Long-term spinal analgesic delivery: a review of the preclinical and clinical literature. Reg Anesth Pain Med. 2000;25(2):117–57.
7. Fonseca G. Intrathecal infusion pumps. In: Cukiert A, editor. Functional neurosurgery. 1st ed. São Paulo: Alaude; 2014. p. 352–73.
8. Gulati A, Puttanniah V, Hung J, Malhotra V. Considerations for evaluating the use of intrathecal drug delivery in the oncologic patient. Curr Pain Headache Rep. 2014;18(2):391.

9. Sol JC, Verdie JC, Lazorthes Y. Intrathecal opiates for cancer pain. In: Lozano AM, Gildenberg PL, Tasker RR, editors. Textbook of stereotactic and functional neurosurgery. 2nd ed. Berlin: Springer; 2009. p. 2171–96.
10. Deer TR, Pope JE, Hayek SM, Lamer TJ, Veizi IE, Erdek M, Wallace MS, Grider JS, Levy RM, Prager J, Rosen SM, Saulino M, Yaksh TL, De Andrés JA, Abejon Gonzalez D, Vesper J, Schu S, Simpson B, Mekhail N. The Polyanalgesic Consensus Conference (PACC): recommendations for intrathecal drug delivery: guidance for improving safety and mitigating risks. Neuromodulation. 2017;20(2):155–76.
11. Bottros MM, Christo PJ. Current perspectives on intrathecal drug delivery. J Pain Res. 2014;7:615–26.
12. Deer TR. A prospective analysis of intrathecal granuloma in chronic pain patients: a review of the literature and report of a surveillance study. Pain Physicisn. 2004;7(2):225–8.
13. Hassenbush S, Burchiel K, Coffey R, et al. Management of intrathecal catheter-tip inflammatory masses: a consensus statement. Pain Med. 2002;3:313–23.
14. Deer TR, et al. 2014. The appropriate use of neurostimulation: avoidance and treatment of complications of neurostimulation therapies for the treatment of chronic pain. Neuromodulation. 2014;17:571–98.
15. Reig E, Abejon D. Continuous morphine infusion: a retrospective study of efficacy, safety, and demographic variables. Neuromodulation. 2009;12:122–9.
16. Coffey RJ, Owens ML, Broste SK, et al. Mortality associated with implantation and management of intrathecal opioid drug infusion systems to treat noncancer pain. Anesthesiology. 2009;111:881–91.
17. Rauck RL, Wallace MS, Leong MS, et al. A randomized, double-blind, placebo-controlled study of intrathecal ziconotide in adults with severe chronic pain. J Pain Symptom Manag. 2006;31:393–406.
18. Hayek SM, Hanes MC, Wang C, Veizi IE. Ziconotide combination intrathecal therapy for noncancer pain is limited secondary to delayed adverse effects: a case series with a 24-month follow-up. Neuromodulation. 2015;18:397–403.

Intracerebroventricular Drug Infusion System Implant: Surgical Technique

Bernardo Assumpcao de Monaco and Joacir Graciolli Cordeiro

Introduction

Systemic opioid administration for cancer pain is frequently associated with partial symptomatic control and limiting side effects. Hence other routes were proposed to mitigate these features, which included epidural, subdural, and intraventricular spaces. Initial preclinical studies with intraventricular morphine date from the 1960s. They were followed by the clinical use of Ommaya reservoirs in which intraventricular morphine was intermittently infused without causing respiratory depression [1].

The first published intraventricular opioid infusion was reported in 1978 by Hosobuchi et al. In the article, beta-endorphin was used, and it promoted analgesia in a group of patients, which was reversible with naloxone [2]. Subsequently, the clinical use of intraventricular infusion of morphine has been corroborated as a safe and effective for cancer pain by a number of studies [1–14].

In the literature one can find different techniques to perform intraventricular drug infusion. The right lateral ventricle is the most commonly site chosen for catheter placement. Intermittent opioid infusion by means of Ommaya reservoir is associated with long-lasting analgesia for days or weeks in some cases [1]. The initial

B. Assumpcao de Monaco (✉)
Division of Functional Neurosurgery, Clinics Hospital, University of Sao Paulo Medicine School, São Paulo, Brazil

Functional Neurosurgery – Association of Assistance to Disabled Children [AACD], São Paulo, Brazil
e-mail: bernardo.monaco@usp.br

J. Graciolli Cordeiro
Division of Functional Neurosurgery – University of Miami/Jackson Memorial Hospital, Miami, FL, USA

T. d. S. Freitas et al. (eds.), *Neuromodulation Techniques for Pain Treatment*,
https://doi.org/10.1007/978-3-030-84778-4_18

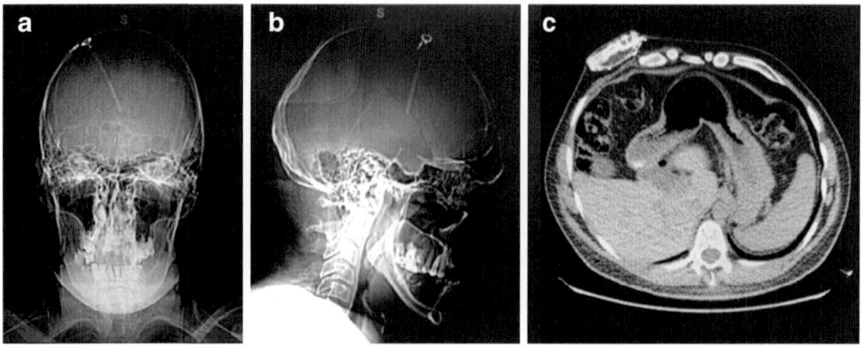

Fig. 1 (**a** and **b**): AP and lateral view of an Ommaya reservoir connected to a distal catheter. (**c**): Drug infusion pump implanted at right chest wall used for on-demand intermittent infusion.

favorable results in cancer pain led to the development of self-controlled implanted devices for drug infusion (Fig.1) [12]. The aim of this chapter is to focus on surgical aspects including details of the implant technique.

Patient Selection

The most common indication for intraventricular drug therapy is refractory oncologic pain encompassing the head, face, and neck [7]. In addition, intraventricular infusion of baclofen was reported to be effective for cases of secondary dystonia [15–19], spasticity [19], and pain [20, 21]. Another potential indication would be patients bearing spinal metastasis in which the intrathecal route is not an option as in severe arachnoiditis, radionecrosis, dehiscence, need for instrumentation, or multilevel tumor-related spinal canal stenosis. In addition, some modalities of neuropathic facial pain could respond to intracerebroventricular opioid infusion [14].

For children with spastic dystonia secondary to cerebral palsy, the intraventricular route showed same efficacy and less complications compared to the intrathecal one [17].

Catheter Placement

There are different ways to place the ventricular catheter. It can be done as a freehand puncture based on anatomic landmarks resembling ventriculoperitoneal (VP) shunt proximal catheter placement. In cases of reduced ventricular dimensions, it is recommended to use some form of navigation. The catheter tip does not need to be placed necessarily on the lateral ventricle. In fact, some authors target the third ventricle as it has shown to be more effective compared to the lateral one, especially for the infusion of less hydrophilic drugs [22].

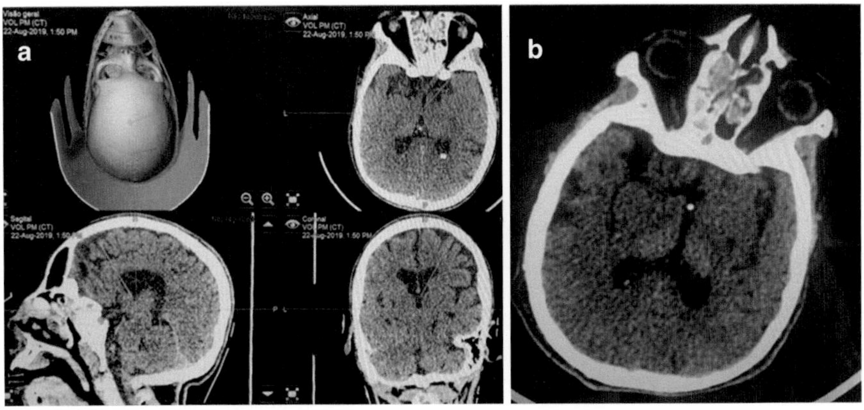

Fig. 2 (**a**) Neuronavigation planning for catheter insertion into the third ventricle. (**b**) Postoperative computed tomography with catheter located at planned site

The most commonly used methods to guide catheter placement are stereotaxy, neuronavigation (Fig. 2), and endoscopy. The frame-based stereotactic method is highly precise, but the frame can be an obstacle for catheter tunneling. Endoscopy is simple and effective and allows direct visualization of the catheter tip positioning through the Monroe foramen into the third ventricle. Endoscopy carries the advantage of providing live information compensating for eventual brain shift due to CSF loss. The initial ventricle puncture can be, however, difficult in case of small ventricles. In such cases its useful to have the endoscope coupled to standard neuronavigation or robotic guidance (e.g., robotic surgical assistant, ROSA™). Optical or electromagnetic neuronavigation (e.g., AxiEM™) alone seems to be a reasonable alternative to the other methods. In this method, the trajectory is planned in advance using a preoperative thin-slice CT. Ultrasound guidance for catheter placement has been also reported with results comparable to the stereotactic method [23].

The implantable proximal catheter from the Medtronic system (i.e., Ascenda™) is very soft; hence an outer cannula is necessary for the ventricle puncture. A regular microelectrode recording (MER) cannula can be used for this purpose as it has a reduced diameter and can also be coupled to the aforementioned guidance modalities. Another option is to use the insertion cannula from AD Tech (Oak Creek, VA, USA) for the ventricular catheter placement. This tool has a side opening which is preferable by some surgeons as it facilitates the cannula removal while holding the ventricular catheter on the other hand. In case of the other cannulas not being available, an alternative option would be to use the insertion needle from the Ascenda™ kit (16-T gauge). It could be intraoperatively trimmed and sanded using sterile surgical sandpaper making it blunt enough for the puncture (Figs. 3 and 4).

Despite the chosen insertion method, we believe it is preferable to use a proximal catheter with the same diameter as the distal one, with a known volume. The reason for that is the experience gathered on previous cases in which a regular VP shunt catheter was used proximally. A regular ventricular catheter can be freehand

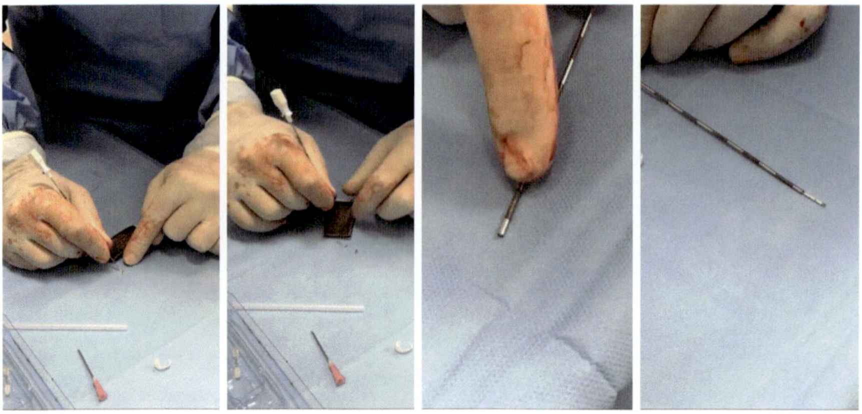

Fig. 3 Insertion needle from the Ascenda™ kit can be intraoperatively trimmed and sanded with sterile surgical sandpaper making it blunt for the ventricle puncture. Note in the last picture on the right that the catheter passes through the needle without resistance

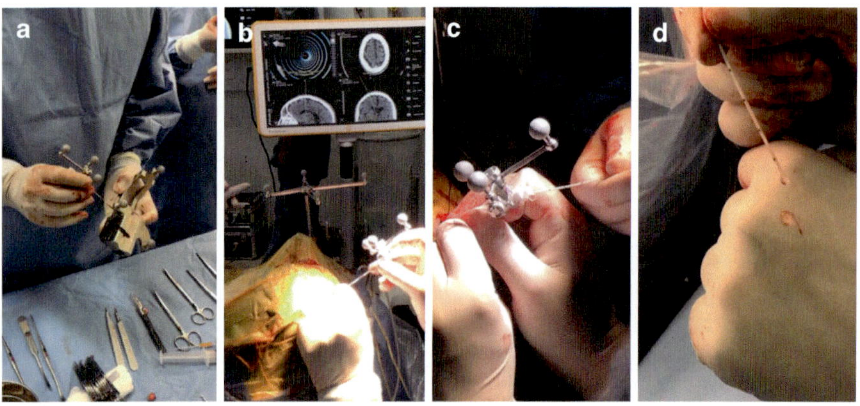

Fig. 4 (**a**) Coupling a navigation tool (BrainLab neuronavigation) to the Ascenda™ catheter 16G insertion blunt needle. (**b**) Navigated ventricle puncture. (**c** and **d**) Navigated needle removal under simultaneous CSF outflow visualization

inserted; however merging catheters with different diameters complicates the total catheter volume calculation. It makes the determination of the initial bolus as well as the bridge boluses less precise, which reduces therapy safety (Fig. 5).

After the proximal catheter is inserted, it can be fixed to the burr hole edge using titan miniplates, methyl methacrylate, or acrylic glue (e.g., Histoacryl® – B. Braun). This step is followed by its connection to the previously tunneled distal catheter. In some cases, the proximal catheter would be long enough to be connected directly to the pump. Nevertheless, we prefer to use a connector to reduce the tension in the system minimizing the risk of catheter migration. In addition, tension could lead to a catheter disconnection from the pump and CSF leak in the distal pocket.

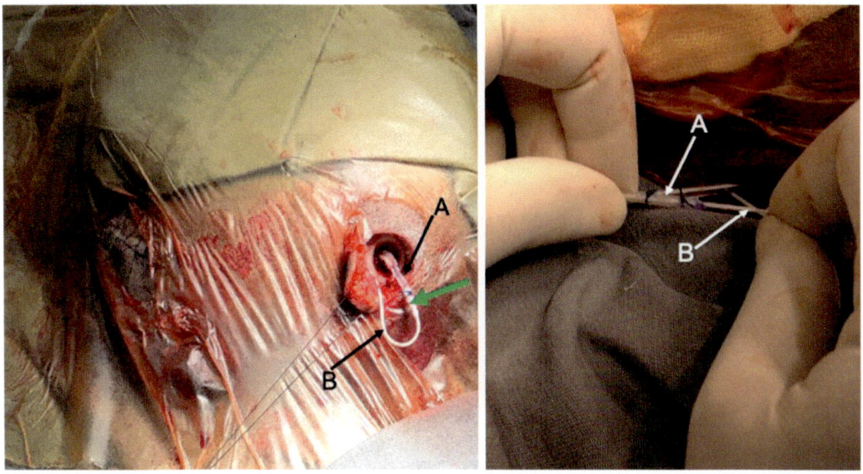

Fig. 5 Left, frontal burr hole depicting the proximal ventricular catheter (A), the connector (green arrow), and the distal catheter (B). Right, another patient demonstrating the use of different catheter sizes being the distal one (B) inserted directly into the proximal one (A) without using a connector

Catheter Tunneling and Pump Implant

The infusion pump is typically implanted on the left abdominal flank as the right side could be used as approach for appendectomies and cholecystectomies. After the incision is performed, the abdominal pocket is created distally wide enough to prevent tension in the suture line. The pump can be placed above or underneath the fascia. It is suggested to use the subfascial plane for implants in children and dystonic and cachectic patients due to the reduced subcutaneous layer. After preparing the subcutaneous pocket, the tunneling cannula is inserted from caudal to cranial, and the catheter passed through it (Fig. 6). If necessary, a retroauricular incision can be made to ease the tunneling process. As in a VP shunt catheter tunneling, it is important to be aware of the sudden change in resistance when crossing the nuchal ligament to avoid adjacent structural damage. Moreover, a too superficial catheter tunneling could make the catheter more vulnerable to exposure due to skin lacerations. We recommend bending the tunneling tool into a wide "C" as it could facilitate its steering during the maneuver.

Once the system is entirely implanted and secured, we suggest checking its patency by puncturing the catheter port on the pump and aspirating CSF. This step will not only confirm CSF flow but also fills the catheters with CSF preventing airlock. Finally, the soft tissue is sutured using 2–0 Vicryl on the cranial galea and 3–0 Vicryl on the abdominal subcutaneous tissue along with Prolene or Monocryl skin closure.

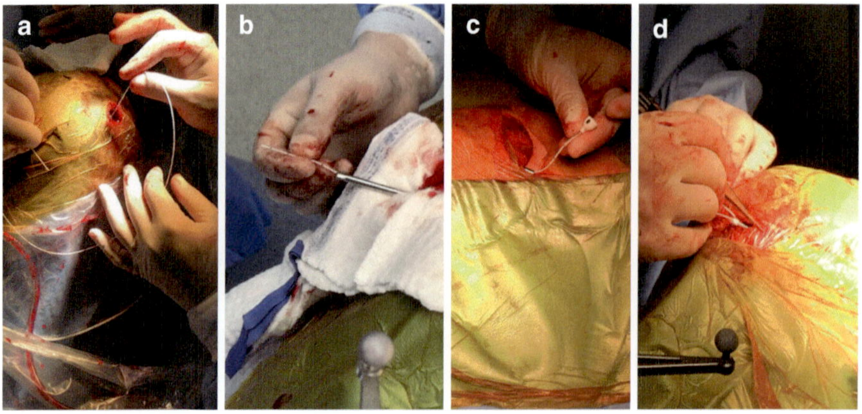

Fig. 6 (**a**) Ventricular catheter being secured to the burr hole with acrylic glue (Histoacryl® – B. Braun). Catheter being tunneled from caudal (**c**) to cranial (**b**). (**d**) Distal catheter being connected with the ventricle catheter using a connector

Table 1 Common intrathecal drugs and their use in intracerebroventricular route

Drug	Initial daily dose	Maximal reported daily dose
Morphine	0,2 mg	24,83 mg [7]
Baclofen	25mcg*	2012mcg [16]
Ziconotide	0,48mcg	2,0mcg [12]
Clonidine	NA	NA
Ropivacaine	1,2 mg	8,16 mg [12]
Bupivacaine	NA	NA
Hydromorphone	0,01 mg	3,27 mg [14]

*For children we suggest start with intrathecal baclofen 1mcg/Kg – until 25Kg. After this, we use 25mcg as starting dose for all the patients
NA not available in humans

Infusion Management

We suggest initiating the intraventricular therapy with lower starting doses rather than the usual intrathecal ones, because the clinical response can be stronger when the drug is infused directly in the ventricle. Table 1 summarizes reports for initial and maximal doses rates. In our experience, adjustments can be done safely every 3 to 5 days, in increments of no more than 15%. We perform the initial bolus in 4 hours, as we know precisely the catheter volume. After this, we start a continuous flow rate. It is recommended maintaining the patient in an intensive care unit for 1 to 2 days after infusion start to observe for side effects as well as possible adverse reactions [7].

Complications

To minimize the occurrence of complications, it's highly recommend following the Polyanalgesic Consensus Conference (PACC): Recommendations for Intrathecal Drug Delivery: Guidance for Improving Safety and Mitigating Risks [24]. Complications can be divided into device-related and pharmacologic. Catheter migration, obstruction, disconnection, and breakage are among the hardware complications. Catheter obstruction by choroid plexus is about 6% [6]. Infection used to be more frequent with the first generation of systems in which repetitive punctures of Ommaya or Rickham reservoir were associated with a high incidence in around 24%. With the current electronic pump systems, it was dramatically reduced. New technologies applied to catheters reduced its related complications as well.

Pharmacologic complications with opioids include mental clouding in 9% of the cases, somnolence in 4%, visual hallucinations in 3%, diaphoresis in 2%, respiratory depression in 1%, gait disturbance in 1%, pruritus in 1%, urinary retention in 1%, and persistent headache 1% [13]. Constipation seems to be rare in intracerebroventricular morphine [5, 6]. Agitation was reported as ziconotide side effect at a level of 0.96 μg/d [12]. Other rare reported complications were hypothermia, hyperglycemia, higher levels of prolactin and growth hormone, decrease of glutathione levels, and seizures [5].

References

1. Obbens EA, Hill CS, Leavens ME, Ruthenbeck SS, Otis F. Intraventricular morphine administration for control of chronic cancer pain. Pain. 1987;28(1):61–8.
2. Hosobuchi Y, Li CH. The analgesic activity of human beta-endorphin in man (1,2,3). Commun Psychopharmacol. 1978;2(1):33–7.
3. Goudas LC, Langlade A, Serrie A, Matson W, Milbury P, Thurel C, et al. Acute decreases in cerebrospinal fluid glutathione levels after intracerebroventricular morphine for cancer pain. Anesth Analg. 1999;89(5):1209–15.
4. Lazorthes YR, Sallerin BA, Verdié JC. Intracerebroventricular administration of morphine for control of irreducible cancer pain. Neurosurgery. 1995;37(3):422–8. discussion 428-429
5. Raffa RB, Pergolizzi JV. Intracerebroventricular opioids for intractable pain. Br J Clin Pharmacol. 2012;74(1):34–41.
6. Cramond T, Stuart G. Intraventricular morphine for intractable pain of advanced cancer. J Pain Symptom Manag. 1993;8(7):465–73.
7. Dennis GC, DeWitty RL. Long-term intraventricular infusion of morphine for intractable pain in cancer of the head and neck. Neurosurgery. 1990;26(3):404–7; discussion 407-408
8. Leavens ME, Hill CS, Cech DA, Weyland JB, Weston JS. Intrathecal and intraventricular morphine for pain in cancer patients: initial study. J Neurosurg. 1982;56(2):241–5.
9. Lee TL, Kumar A, Baratham G. Intraventricular morphine for intractable craniofacial pain. Singap Med J. 1990;31(3):273–6.
10. Lobato RD, Madrid JL, Fatela LV, Rivas JJ, Reig E, Lamas E. Intraventricular morphine for control of pain in terminal cancer patients. J Neurosurg. 1983;59(4):627–33.

11. Nurchi G. Use of intraventricular and intrathecal morphine in intractable pain associated with cancer. Neurosurgery. 1984;15(6):801–3.
12. Staquet H, Dupoiron D, Nader E, Menei P. Intracerebroventricular pain treatment with analgesic mixtures including Ziconotide for intractable pain. Pain Physician. 2016;19(6):E905–15.
13. Karavelis A, Foroglou G, Selviaridis P, Fountzilas G. Intraventricular administration of morphine for control of intractable cancer pain in 90 patients. Neurosurgery. 1996;39(1):57–61. discussion 61-62
14. Lee DJ, Gurkoff GG, Goodarzi A, Muizelaar JP, Boggan JE, Shahlaie K. Intracerebroventricular opiate infusion for refractory head and facial pain. World J Clin Cases. 2014;2(8):351–6.
15. Albright AL. Intraventricular baclofen infusion for dystonia. Report of Two Cases. J Neurosurg. 2006;105(1 Suppl):71–4.
16. Albright AL, Ferson SS. Intraventricular baclofen for dystonia: techniques and outcomes. Clinical article. J Neurosurg Pediatr. 2009;3(1):11–4.
17. Rocque BG, Leland AA. Intraventricular vs intrathecal baclofen for secondary dystonia: a comparison of complications. Neurosurgery. 2012;70(2 Suppl Operative):321–5. discussion 325-326
18. Ruggiero C, Meccariello G, Spennato P, Mirone G, Graziano S, Gilone M, et al. Early intraventricular baclofen therapy (IVB) for children with dystonic and dysautonomic storm. Childs Nerv Syst ChNS. 2019;35(1):15–8.
19. Turner M, Nguyen HS, Cohen-Gadol AA. Intraventricular baclofen as an alternative to intrathecal baclofen for intractable spasticity or dystonia: outcomes and technical considerations. J Neurosurg Pediatr. 2012;10(4):315–9.
20. Liebman JM, Pastor G. Antinociceptive effects of baclofen and muscimol upon intraventricular administration. Eur J Pharmacol. 1980;61(3):225–30.
21. Monaco BA, Alho EJL, Okuda FAF. Dystonic-spastic vulvodynia-related treatment with intraventricular baclofen in a cerebral palsy patient. Neuromodulation. 2020;23(3):14536.
22. Albright AL. Technique for insertion of intraventricular baclofen catheters. J Neurosurg Pediatr. 2011;8(4):394–5.
23. Wilson TJ, Stetler WR, Al-Holou WN, Sullivan SE. Comparison of the accuracy of ventricular catheter placement using freehand placement, ultrasonic guidance, and stereotactic neuronavigation. J Neurosurg. 2013;119(1):66–70.
24. Deer TR, Pope JE, Hayek SM, Lamer TJ, Veizi IE, Erdek M, et al. The Polyanalgesic Consensus Conference (PACC): recommendations for intrathecal drug delivery: guidance for improving safety and mitigating risks. Neuromodulation. 2017;20(2):155–76.

Peripheral Nerve Stimulation: Fluoroscopic Implant Techniques

Ryan B. Kochanski and Konstantin V. Slavin

Abbreviations

CT	computed tomography
IPG	implanted pulse generator
ONS	occipital nerve stimulation
PNFS	peripheral nerve field stimulation
PNS	peripheral nerve stimulation

Introduction

Following the original work by Wall and Sweet in 1967 demonstrating the efficacy of peripheral nerve stimulation (PNS), the early PNS devices consisted of a paddle electrode placed along the nerve which necessitated open surgical dissection/exposure and thus restricted the procedure to orthopedic, plastic, and neurological surgeons specializing in peripheral nerve surgery [1, 2]. In 1999, the first description of a percutaneous implantation technique for occipital nerve stimulation (ONS) completely revolutionized the field, opening the door for implantation to nonsurgical specialists while also expanding indications and reducing the invasive nature of the procedure [2, 3]. As opposed to open dissection and neurolysis, emphasis shifted toward reliance on anatomical landmarks and imaging such as fluoroscopy and/or

R. B. Kochanski
Department of Neurosurgery, University of California, San Francisco, CA, USA

K. V. Slavin (✉)
Department of Neurosurgery, University of Illinois at Chicago, Chicago, IL, USA
e-mail: kslavin@uic.edu

T. d. S. Freitas et al. (eds.), *Neuromodulation Techniques for Pain Treatment*,
https://doi.org/10.1007/978-3-030-84778-4_19

ultrasound for percutaneous implantation. The application of percutaneous techniques has evolved to include stimulation of various somatic nerves, including trigeminal branches and peripheral nerves of the trunk and extremities [4]. This technique has gained in popularity due to its low invasiveness and technical ease, obviating the need for open surgical dissection and nerve exposure [5].

When percutaneous technique is used, the trial electrodes are often discarded upon trial completion, therefore requiring insertion of new electrodes during the second stage of the PNS procedure, the so-called permanent implantation. In this scenario, reliance is placed on standard anatomical landmarks based on limited variability in the nerve course and an ability to capture the nerve with multiple contacts of the stimulating electrode. In addition, both fluoroscopy and ultrasound are useful intraoperatively to check the direction of electrode path and the position of the targeted nerve, respectively [5]. While fluoroscopy is useful in visualizing lead location in relation to bony anatomical landmarks, it does not visualize nerves and blood vessels. Thus, other means of image guidance, such as ultrasound, serve as a useful adjunct to ensure optimal electrode positioning and help to avoid nearby vessels [6]. This chapter will focus specifically on the use of intraoperative fluoroscopy to guide and confirm the placement of percutaneous PNS electrodes.

Fluoroscopically Guided Procedures and Workflow

The general workflow to fluoroscopic lead placement for both PNS and peripheral nerve/field stimulation (PNFS) has been previously described [7] and is detailed below.

The patient is positioned to allow for optimal access to the region of interest. Careful consideration should be made to allow for optimal fluoroscopic access and image acquisition of the target site. Performing the procedure under conscious sedation provides adequate patient comfort and anxiolysis during electrode placement while also allowing for intraoperative confirmation of acceptable paresthesia coverage described by the patient. Perioperative antibiotics are administered, and standard surgical preparation and draping are performed with the entire planned path of the electrode visible within the sterile surgical field. The general workflow for a percutaneous PNS lead placement trial is then performed via the following sequential steps:

1. After infiltration of the entry point with local anesthetic, a small stab incision is made.
2. A straight or slightly curved Tuohy needle is slowly advanced into the subcutaneous space overlying the nerve. The trajectory of the needle may be in parallel to the target nerve or at an angle. PNFS electrodes are arranged variably to provide optimal coverage of the entire painful area.
3. The inner stylet of the Tuohy needle is withdrawn, and the electrode lead is threaded through the needle and its position is confirmed with fluoroscopy.
4. The Tuohy needle is then removed leaving the electrode lead in place.

5. The electrode lead is connected to a temporary testing cable. The patient's sedation is lightened so that any perceived paresthesias are reported. The optimal stimulation coverage can be ascertained by changing the combination of anode and cathode contacts and varying amplitude, frequency, and pulse width. If these alterations do not result in optimal coverage of the target area, then the electrode can be repositioned.
6. After optimal electrode position is confirmed, it is secured at the entry site with a single stitch. The site is further dressed with a sterile occlusive dressing. The externalized trial electrode is then connected to the trial stimulator system. Fluoroscopic images or plain radiographs should be obtained to document final electrode position.
7. These steps are repeated for each additional electrode planned. For most PNS cases, 1 or 2 electrodes are used. For PNFS, multiple electrodes may be needed to provide adequate coverage.

The specific types of PNS stimulation for which fluoroscopic implantation techniques are utilized are described below.

Occipital Nerve Stimulation

The electrodes are generally implanted perpendicular to the course of the greater occipital nerves on one or both sides of the patient's head at the level of craniovertebral junction [5]. The direction of insertion and the anchoring points vary among those who perform the procedure. The senior author prefers to anchor the occipital PNS electrodes in the retromastoid region while tunneling them toward the implanted pulse generator (IPG) located in the infraclavicular region [8]. A thorough description of the procedure by the senior author has been previously described in detail [9]. For permanent device and bilateral lead implantation, the patient is placed supine with the head turned maximally away from the infraclavicular side chosen for IPG insertion. The head is positioned on a small cushion, allowing access to the dependent occipital region and mastoid process. The occipital area, neck, and upper chest on the ipsilateral side are prepped and draped in the usual sterile fashion. The C-arm fluoroscopy machine is oriented perpendicularly around the patient's head, such that sufficient space allows for the implanter to stand within the C-arm during implantation (Fig. 1). For lead implantation, a 2.5 cm straight, vertically oriented retromastoid incision is made to the fascia, and the tissues medial and lateral are undermined in order to create an anchoring pocket and to allow for creation of a strain relief loop. Next, a stab incision is made in the midline at the level of C1 for percutaneous placement of the contralateral electrode. The inserting needle is advanced toward the contralateral mastoid process under fluoroscopic guidance. For the ipsilateral side, the inserting needle is advanced through the ipsilateral retromastoid incision toward to the midline within the epifascial plane under fluoroscopic guidance. The stylets are removed and the electrodes are inserted through each

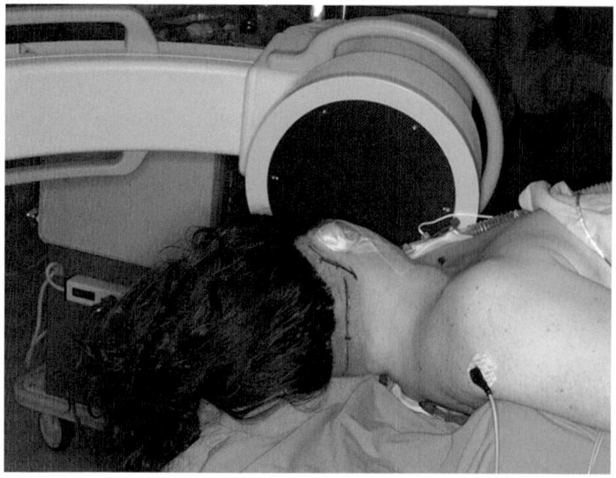

Fig. 1 Patient and C-arm fluoroscopy positioning for ONS electrode implantation

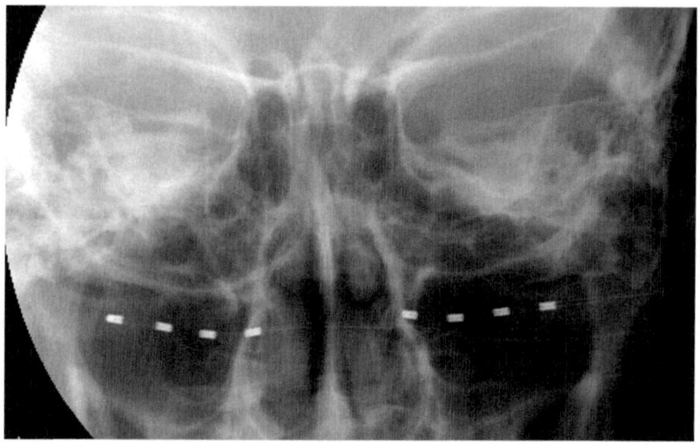

Fig. 2 Intraoperative fluoroscopic image confirming adequate placement of bilateral ONS electrodes

needle, again under fluoroscopic guidance with the ipsilateral electrode traveling from retromastoid incision toward midline and the contralateral electrode traveling from midline to contralateral mastoid process. The leads are tunneled subcutaneously using the same insertion needles with the stylets removed and are anchored within the retromastoid incision with strain relief loops next to each anchor. These leads are then subcutaneously tunneled to an infraclavicular pocket made for the IPG. Final fluoroscopic images are taken to ensure that the placement of the leads remains adequate after tunneling (Fig. 2).

Trigeminal Branch Stimulation

Percutaneous techniques for trigeminal branch stimulation (supraorbital, supratrochlear, infraorbital, auriculotemporal, and, most recently, the mental and inferior alveolar branches of the mandibular nerve) are technically similar to occipital PNS. Electrodes are placed based on anatomical landmarks crossing the course of

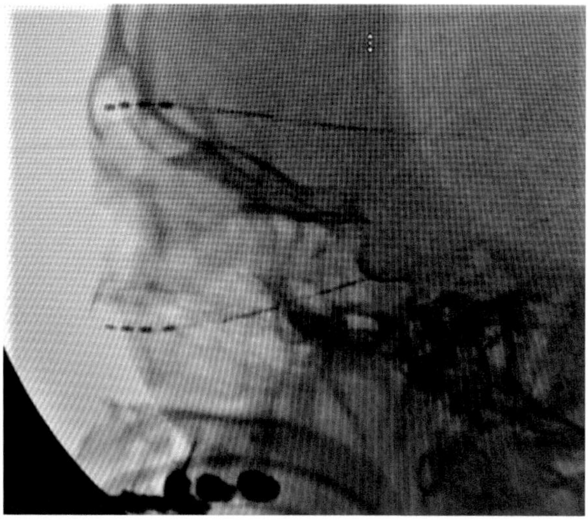

Fig. 3 Intraoperative fluoroscopic image confirming adequate placement of trigeminal branch electrodes

the targeted nerve(s) [5]. A stab incision is made over the zygoma at the temporal pre-auricular hairline, and a contoured 12- to 14-gauge Tuohy needle is advanced within the epifascial plane toward the painful region. Once the needle tip is in place, a four or eight contact electrode is advanced through it all the way to the target under fluoroscopic guidance [10]. Typical landmarks used for fluoroscopic guidance include the supraorbital groove/foramen, the infraorbital foramen, the floor of the orbit, etc. [10, 11]. It is crucial that the electrodes are advanced within the epifascial plane which provides sufficient depth to avoid electrode erosion postoperatively. The anchoring point for these electrodes is usually placed in the retroauricular region, and, from there, the electrode or extension cable is tunneled toward the infraclavicular IPG [5]. Final lead location is confirmed with intraoperative fluoroscopy (Fig. 3).

Trigeminal Ganglion Stimulation

Percutaneous lead implantation into the Gasserian ganglion for treatment of intractable neuropathic facial pain has been previously described by the Belgian group of Van Buyten and colleagues using three-dimensional (3D) fluoroscopic techniques [12, 13]. Their technique utilizes an intraoperative three-dimensional computed tomography (3D CT) scan using the O-arm®-coupled electromagnetic neuronavigational system (Axiem, Medtronic) in order to guide electrode placement into the foramen ovale. In the operating room, the patient is first positioned supine on a radiolucent Table. A 3D CT scan using O-arm® is then performed. The obtained images are used to calculate the trajectory to the Gasserian ganglion through the foramen ovale. A small stab incision is made lateral to the labial commissure, and a 15-gauge needle, guided by 3D real-time electromagnetic tip tracking, is inserted into the foramen ovale. Under continuous fluoroscopy, the electrode is inserted until its tip reaches the clivus. Once the electrode contacts reach the target, the patient is awakened, and test stimulation is performed until the patient endorses paresthesia within the area of neuropathic facial pain. The needle is then withdrawn under continuous fluoroscopy so as to assure that the electrode remains in place, and a suture is placed on the electrode at the entry site. No anchor is used. The patient is then re-sedated and the electrode is tunneled subcutaneously between the maxilla and mandibular region [12].

Peripheral Nerve Field Stimulation

PNFS involves the targeting of small distal branches of peripheral nerves within the subcutaneous space by placing one or more electrodes into the region of maximal pain [7, 14]. Field stimulation produces paresthesias within diffuse painful areas that may not necessarily correlate with a single dermatome or is otherwise poorly defined dermatomally. Thus, body regions rather than nerves are used to describe the location of PNFS (i.e., low back, trunk, joint). The technique was outlined by the Australian implanters Verrills and Russo [15].

Octopolar leads are placed subcutaneously within the area of maximal pain using a 14-gauge vascular access catheter under live C-arm fluoroscopy. The ideal depth for the placement of the electrode that provides optimal stimulation of the affected nerves is not well defined between specific patients. More superficial implantation into the dermal layers can result in painful stimulation, while deeper subfascial placement can result in muscle recruitment and uncomfortable sensations [15]. A previously described "pin-drop" technique uses a device with multiple freely moving pins that sits directly on the skin above the desired implantation site. Using fluoroscopic imaging at 30° cephalad and caudad, the depth of each lead can be estimated by measuring the distance between the contacts and the reference pins. Using this technique in 17 patients, its Australian inventors found that the distribution of electrode depth providing adequate stimulation ranged between 4 and 19 mm, with an average depth of 10.5 mm [15]. Once the leads are determined to be at adequate depth and location, on-table stimulation is performed to determine that paresthesia is felt in the area of pain and that it is comfortable. The leads are then sutured to the skin and dressings applied.

Conclusion

Since the introduction of the percutaneous fluoroscopically guided technique in the late 1990s, the use of percutaneous PNS or PNFS electrodes has steadily increased. Fluoroscopy is a useful intraoperative adjunct to both guide and confirm percutaneously placed electrodes in relation to bony anatomic landmarks. When used alone or in conjunction with other intraoperative image-guidance modalities such as ultrasound, fluoroscopy improves both the safety and efficiency of these procedures.

References

1. Wall PD, Sweet WH. Temporary abolition of pain in man. Science. 1967;155:108–9.
2. Slavin KV. History of peripheral nerve stimulation. Prog Neurol Surg. 2011;24:1–15.
3. Weiner RL, Reed KL. Peripheral neurostimulation for control of intractable occipital neuralgia. Neuromodulation. 1999;2:217–21.
4. Slavin KV. Technical aspects of peripheral nerve stimulation: hardware and complications. Prog Neurol Surg. 2011;24:189–202.
5. Slavin KV. Chapter 5 - peripheral nerve. In: Arle JE, Shils JL, editors. Essential Neuromodulation. San Diego: Academic Press; 2011. p. 95–106.
6. Chan I, Brown AR, Park K, Winfree CJ. Ultrasound-guided, percutaneous peripheral nerve stimulation: technical note. Neurosurgery. 2010;67:136–9.
7. Petersen EA, Slavin KV. Peripheral nerve/field stimulation for chronic pain. Neurosurg Clin N Amer. 2014;25:789–97.
8. Trentman TL, Slavin KV, Freeman JA, Zimmerman RS. Occipital nerve stimulator placement via a retromastoid to infraclavicular approach: a technical report. Stereotact Funct Neurosurg. 2010;88:121–5.
9. Slavin KV, Yin D. Peripheral nerve stimulation for pain relief: primer on occipital nerve stimulation. In: Gross RE, Boulis NM, editors. Neurosurg Oper Atlas Funct Neurosurg. 3rd Edition. Thieme/AANS; 2018. p. 253–257.
10. Keifer Jr. O, Gutierrez J, Tora M, Boulis NM. Neurosurgical interventions for neuropathic craniofacial pain. In: Gross RE, Boulis NM, editors. Neurosurg Oper Atlas Funct Neurosurg. 3rd Edition. Thieme/AANS; 2018. p. 264–272.
11. Lenchig S, Cohen J, Patin D. A minimally invasive surgical technique for the treatment of posttraumatic trigeminal neuropathic pain with peripheral nerve stimulation. Pain Physician. 2012;15:E725–32.
12. Van Buyten J-P. Trigeminal ganglion stimulation. Prog Neurol Surg. 2015;29:76–82.
13. Van Buyten J-P, Smet I, Van de Kelft E. Electromagnetic navigation technology for more precise electrode placement in the foramen ovale: a technical report. Neuromodulation. 2009;12:244–9.
14. Levy RM. Differentiating the leaves from the branches in the tree of neuromodulation: the state of peripheral nerve field stimulation. Neuromodulation. 2011;14:201–5.
15. Verrills P, Russo M. Peripheral nerve stimulation for back pain. Prog Neurol Surg. 2015;29:127–38.

The Value of Intraoperative Neuromonitoring for Neuromodulation

Steven Falowski

Introduction

Spinal cord stimulation (SCS) has been employed for the treatment of intractable pain most commonly for failed back surgery syndrome (FBSS) and complex regional pain syndromes (CRPS) [1, 2]. It is generally accepted that for successful SCS treatment there is the superposition of SCS-induced paresthesias overlapping the regions of perceived pain. This has become true for both paresthesia-based and paresthesia-free stimulation as physiologic placement is paramount. This is especially true when utilizing traditional tonic stimulation which has become an option on each SCS system.

The most straightforward way to confirm pain paresthesia during lead implantation is via verbal feedback from the conscious patient. In this way, the implanter can achieve optimal lead placement by adjusting the lead location within the epidural space based on the patient's report of perceived paresthesia. However, there is stress/discomfort with awake procedures, there is risk of over-sedation in a prone non-intubated patient, and sometimes it is not possible to perform interventions in an awake patient. Although there is a common acceptance within the field for awake placement, there is no published data specifically investigating awake placement. It generally became accepted because an awake patient gives you a marker of safety and confirmation of lead positioning in the placement of spinal cord stimulators. The difficulty also arises in that noncooperative patients for awake procedures are often sedated which removes the ability to have these two factors.

For these reasons, there is the option of placing the patient under general anesthesia; this may be especially true for surgical lead placement because a laminotomy is required but also for percutaneous placement as well. In this scenario it is imperative to have a method of cord protection for which neuromonitoring has been

S. Falowski (✉)
Neurosurgical Associates of Lancaster, Lancaster, PA, USA

T. d. S. Freitas et al. (eds.), *Neuromodulation Techniques for Pain Treatment*,
https://doi.org/10.1007/978-3-030-84778-4_20

widely accepted in spinal surgery [1–4]. Asleep lead placements, however, do not allow for verbal feedback from the patient during the procedure and could therefore contribute to suboptimal lead placement. It has been shown that anatomic midline does not correlate with physiologic midline at least 40% of the time [5, 6]. It has also been shown that placing a paddle lead without mapping will lead to revisions 20% of the time [7]. This number can be expected higher with percutaneous leads given the smaller range of coverage. Given these findings, protocols have been established to use neuromonitoring in asleep patient to also confirm lead placement and perform physiological mapping [8]. First papers were written over 10 years ago and have been improved upon [9, 10]. At present, there are numerous retrospective and prospective studies demonstrating its efficacy and sometimes superiority to awake placements [1, 2, 7–12]. In addition, protocols have been established and published. Perhaps the most landmark study was a prospective multicenter study directly comparing awake to asleep placement with neuromonitoring ("NAPS") that demonstrated the use of neuromonitoring improved time efficiency by 25%, had superior paraesthesia coverage, and had a fifth of the adverse events [12].

The Neurostimulation Appropriateness Consensus Committee (NACC) guidelines state: "Confirmation of correct lead placement has been advocated with either awake intraoperative confirmation of paresthesia coverage or use of neuromonitoring in asleep placement, such as EMG responses or SSEP collision testing" [13]. The observation of compound motor action potentials (CMAPs) or somatosensory-evoked potentials (SSEPs) within the painful dermatome(s) in response to intraoperative SCS can be used as a proxy for verbal confirmation of paresthesia coverage [8–12]. CMAPs use myotomal coverage as a marker for dermatomal coverage. The NACC guidelines, combined with published evidence, have led to an increase in its use that not only includes surgeons but also interventional pain physicians.

Description of Neuromonitoring Protocol

Muscle coverage for EMG responses is the primary concern in utilizing neuromonitoring for placement of SCS electrodes when done under general anesthesia [8]. In addition, it allows for monitoring of the spinal cord in case of injury during placement of an electrode. Monitoring for safety of the cord will include somatosensory evoked potentials (SSEP) as a baseline but may also include transcranial motor evoked potentials (TceMEP).

Sterile, 1.3 cm, 27-gauge subdermal needle electrodes are placed in pairs for bilateral coverage. Symmetrical placement of the monitoring leads is imperative given that the basis for the neurophysiologic mapping resides in response amplitude comparisons. EMG responses are determined with the addition of physician interpretation of the placement of the electrode, as well as fluoroscopy for confirmation. This interpretation will then be utilized to determine the physiological midline, laterality and orientation of the electrode, and myotomal coverage as a marker for anticipated dermatomal paresthesia.

For thoracic cord placement, the surgeon will usually perform a laminectomy at the lower thoracic levels, or percutaneous leads will be placed by a usual lumbar epidural access technique. Coverage for local thoracic nerve roots is desirable. Monitoring electrodes are placed in the periumbilical rectus abdominis muscles for mid-lower thoracic electrode placement to achieve sensitivity in the T8/12 spinal nerve root distributions. We also display the iliopsoas, adductor-quadriceps, tibialis anterior, and medial gastrocnemius channels in EMG mode.

Determine electrode area that is being used to stimulate, such as "middle middle" or "top right" which is dependent on the type of lead placed. This can vary from percutaneous or single column leads to multicolumn paddle electrodes. A bipole configuration with a single cathode and anode is most commonly used. During testing, you will see stimulus artifact at low levels of stimulation and then stimulus artifact accompanied by time-locked compound muscle action potential responses at higher levels. Typical stimulation parameters are frequencies of 10 Hz (range from 4 to 20), 200 μsec pulse width (varies from 100 to 500), and level increasing from 0 to approximately 10–12 mA. When viewed in the 200 msec/div sweep sEMG window, both the stimulation artifact and compound muscle action potential will appear as spikes; in the 10 msec/div sweep tEMG window, the stimulation artifact spike and compound muscle action potential will appear distinctly different in morphology. Comparing amplitude, shape of the compound muscle action potential, and symmetry will allow for interpretation of lead positioning (Figs. 1 and 2).

Monitoring for cervical SCS placement (Fig. 3) can be done in a similar fashion. The main difference is the selection of muscles used for EMG. Although the stimulation parameters are the same as thoracic stimulator placement, the thresholds for responses are usually lower in the cervical spine. Therefore lower pulse widths and amplitudes should be attempted initially. Evaluation and interpretation of data is otherwise similar to thoracic stimulator placement.

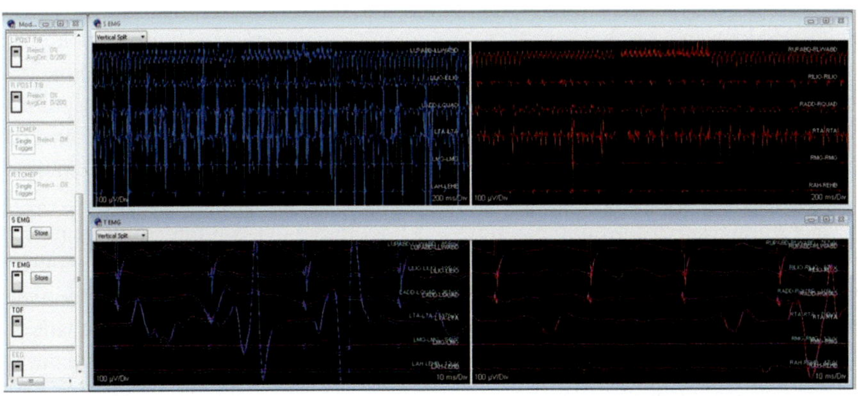

Fig. 1 This is an example of bilateral coverage from a thoracic midline placement with slightly stronger signals on the left

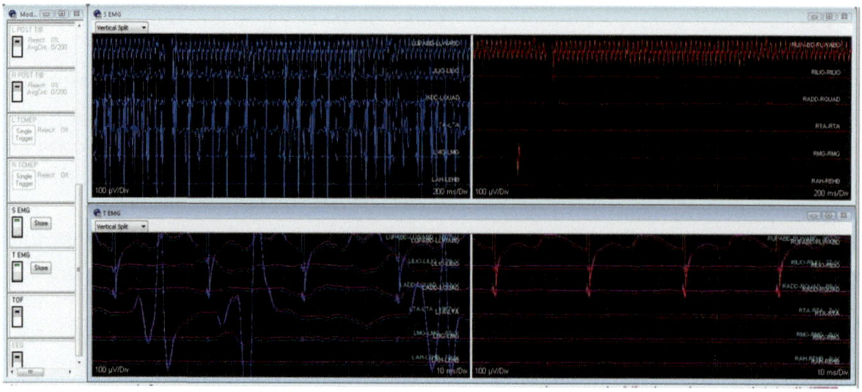

Fig. 2 This is an example of left predominant coverage in a thoracic SCS placement

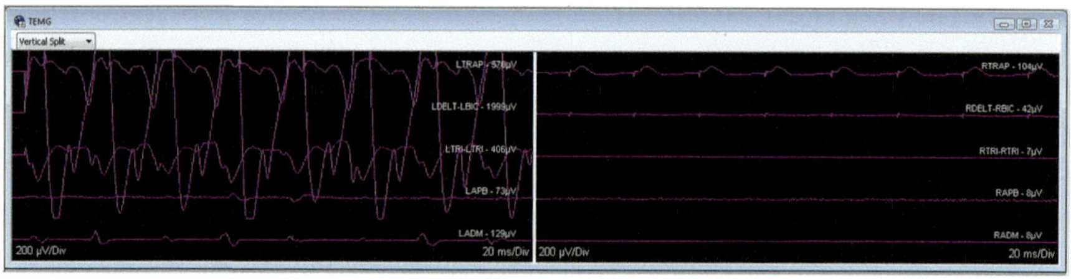

Fig. 3 This is an example of left predominant coverage in a cervical SCS placement

Physician Interpretation of Data

Neuromonitoring can be used to determine differences in anatomic midline and physiologic midline, as well as determine myotomal coverage as a marker for dermatomal coverage [8]. The physician will make adjustments in positioning of the lead based on the feedback from neuromonitoring to optimize symmetry and/or coverage. Stimulation artifact will first be elicited at lower levels of stimulation and will then be followed by time-locked compound muscle action potential responses as the levels increase. Stimulation artifact can be a good marker for determining coverage but should only be loosely interpreted until there are time-locked true motor responses.

Determination of physiologic midline is imperative in obtaining accurate paresthesia coverage with coverage obtained with neuromonitoring being shown to be superior to awake testing [12]. Stimulation artifact will initially be seen in thoracic nerve roots. Regardless of placement it is expected that bilateral stimulation will be seen in nerve roots secondary to current spread and the ease of exciting the nerve roots. It is therefore suggested to only loosely use this data for symmetry. This same holds true for activation of the abdominal muscles and iliopsoas muscles. Although true muscle responses can be expected, absolute symmetry and interpretation may be difficult. First symmetry interpretation is from the adductor quadriceps and distal when determining midline. Lastly an additional marker of symmetry and physiologic midline is to determine the timing of firing on both sides. It may be visualized that the amplitude on both sides is symmetric, but a slight preference off midline can be determined by monitoring which side and muscle groups fired first. This equates to an exact determination of placement and precise stimulation (Figs. 1, 2, and 3).

Advances in technology have led to paddle electrodes with complex arrays. It is because of this complexity that proper placement is of importance for use of an entire electrode array. However, the increased length and width of these paddle arrays has led to the added complexity of ensuring the array is lying flat and flush in the canal. Neuromonitoring can be utilized to ensure that the lead is not canted or tilted. This is done by determining the amplitudes at which responses are first generated. This should be consistent across the lead. If there is large discrepancies across or within columns, it may be a sign that the lead is tilted or canted since the distance from the contact to the spinal cord is varying.

Determination of myotomal coverage as a marker for dermatonal coverage can be used to ensure proper paresthesia coverage as well. Anatomy and somatotopy may differ slightly among patients and therefore the lead may be moved either cranial/caudal or medial/lateral in an attempt to activate specific fibers and generate coverage on the neuromonitoring.

Specific IONM for Dorsal Root Ganglion (DRG) Stimulation

Similar needs exist in placing DRG stimulators as with SCS, such as safety, and confirmation of lead placement. More important though in reference to placing DRG stimulators is the added discomfort in placing these leads as you brush or cross the DRG in the foramen. This discomfort is very difficult for awake patients to tolerate and can also lead to nerve injury. Ultimately, this leads to sedating patients which is not in line with our current published guidelines [13, 14]. There is therefore more of a need for the use of IONM in DRG stimulation even compared to SCS.

Performing the procedure using neuromonitoring differs from the traditional awake-patient technique in that the patient remains anesthetized throughout the procedure, and the accuracy of the placement and expected sensory and motor thresholds for stimulation are determined objectively using a combination of SSEP and Free-run EMG testing [15]. The electrode is placed utilizing fluoroscopic imaging, and then the device is connected to the neuromonitoring system with an adapter that allows the electrode contacts to be supplied with electrical stimulation from the constant-current stimulator that also runs the traditional SSEP modes.

Monitoring for the surgery consists of SSEPs and Free-run EMG for muscles representing the appropriate nerve level(s) for the stimulator placements. SSEPs and EMG are monitored as for any typical spine surgery. Specific nerve root level

EMG activation can be used as the marker of safety with placement. In reference to confirmation of lead placement, both SSPEP and EMG will be utilized with determination of their respective thresholds. A sensory threshold that is equal to or even greater than the motor threshold indicates a potential ventral placement of the electrode and should prompt repositioning.

At this point, there has been the abovementioned single case series that looked at the adaption of IONM for both safety and lead placement in DRG stimulator placement [15], as well as several small prospective studies confirming the accuracy in its use for both lead placement and guiding postoperative programming [16–18].

Overview of Existing IONM Opportunities

At present IONM companies are available to cover spinal procedures and SCS. There are large national companies, as well as numerous smaller regional companies. These companies can bring in their own equipment which includes needles, technical setup, and the neuromonitoring machine, as well as the technician.

Financial relationships with these services include paying a set fee for the services either per case, per hour, or per day. This covers the cost of technician to deliver the services. The neuromonitoring company will then bill/code for their services to the insurance company. That cost will also include physician oversight remotely of the neuromonitoring data. The upside for this model is it allows the hospital or physician to be separate from the services, not need their own equipment, and not take the risk of lack of reimbursement. It should also be known that Medicare, Medicaid, and government plans consider IONM as part of the bundled procedure.

The downside to this model is potential lost revenue, relying on a technician and companies' resources, and the need to bring in the equipment for each case. Another model is running all the services in house and billing/coding for it. This would require hiring your own technician, owning the equipment, and setting up an interpreting physician of the data outside the OR. This is also a model that is run by hospitals and surgery centers, which ultimately saves costs overtime. Private practice physicians will also sometimes employ this model.

References

1. Falowski S, Sharan A. A review on spinal cord stimulation. J Neurosurg Sci. 2012;56(4):287–98.
2. Falowski S, Celii A, Sharan A. Spinal cord stimulation: an update. Neurotherapeutics. 2008;5(1):86–99.
3. Tsirikos AI, Duckworth AD, Henderson LE, Michaelson C. Multimodal intraoperative spinal cord monitoring during spinal deformity surgery: efficacy, diagnostic characteristics, and algorithm development. Med Princ Pract. 2020;29(1):6–17. https://doi.org/10.1159/000501256.
4. Biscevic M, Sehic A, Krupic F. Intraoperative neuromonitoring in spine deformity surgery: modalities, advantages, limitations, medicolegal issues - surgeons' views. EFORT Open Rev. 2020;5(1):9–16. Published 2020 Jan 29. https://doi.org/10.1302/2058-5241.5.180032.

5. Barolat G. Epidural spinal cord stimulation: anatomical and electrical properties of the intraspinal structures relevant to spinal cord stimulation and clinical correlations. Neuromodulation. 1998;1(2):63–71. https://doi.org/10.1111/j.1525-1403.1998.tb00019.x.
6. Struijk JJ, Holsheimer J, van Veen BK, Boom HB. Epidural spinal cord stimulation: calculation of field potentials with special reference to dorsal column nerve fibers. IEEE Trans Biomed Eng. 1991;38(1):104–10. https://doi.org/10.1109/10.68217.
7. Shils JL, Arle JE. Neuromonitoring for spinal cord stimulation Lead placement under general anesthesia. J Clin Neurol. 2018;14(4):444–53. https://doi.org/10.3988/jcn.2018.14.4.444.
8. Falowski S, Dianna A. Neuromonitoring protocol for spinal cord stimulator cases with case descriptions. Int J Acad Med. 2016;2(2):132–44.
9. Mammis A, Mogilner AY. The use of intraoperative electrophysiology for the placement of spinal cord stimulator paddle leads under general anesthesia. Neurosurgery. 2012;70(ONS Suppl 2):ONS230-236.
10. Falowski SM, Celii A, Sestokas AK, Schwarz DM, Matsumoto C, Sharan A. Awake vs. asleep placement of spinal cord stimulators: a cohort analysis of complications associated with placement. Neuromodulation. 2011;14(2):130–5.
11. Lad SP, Petersen E, Marky A, Deer TR, Levy RM, Feler CA. Stimulation of the spinal cord by placement of surgical-based paddle leads. In: Deer TR, Pope JE, editors. Atlas of implantable therapies for pain management. New York: Springer; 2016. p. 41–7.
12. Falowski SM, Sharan A, McInerney J, Jacobs D, Venkatesan L, Agnesi F. Nonawake vs awake placement of spinal cord stimulators: a prospective, multicenter study comparing safety and efficacy. Neurosurgery. 2019;84(1):198–205. https://doi.org/10.1093/neuros/nyy062.
13. Deer TR, Lamer TJ, Pope JE, et al. The neurostimulation appropriateness consensus committee (NACC) safety guidelines for the reduction of severe neurological injury. Neuromodulation. 2017;20(1):15–30.
14. Deer TR, Pope JE, Lamer TJ, Grider JS, Provenzano D, Lubenow TR, et al. The neuromodulation appropriateness consensus committee on best practices for dorsal root ganglion stimulation. Neuromodulation. 2019;22(1):1–35.
15. Falowski SM, Dianna A. A prospective analysis of neuromonitoring for confirmation of lead placement in dorsal root ganglion stimulation. Oper Neurosurg (Hagerstown). 2018;14(6):654–60. https://doi.org/10.1093/ons/opx172.
16. Falowski S, Conti K, Mogilner A. Analysis of S1 DRG programming to determine location of the DRG and ideal anatomic positioning of the electrode. Neuromodulation. 2019. https://doi.org/10.1111/ner.13039. [Epub ahead of print].
17. Falowski S, Pope JE, Raza A. Early US experience with stimulation of the dorsal root ganglia for the treatment of peripheral neuropathy in the lower extremities: a multicenter retrospective case series. Neuromodulation. 2019 Jan;22(1):96–100.
18. Falowski SM. A prospective analysis of the use of intraoperative neuromonitoring for mapping the S1 dorsal root ganglion location to determine ideal lead positioning and predict postoperative programming [published online ahead of print, 2020 Apr 13]. Neuromodulation. 2020. https://doi.org/10.1111/ner.13156.

Sacral Neuromodulation for Urinary and Fecal Incontinence: Surgical Technique

Sérgio Adrian Fernandes Dantas, Francisco Irochima Pinheiro, and César Araújo Britto

Abbreviations

FDA	Food and Drug Administration
FI	Fecal incontinence
IPG	Internal pulse generator
SNS	Sacral nerve stimulation
UI	Urinary incontinence

Introduction

Urinary incontinence (UI) and fecal incontinence (FI) are prevalent conditions with a profound influence on well-being and quality of life causing low self-esteem, restriction of social and sexual activities and depression, as well as being of immense economic importance for the health service [1, 2].

Based on the results of the EPIC study, the global prevalence of UI was estimated to be 8.7% worldwide, with over 421 million people affected [3]. The prevalence of FI is 1.4–1.9% [4, 5].

Clinically, urge incontinence is an involuntary loss of urine upon a sudden urge. Urgency-frequency is an uncontrollable urge to void, resulting in frequent, small volume voids, and is often associated with interstitial cystitis and chronic pelvic pain.

S. A. F. Dantas (✉)
Department of Neurosurgery, Onofre Lopes University Hospital, Natal, Brazil

F. I. Pinheiro
Department of Oftalmology, Onofre Lopes University Hospital, Natal, Brazil

C. A. Britto
Department of Urology, Onofre Lopes University Hospital, Natal, Brazil

T. d. S. Freitas et al. (eds.), *Neuromodulation Techniques for Pain Treatment*,
https://doi.org/10.1007/978-3-030-84778-4_21

Urinary retention is the inability to void despite having the urge to void; it can be caused by a hypocontractile detrusor or urethral overactivity. Fecal incontinence is a loss of voluntary control of the passage of stool. About three-quarters of these patients will be successfully treated with conservative measures which include biofeedback, pelvic floor exercises, intermittent catheterization, and pharmacotherapy (anticholinergic drugs, smooth muscle relaxants, and tricyclic antidepressants). If conservative therapies are all unsuccessful, surgical alternatives for UI include enterocystoplasty, bladder denervation, detrusor myectomy, and permanent indwelling catheterization and for FI include sphincter repair, dynamic graciloplasty, artificial bowel sphincter, and the most extreme, colostomy. These procedures, however, may have variable efficacy besides being associated with adverse effects and complications [6, 7].

Sacral nerve stimulation (SNS) is a reversible procedure, in that the device can be removed without permanent injury, being considered as a less invasive alternative for patients to whom prior conservative therapeutics failed and who are not ready for irreversible surgery [8].

The technique of SNS was published by Tanagho [9]. In 1997, the Food and Drug Administration (FDA) approved this technique for treatment of refractory urge incontinence. In 1999, it was approved for use in urge/frequency syndrome and idiopathic obstructive urinary retention management. In 2002, it was approved for treatment of refractory overactive bladder. Matzel introduced SNS to treat FI in 1995 [10]. It was approved by FDA in 2006 to treat severe constipation and FI.

Emerging "off-label" indications include interstitial cystitis, chronic pelvic pain syndrome, neurogenic lower urinary tract symptoms, and pediatric voiding dysfunction [11].

Mechanisms of Action

The exact neurophysiological basis that explains the action of the electrical stimulation of sacral nerves is still unknown. Some authors suggest that the effect is due to the stimulation of both afferent and efferent neural circuits in the pelvic viscera and connections with spinal interneurons [12].

Surgical Technique

The surgical procedure for electrical stimulation of sacral nerves is performed in two phases.

Phase 1: Test Stimulation

The objective of this first phase is to evaluate the effectiveness of the stimulation to select which patients will undergo the definitive implant.

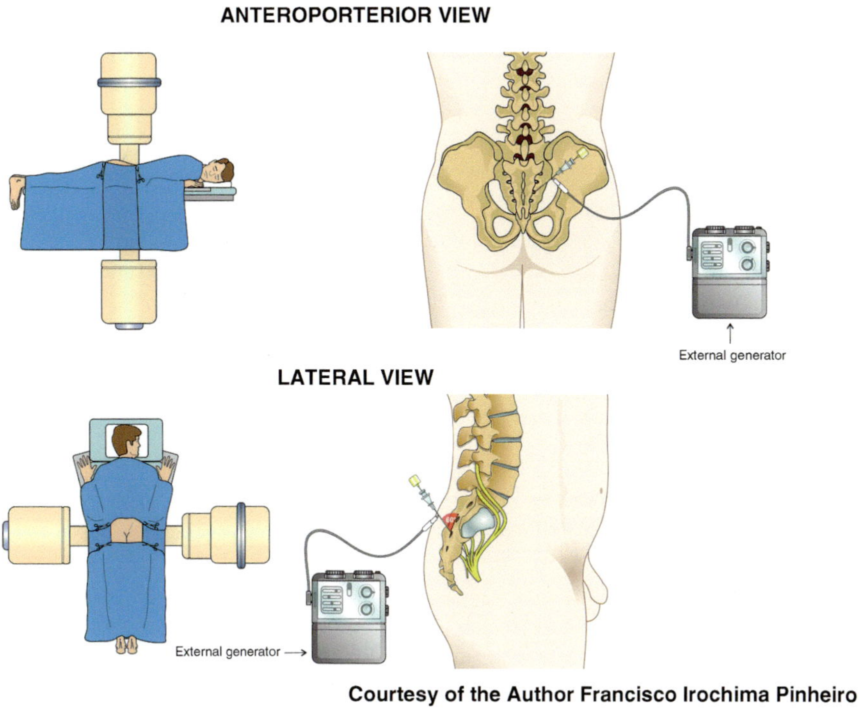

Fig. 1 The patient is positioned in a prone position. A test needle is inserted into the sacral foramen (usually S3), preferably under local anesthesia and fluoroscopy guidance. Then, the needle is connected to an external generator and the percutaneous nerve evaluation test is done

The patient is positioned in a prone position, under local anesthesia; a needle is inserted into the sacral foramen (usually S3) with fluoroscopy guidance. Once the needle is in place, it is connected to an external generator, and the electrophysiological evaluation is started (Fig. 1). The typical motor and sensory responses to lead placement in the S3 foramen are anal contractions, great toe dorsiflexion, and perineal paresthesia in the rectum, scrotum, or vagina [13]. Then, the definitive quadripolar electrode is implanted in the chosen foramen and, through a subcutaneously tunneled extension cable, connected to an external pulse generator (Figs. 2, 3, 4, and 5).

This test period is 3–7 days for a patient with urinary dysfunction and 2–3 weeks if the patient has FI. Improvement of at least 50% of symptoms (voiding diary, pad test record, continence scores) indicates a good response and is followed by phase 2 which consists of the implantation of the permanent pulse generator. In case of unsatisfactory response, the electrode is explanted.

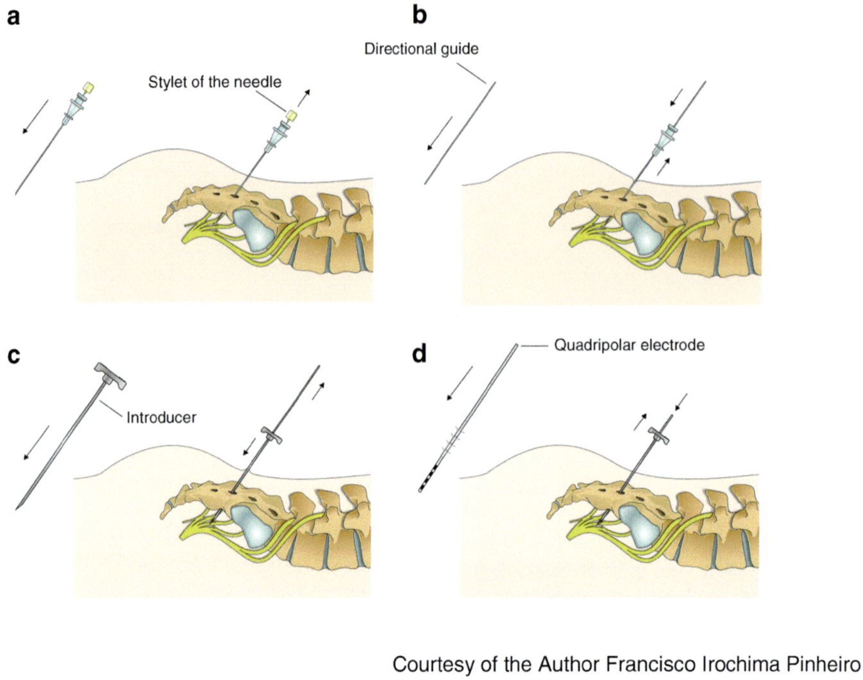

Fig. 2 (**a**) The stylet of the needle is removed. (**b**) A directional guide wire is placed through the foramen needle. Holding the directional guide in place, the foramen needle is removed. (**c**) The introducer (dilator and introducer sheath) is placed over the directional guide and positioned into the foramen. Then, the directional guide and dilator are removed leaving the introducer sheath in place. (**d**) The quadripolar electrode is placed through the introducer sheath until all the electrode poles enter the foramen. After confirmation of correct electrode placement by fluoroscopy, the lead stylet and introducer sheath are carefully removed

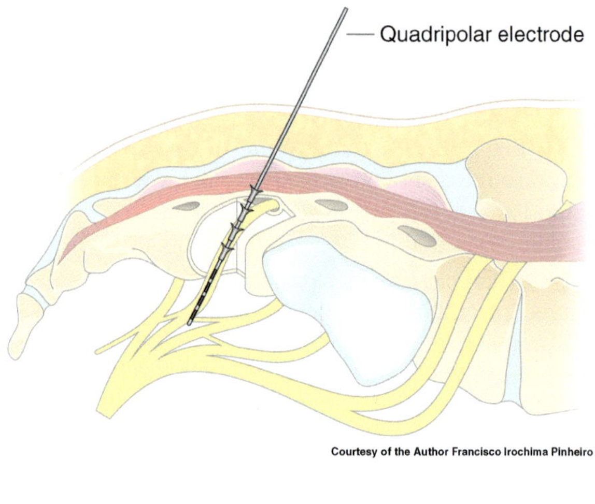

Fig. 3 Quadripolar electrode implanted in the sacral foramen

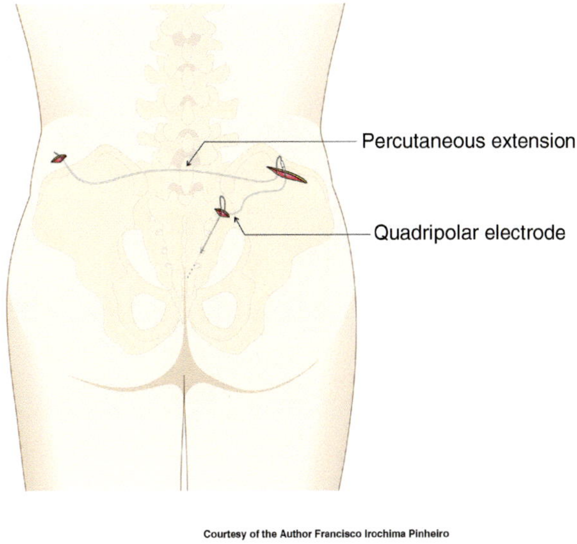

Fig. 4 The electrode is tunneled subcutaneously for a small incision in the upper part of the buttock, connected to the percutaneous extension that is tunneled to the contralateral side, externalizing through a small stab incision

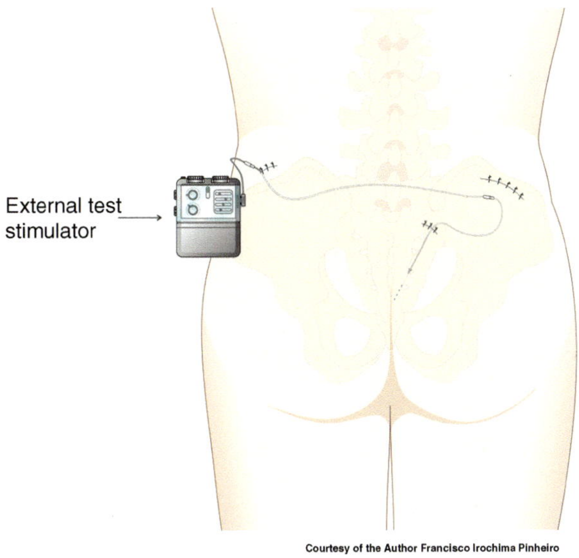

Fig. 5 The percutaneous extension is connected to the external test stimulator

Phase 2: Implantation of Internal Pulse Generator (IPG)

At this stage, the external extension cable used in the test phase is removed, and the IPG is implanted in a subcutaneous pocket created on the upper part of the buttock on the same side of the sacral electrode which will be connected to the IPG (Figs. 6 and 7).

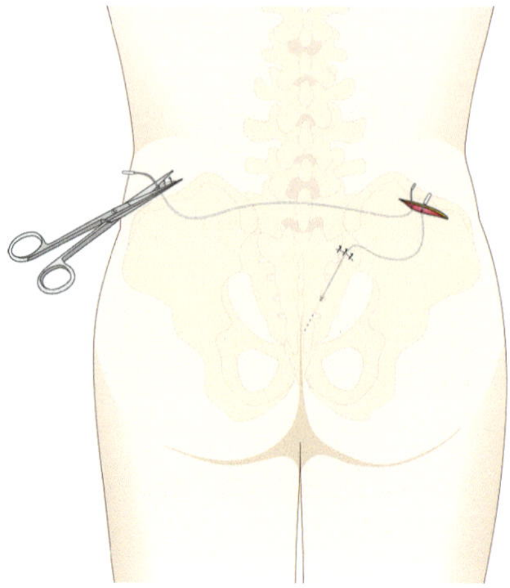

Courtesy of the Author Francisco Irochima Pinheiro

Fig. 6 After the successful test period, the percutaneous extension is pulled out slightly and cut. The incision at the connection level is enlarged; the electrode is disconnected from the rest of the percutaneous extension that is explanted. A subcutaneous pocket is created

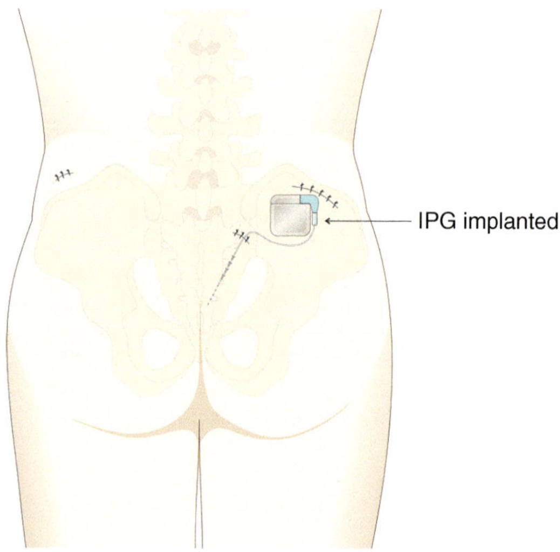

Courtesy of the Author Francisco Irochima Pinheiro

Fig. 7 The IPG is connected to the electrode and implanted in the subcutaneous pocket

Illustration of Surgical Steps

Complications

- Pain perceived at the site of the IPG
- Undesirable change in stimulation
- Implant infection
- Lead fracture and displacement
- IPG failure

References

1. Ekelund P, Grimby A, Milsom I. Urinary incontinence. Social and financial costs are high. BMJ. 1993;306(6888):1344.
2. Irwin DE, Kopp ZS, Agatep B, Milsom I, Abrams P. Worldwide prevalence estimates of lower urinary tract symptoms, overactive bladder, urinary incontinence and bladder outlet obstruction. BJU Int. 2011;108(7):1132–8.
3. Irwin DE, Milsom I, Hunskaar S, Reilly K, Kopp Z, Herschorn S, et al. Population-based survey of urinary incontinence, overactive bladder, and other lower urinary tract symptoms in five countries: results of the EPIC study. Eur Urol. 2006;50(6):1306–14; discussion 1314-1315.
4. Perry S, Shaw C, McGrother C, Matthews RJ, Assassa RP, Dallosso H, et al. Prevalence of faecal incontinence in adults aged 40 years or more living in the community. Gut. 2002;50(4):480–4.
5. Walter S, Hallböök O, Gotthard R, Bergmark M, Sjödahl R. A population-based study on bowel habits in a Swedish community: prevalence of faecal incontinence and constipation. Scand J Gastroenterol. 2002;37(8):911–6.
6. Oerlemans DJAJ, van Kerrebroeck PEV. Sacral nerve stimulation for neuromodulation of the lower urinary tract. NeurourolUrodyn. 2008;27(1):28–33.
7. Wong WD, Congliosi SM, Spencer MP, Corman ML, Tan P, Opelka FG, et al. The safety and efficacy of the artificial bowel sphincter for fecal incontinence: results from a multicenter cohort study. Dis Colon Rectum. 2002;45(9):1139–53.
8. van der Pal F, Heesakkers JPFA, Bemelmans BLH. Current opinion on the working mechanisms of neuromodulation in the treatment of lower urinary tract dysfunction. Curr Opin Urol. 2006;16(4):261–7.
9. Tanagho EA, Schmidt RA. Electrical stimulation in the clinical management of the neurogenic bladder. J Urol. 1988;140(6):1331–9.
10. Matzel KE, Stadelmaier U, Hohenfellner M, Gall FP. Electrical stimulation of sacral spinal nerves for treatment of faecal incontinence. Lancet. 1995;346(8983):1124–7.
11. Moore CK, Rueb JJ, Derisavifard S. What is new in neuromodulation? Curr Urol Rep. 2019;20(9):55.
12. Malde S, Fry C, Schurch B, Marcelissen T, Averbeck M, Digesu A, et al. What is the exact working mechanism of botulinum toxin A and sacral neuromodulation in the treatment of overactive bladder / detrusor overactivity? ICI-RS 2017. Neurourol Urodyn. 2018;37(S4):S108–16.
13. Hubsher CP, Jansen R, Riggs DR, Zaslau S. Sacral nerve stimulation for neuromodulation of the lower urinary tract. Can J Urol. 2012;5:6480–4.

Motor Cortex Stimulation: Neural Circuits and Practical Approach on Electrode Implantation Technique

Erich Talamoni Fonoff, Kleber Carlos de Azevedo Junior, and Eduardo Joaquim Lopes Alho

The electric stimulation of the human motor cortex to treat pharmacoresistant neuropathic pain has been reported in the early 1990s by Tsubokawa et al. [1, 2], and since then, the encouraging results [3–6] have led to an increasing use of motor cortex stimulation (MCS) as treatment option to drug-resistant neuropathic pain in the past three decades. Although the efficacy of MCS has been questioned because of variable results, hundreds of patients around the world have benefited by this technique in the treatment of refractory pain. It is important to highlight that most of patients referred to MCS are treatment-resistant to most techniques available in therapeutic resource presently. Patients suffering from various pain syndromes, such as trigeminal neuralgia, trigeminal neuropathy [7, 8], phantom limb pain [9], post-stroke pain [2], and complex regional pain syndrome [5, 10], among other deafferentation syndromes, have experienced alleviation of pain over the past decades. The technique consists in implanting an epidural electrode over the contralateral motor cortex connected to a battery-powered implantable pulse generator to drive transdural electrical pulses onto the neural circuits located in the primary motor cortex. As observed in most therapies in functional neurosurgery, the technical variations are always present and frequently are matter of debate. In this article the authors highlight their practical experience in the technique of MCS electrode implantation, using widely available surgical tools to solve methodological hitches while applying this ingenious treatment in refractory pain syndromes. They also give an overview and illustrations on pathways that possibly mediate the effects of MCS in alleviating pain.

E. Talamoni Fonoff (✉) · K. C. de Azevedo Junior · E. J. Lopes Alho
Department of Neurology, School of Medicine, University of São Paulo, São Paulo, Brazil

T. d. S. Freitas et al. (eds.), *Neuromodulation Techniques for Pain Treatment*,
https://doi.org/10.1007/978-3-030-84778-4_22

Overview on Neural Circuits

Although the precise mechanisms and circuits involved in pain relief by MCS remain unclear, some studies in humans [11] and in animal models [12–15] indicate the role of ventrolateral and medial thalamic nuclei, anterior cingulate and orbitofrontal cortices, periaqueductal gray matter (upper brainstem structures), and insula as major structures involved in chronic neuropathic pain modulation and also in the emotional aspects of pain [12, 16–18].

In this section, the objective is to give an overview of the anatomic structures classically involved in pain circuits and its possible relationships with motor cortex, based on the models found in the current literature.

Therefore, histological sections processed as described and analyzed to develop tridimensional reconstructions of the anatomical structures involved in pain in order to give the reader a true 3D impression of size, topography, and interrelation of nuclei and cortical regions engaged in neurophysiological processing of painful stimuli [19–21].

The neural circuits that are responsible for conduction, modulation, and interpretation of painful stimuli can be divided into afferent or ascending systems, efferent or descending systems, and pathways that connect different supraspinal centers.

Afferent Systems (See Fig. 1)

→

Fig. 1 *Afferent or Ascending Systems for Pain, Itch and Temperature.* The three ascending systems are shown here. The red system represents the spinothalamic tract (STT) since its origin in spinal cord gray matter (laminae I and IV to VIII), passing through its thalamic connections (MD, intralaminar nuclei, VMpo, and VPL), and finally the cortical projections (anterior cingulate cortex and anterior insula). The nuclei and cortex known to play a role in painful stimuli perception are shown in orange. The system shown in black lines is the anterolateral fascicle and its projections to principal and accessory olives, PAG, tectal structures, medial geniculate body, hypothalamus, and amygdala directly and indirectly by synapses with the A1 noradrenergic cell group and parabrachial nucleus. The synapses of the anterolateral fasciculus with the multisynaptic medial pain system in the reticular formation, parabrachial nucleus, and A1 and their projections to the thalamic intralaminar nuclei are also represented by black lines. The blue arrow represents the projection from VPL to S1. The structures represented in blue are known to have a discriminative perception of the painful stimuli, and the structures represented in green have a modulatory role in them. Full circles represent neuronal perikarya, the inverse arrowheads represent synapses, and the arrowheads represent final connections (*further details inside the text*). *In orange*: medial and lateral parabrachial nuclei (Pb); ventrocaudal medial dorsal nucleus (MD); ventromedial posterior nucleus (VMpo); intralaminar thalamic nuclei (I) insula; amygdala (Amy); and anterior cingulate cortex (ACC). *In green:* nucleus raphe magnus (RM); A1 noradrenergic cell group (A1); coeruleus and subcoeruleus complex (A6); periaqueductal gray matter (PAG); primary motor cortex (M1). *In blue*: anterior mediodorsal nucleus (MD); ventral posterior complex, with ventral posterolateral nucleus (VPL); and ventral posteromedial nucleus (VPM). *In gray:* olivary complex (O) and brainstem reticular formation (FR)

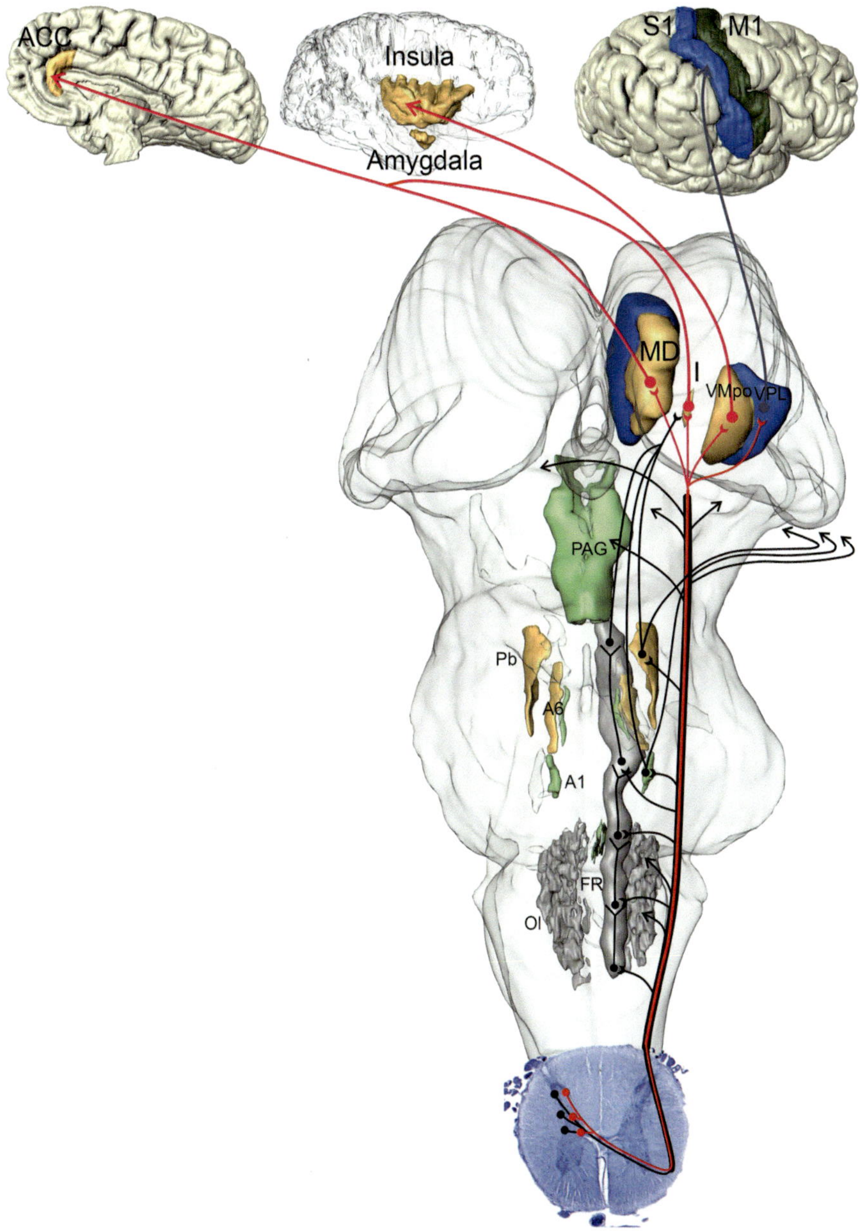
ACC
Insula
Amygdala
S1
M1
MD
I
VMpo
VPL
PAG
Pb
A6
A1
FR
OI

So far three ascending systems have been recognized, comprising:

1. The spinothalamic tract (STT) in the anterolateral fascicle.
2. Other ascending fibers from neurons located in superficial and deeper laminae of the dorsal horn of the spinal cord that also course in the anterolateral fascicle (ALF). They are difficult to disentangle from the ascending STT.
3. A multisynaptic medial pain system [22].

The spinothalamic tract is the best characterized of them. The name indicates its topography in the spinal cord. Most of the STT axons begin in lamina I, and three morphological and functional groups of neurons can be there distinguished: fusiform, pyramidal, and multipolar cells. These cells can be activated by pinch or noxious heat. The pyramidal cells are thermoceptive and are activated by innocuous cooling; multipolar neurons are a mixture of polymodal (heat, pinch, and cold sensitive) and nociceptive-specific neurons [23–25]. An additional population of lamina I spinothalamic cells, sensitive to histamine and involved in the perception of itch, was also identified [23]. The polymodal neurons of lamina I do not project to the thalamus but are involved in spinal motor or sympathetic reflex pathways [26]. The specific nociceptive fusiform and thermoceptive pyramidal cells of lamina I contribute to the spinothalamic tract. After crossing, the fibers course in the ventral white funiculus of the spinal cord. Caudal segmental fibers are shifted laterally by succeeding increments of more rostral fibers in a kind of topical lamination. During its ascending course through the brainstem, the spinothalamic tract is less well demarcated than the medial lemniscus. In general it can be found lateral to the latter and hence more superficial with respect to the surface of the spinal cord. They end in the thalamic VMPo (ventromedial posterior nucleus) and the ventrocaudal medial dorsal nucleus (MD). Other components of the STT derive from layer IV to layer VIII neurons and end in the thalamic VPL (ventral posterolateral nucleus) and in intralaminar thalamic nuclei (I).

The anterolateral fascicle (fascicle of Gowers) comprises ascending fibers arising from different laminae of the spinal gray matter and heading to the hypothalamus, the central nucleus of the amygdala, and to the intralaminar thalamic nuclei. They collateralize or end in brain stem centers including the medullary and pontine reticular formation, the olives, A1 noradrenergic cell group, parabrachial nuclei, coerulean/subcoerulean complex, mesencephalic periaqueductal gray, dorsally located tectal structures, and the diencephalic medial geniculate body. Direct hypothalamic endings parallel to efferents from A1 likewise end in the hypothalamus. Spinothalamic fibers from lamina I spinal cord neurons mainly terminate in a somatotopical fashion in the thalamic VMPo and in the ventrocaudal medial dorsal nucleus. Fiber endings subserving pain, itch, and temperature remain segregated within the VMPo. Fibers originating from deeper dorsal horn laminae end diffusely in the centrolateral intralaminar nucleus, in the adjoining lateral paralaminar region of the mediodorsal nucleus, and more sparsely in other intralaminar and midline nuclei of the thalamus [27].

The medial multisynaptic pain system is an ascending pathway parallel to STT. The neurons from spinal gray matter laminae VII and VIII via ALF send collaterals to the brainstem reticular formation and periaqueductal gray (PAG). In the reticular formation, the signal is transmitted in a multisynaptic way. Both supraspinal centers are connected to thalamic intralaminar nuclei. This kind of transmission could represent the morphological basis of the behavioral, emotional-affective, autonomic, and endocrine aspects of pain sensation.

The thalamocortical projections and hence the cortical role in pain perception are still a matter of debate. VMpo projections are directed to the posterior insular cortex. Neurons in the ventrocaudal medial dorsal nucleus together with neurons from the intralaminar nucleus target the cortex of the anterior cingulate gyrus (ACC).

Other spinothalamic fibers end in VPM (ventral posteromedial nucleus) and VPL. Efferents from these nuclei project to S1 (primary somatosensory cortex or Brodmann areas 1, 3, and 2).

Cingulate and insular cortical regions are considered to play a role in emotional and affective assessment of pain, whereas S1 should play a role in its sensory-discriminative aspects [11].

Efferent Systems (See Fig. 2)

The primary motor cortex (Brodmann area 4 or M1) is the target of transcranial magnetic stimulation and direct electrical stimulation by epidural electrodes to treat neuropathic pain [28]. Descending axons from the primary motor cortex are long known to inhibit the activity of layer I dorsal horn neurons [29]. This is at odds with MCS-induced pain relief, which occurs after prolonged time intervals.

Several supraspinal structures are involved in the control of neuronal transmission of painful stimuli. Most of the superordinate cortical and subcortical structures converge directly or collaterally onto the mesencephalic periaqueductal grey (PAG). The periaqueductal grey is connected to aminergic brainstem nuclei including the serotoninergic raphe magnus, A1 noradrenergic cell group, and the noradrenergic coeruleus/subcoeruleus complex. These aminergic nuclei emit descending axons to the posterior horn of the spinal cord and are likely to modulate pain transmission in long-term periods. Stimulation of the mesencephalic periaqueductal gray matter activates encephalin-releasing neurons [30] that project to the nucleus raphe magnus and adjacent raphe nuclei in the brainstem [31]. The nucleus raphe magnus (RM) is located directly rostral to the raphe obscurus and receives afferent axons from the spinal cord and cerebellum connected to the motor system. The RM receives descending afferents not only from the periaqueductal gray matter but also from the paraventricular hypothalamic nucleus, central nucleus of the amygdala, lateral hypothalamic area, parvocellular reticular nucleus, and the prelimbic, infralimbic, medial, and lateral precentral cortices in rats [32].

In response to raphe nuclei stimuli, serotonin is released to the dorsal horn of the spinal cord where it forms excitatory connections with the inhibitory interneurons located in lamina II (substantia gelatinosa). When activated, these interneurons release either encephalin or dynorphin, which bind to μ-opioid on the axons of incoming C and

A-δ fibers carrying pain signals from nociceptors activated in the periphery [33]. The activation of the μ-opioid receptor inhibits the release of substance P from these incoming first-order neurons and, in turn, inhibits the activation of the second-order neuron that is responsible for transmitting the pain signal via the spinothalamic tract to the thalamus and brainstem structures. The nociceptive signal is blocked before it is able to reach the cortical areas that interpret the signal as pain (such as the anterior cingulate and posterior insula). This is sometimes referred to as the gate control of pain, as first described by Melzack and Wall [34] and is supported by the fact that electrical stimulation of the PAG results in profound analgesia [35]. Four known kinds of opioid receptors have been identified: μ (mu), κ (kappa), σ (sigma), and δ (delta). Synthetic opioid and opioid-derivative drugs activate these receptors (possibly by acting on the PAG directly, where these receptors are densely expressed) to produce analgesia [36]. The neurons from noradrenergic A1 group and the noradrenergic coeruleus/subcoeruleus complex emit also descending axons to the posterior horn of the spinal cord and modulate pain transmission at this level.

Pathways Connecting Different Supraspinal Centers (See Fig. 2)

Thalamic connection patterns with motor, premotor, and supplementary motor areas of primate cortex indicate that VLa (ventral lateral nucleus, anterior subdivision) and VLp (ventral lateral nucleus, posterior subdivision) are the principal motor

Fig. 2 *Efferent or Descending Systems*. The red system is still the STT ascending system described in Fig. 1, in order to show its relationship with the descending systems and with the pathways connecting different supraspinal centers. The descending systems are shown in green, heading from M1 directly to the posterior horn of the spinal cord or terminating in the thalamic nuclei. The descending pathways from PAG to raphe magnus and from A1 noradrenergic cell group, subcoerulean region, and raphe magnus to the posterior horn are also shown in green. The arrows in gray represent the pathways connecting the anterior insula and amygdala to PAG, parabrachial nucleus and PAG to the hypothalamus, and anterior cingulate cortex to PAG. In the spinal cord section detail, these are represented: the peripherally incoming axons from C (thinner axon in black) and A-δ (thicker axons in black) fibers, the inhibitory interneuron in lamina II (small neuron in red), and the modulatory descending system from M1, PAG via raphe magnus and noradrenergic A1 and subcoeruleus (in green). Full circles represent neuronal perikarya, the inverse arrowheads represent synapses, and the arrowheads represent final connections (*further details inside the text*). *In orange*: medial and lateral parabrachial nuclei (Pb); ventrocaudal medial dorsal nucleus (MD); ventromedial posterior nucleus (VMpo); intralaminar thalamic nuclei (I); insula; amygdala (Amy); and anterior cingulate cortex (ACC). *In green:* nucleus raphe magnus (RM); A1 noradrenergic cell group (A1); coeruleus and subcoeruleus complex (A6); periaqueductal grey matter (PAG); primary motor cortex (M1). *In blue*: anterior mediodorsal nucleus (MD); ventral posterior complex, with ventral posterolateral nucleus (VPL); and ventral posteromedial nucleus (VPM). *In gray:* olivary complex (O) and brainstem reticular formation (FR)

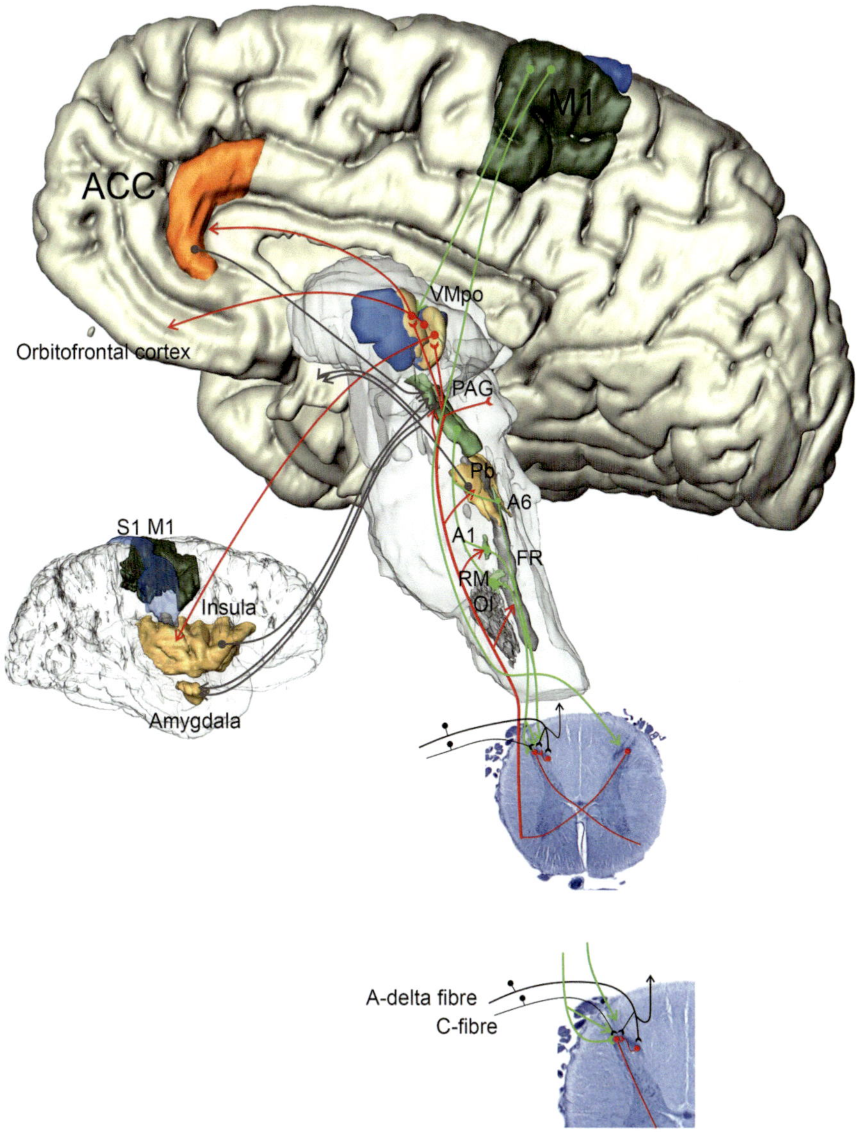
M1
ACC
VMpo
Orbitofrontal cortex
PAG
Pb
A6
S1 M1
A1
FR
RM
OI
Insula
Amygdala
A-delta fibre
C-fibre

nuclei, with VLp contributing dense inputs to M1 but also to PMV (ventral premotor cortex), PMD (dorsal premotor cortex), and SMA (supplementary motor area). VLa projects moderately to M1 and SMA while projecting densely to PMD. Furthermore, neurons from the primary motor cortex are reciprocally linked to the thalamic VPLo (ventroposterior lateral nucleus, pars oralis) and small contingent fibers to the caudal part of MD (medial dorsal nucleus) and the adjacent intralaminar nuclei [27]. These thalamic nuclei are also connected to the orbitofrontal cortex, to the insula, and to the cortex of the anterior cingulate gyrus. In addition, by feed-forward cortical connections, the motor cortex has access via premotor, supplementary motor, and cingulate motor fields to orbitofrontal and anterior cingulate regions.

These neuronal loops and intersections between M1, PM (premotor cortex), and SMA with the thalamic relays involved in pain circuits are probably engaged in pain relief by motor cortex stimulation. The connection between motor areas with the orbitofrontal and anterior cingulate cortices seems to play a defining role too, since they are linked to the mesencephalic periaqueductal gray. Other loops that may be important are the connections from anterior insula and amygdala to PAG, parabrachial nucleus and PAG to the hypothalamus, parabrachial nucleus to amygdala, and anterior cingulate cortex to PAG.

Techniques for Implantation of MCS Electrodes

Although the best approach to determine the site for implanting MCS electrodes is still a matter of debate, if the intention is to stimulate the primary motor cortex by applying transdural electrical pulses, whatever method applied has got to the make sure this occurs efficiently in all patients. The effective delivery of electrical pulses in a particular site or region of the nervous system is a common key starting point neuromodulation and should always be the core objective when choosing electrode type and method of implant. Currently, most of the authors perform the implantation procedure under general anesthesia, using different methods for the localization of motor cortex. Reports include either localization of precentral gyrus based merely on anatomic landmarks or added to intraoperative sensory evoked potentials (SEP) for functional localization. Intraoperative SEP is oriented for the localization of central sulcus, by inverted SEP wave, what indirectly leads to the precentral gyrus located immediately anteriorly. The combination of those techniques provides the functional localization of the mid-precentral gyrus, which normally corresponds to the primary motor cortex itself. However the use of SEP is limited to patients who present sensory pathways which are at least partially preserved ensuring that SEPs can be elicited by applying electrical current in median nerve and capturing evoked potentials over the central sulcus. On the other hand, there are deafferentation pain syndromes (e.g., brachial plexus avulsion or amputation) in which the peripheral sensory pathways are severely or totally injured, precluding the intraoperative use of SEP as a target refining method.

In our experience, a different and much simpler technique has been used with much success. It provides detailed functional and spatial information for target refining during implantation of electrodes capable to stimulate the motor cortex stimulation efficiently. It is totally capable of eliciting evoked motor potentials at higher current intensity and even to evoke complex segmental limb movement depending on the stimulation frequency. Although therapeutic stimulation applied in the motor cortex is always under the motor threshold, the best electrode location is the one closest to the site that makes MEPs (motor evoked potentials) occur at lowest threshold. While most of the procedures are performed under sedation, the core technique for mapping the motor cortex should be performed with patients awake and responsive. This method does not require that patients to be awake during the whole procedure but only a few minutes during the cortical mapping procedure. Having the anatomical location of the mid-precentral gyrus, more specifically the "hand knob" as a starting point situated by either image-guided navigation system to point the center of a nummular craniotomy leaving the dura completely intact. Although MEPs can be routinely elicited in patients under light sedation, the same procedure performed in an awake patient allows lower MEP thresholds and provides the possibility of mapping the motor cortex in amputees or in severely injured brachial plexus patients, as described further on this chapter.

As above cited this technique relies on stereotactic localization of the hand knob in the posterior aspects of the precentral gyrus pinpointed in MRI to guided navigation followed by intraoperative target refining by transdural stimulation of the cerebral cortex in awake patients. Standard frameless navigation system fed by volumetric MR images in dedicated software guides the localization of the precentral gyrus in each individual patient. During targeting in navigation system, the surgeon should aim at the center of the omega-shaped knob on the posterior border of the pre-central gyrus within the central sulcus, which lines up perpendicularly with the posterior ending of the superior frontal sulcus used as anatomical landmark used to guide the center of the craniotomy. This is usually the initial point in the surface of dura for the following procedure mapping the cerebral cortex. As suggested by Yousry et al. [37], the image generated by this knob in the horizontal MR images is highly specific to indicate the primary motor area of hand in normal subjects. However, this point is usually 1.5–2 cm deep into the central sulcus and 3.5 cm from midline, consequently not visible at the cortical surface. So this targeting method provides a point deep seated in the central sulcus, not the final target itself, which is immediately above at a point on the surface of cerebral cortex. However, the technique of MCS does not require dural opening, so during the procedure only anatomical landmarks guided by imaging guided navigation are the only way to ensure the target starting point in epidural space, and the final site and orientation for electrode implantation is then specified by the intraoperative cortical mapping.

So the coordinates of the hand knob are then perpendicularly projected onto the surface of the scalp to guide the skin incision, further projected onto the surface of the skull to point the center of the craniotomy, and finally the same projection was made onto the dural surface in order to provide the initial point for cortical mapping by transdural electrical stimulation. A small craniotomy (3 cm) encompassing the region of the anatomical target can be performed under local anesthesia and light sedation. After the craniotomy is performed, sedation can be completely withdrawn so the patient is found completely awake and responsive. Transdural bipolar stimulation of the cortex can be conducted at current amplitudes up to 4–6 mA, 1 ms, and 30–60 Hz using a bipolar stimulator. Our largest experience is using bipolar probes with tips 7–10 mm apart, although a monopolar probe can also be used with a distant reference plate. Usually protocols that include MEP peripheral myograms evoked by focalized cortical simulation do not require patients to be awake, as described elsewhere [38] and mentioned above. However, patients who suffer from severe deafferentation or amputees do not benefit from this technique because MEPs record from muscles cannot be performed either due to severe sensorimotor or, in case of proximal amputation, absence of the limb itself. So the technique described earlier in this text was designed for patients with severe injuries in the affected limb. In our experience stimulation of the motor cortex does evoke movements as early descriptions of Wilder Penfield and many other authors; however in severely injured patients, movements cannot be recorded. In the last few years, our team operated close to 50 patients for implanting MDS electrode. Some of them had severe brachial plexus injury and some were amputees. So in those patients we had a different protocol. The most effective method to map the cortex was to have the patients describe in details the sensation after each stimulation pulse. Patients describe very well sensations of pressure or paresthesias with consequent interpretations of stimulation the sensory cortex, while descriptions of sensation of movements in the inexistent or flail limb with no actual muscle activity are clearly described by patients. The consequent interpretation in this case is that stimulations have been applied over the primary motor cortex. So during the stimulation session, the patient was required to describe any sensation different from the resting state, after each short period of stimulation (1–2 s). Stimulation can be then repeated in targets that generate any sensation of interest over a longer period (2–5 s). The repeated stimulation allowed patients to improve the description of the sensation in a more detailed manner, including the part of the limb involved and the type of movement. To help the description of movements and the joints involved, as well as the speed and repetition of the entire movement, the patient used the contralateral limb to mimic the sensation of movement on the affected side. In patients with severe brachial plexus injuries or amputees, electrical stimulation at 4.0–6.0 mA, 30–60 Hz, and 1 ms of pulse width evokes a vivid sensation of movement in the nonexistent hand, forearm, and arm. The sensation of wrist flexion is usually elicited in all patients, while two-thirds of patients can make clear distinction of thumb and index movements and differentiate from the wrist flexion and from the other fingers' movements. Phantom movements of the remaining fingers (third to fifth) are usually describes in one-third of patients. The cortical area responsive to thumb tends to occupy a lateral position related to the areas of the other fingers, following the maps of normal homunculus. The evoked sensation is restricted to the period of stimulation, and it stopped as soon as that was discontinued. However some of the patients refer intense emotions because the sensation of movements can be quite vivid and the feeling of the sensation of inexistent of severely injured limb is compared as if it became healthy and active again. All patients are warned that sensations like those may be evoked and that it does not mean that the limb can be recovered unfortunately.

Once mapping was finished, an epidural paddle electrode can be implanted following the map generated over the area of the greatest evoked motor sensation. The center contacts of the paddle electrode are then placed over the area, which elicited sensation of movement, related to the area affected by the pain syndrome. The contacts in the two extremities of the electrode covered adjacent areas of the motor cortex also elicited by stimulation, the forearm, arm, face, and so on. Eventually, two stripes of electrodes are implanted in order to expand the spatial combinations and topographically refine the therapeutic stimulation. Currently, new types of electrodes with multiple are available, so the possible combinations are numerous.

Based in our experience, this technique was useful for target refining during of implantation of electrode for motor cortex stimulation. However, comparative studies are required to investigate whether target refining by intraoperative mapping significantly improves the results of therapeutic MCS for refractory pain.

References

1. Tsubokawa T, Katayama Y, Yamamoto T, Hirayama T, Koyama S. Treatment of thalamic pain by chronic motor cortex stimulation. Pacing Clin Electrophysiol. 1991;14:131–4.
2. Tsubokawa T, Katayama Y, Yamamoto T, Hirayama T, Koyama S. Chronic motor cortex stimulation in patients with thalamic pain. J Neurosurg. 1993a;78:393–401.
3. Nguyen JP, Lefaucher JP, Le Guerinel C, Eizenbaum JF, Nakano N, Carpentier A. Motor cortex stimulation in the treatment of central and neuropathic pain. Arch Med Res. 2000;31:263–5.
4. Fonoff ET, Hamani C, Andrade DC, Yeng LT, Marcolin MA, Teixeira MJ. Pain relief and functional recovery in patients with complex regional pain syndrome after motor cortex stimulation. Stereotact Funct Neurosurg. 2011;89:167–72.
5. Parravano DC, Ciampi DA, Fonoff ET, Monaco B, Navarro J, Yeng LT, Teixeira MJ, Hamani C. Quality of life after motor cortex stimulation: clinical results and systematic review of the literature. Neurosurgery. 2019;84(2):451–6. https://doi.org/10.1093/neuros/nyy060. PMID: 29547990.
6. Lopez WO, Barbosa DC, Teixera MJ, Paiz M, Moura L, Monaco BA, Fonoff ET. Pain relief in CRPS-II after spinal cord and motor cortex simultaneous dual stimulation. Pain Physician. 2016;19(4):E631–5. PMID: 27228530.
7. Meyerson BA, Lindblom U, Linderoth B, Lind G, Herregodts P. Motor cortex stimulation as treatment of trigeminal neuropathic pain. Acta Neurochir Suppl (Wien). 1993;58:150–3.
8. Nguyen JP, Lefaucheur JP, Decq P, Uchiyama T, Carpentier A, Fontaine D, Brugieres P, Pollin B, Feve A, Rostaing S, Cesaro P, Keravel Y. Chronic motor cortex stimulation in the treatment of central and neuropathic pain. Correlations between clinical, electrophysiological and anatomical data. Pain. 1999;82:245–51.
9. Saitoh Y, Hirano S, Kato A, Kishima H, Hirata M, Yamamoto K, Yoshimine T. Motor cortex stimulation for deafferentation pain. Neurosurg Focus. 2001;11:E1.
10. Velasco F, Carrillo-Ruiz JD, Castro G, Argüelles C, Velasco AL, Kassian A, Guevara U. Motor cortex electrical stimulation applied to patients with complex regional pain syndrome. Pain. 2009;147:91–8.
11. Garcia-Larrea L, Peyron R. Motor cortex stimulation for neuropathic pain: from phenomenology to mechanisms. Neuroimage. 2007;37 suppl 1:S71–9.

12. Pagano RL, Assis DV, Clara JA, Alves AS, Dale CS, Teixeira MJ, Fonoff ET, Britto LR. Transdural motor cortex stimulation reverses neuropathic pain in rats: a profile of neuronal activation. Eur J Pain. 2011;15(3):268.e1–14. https://doi.org/10.1016/j.ejpain.2010.08.003. PMID: 20817578.
13. Pagano RL, Fonoff ET, Dale CS, Ballester G, Teixeira MJ, Britto LR. Motor cortex stimulation inhibits thalamic sensory neurons and enhances activity of PAG neurons: possible pathways for antinociception. Pain. 2012;153(12):2359–69. https://doi.org/10.1016/j.pain.2012.08.002. Epub 2012 Sep 25. PMID: 2301729.
14. Campos ACP, Kikuchi DS, Paschoa AFN, Kuroki MA, Fonoff ET, Hamani C, Pagano RL, Hernandes MS. Unraveling the role of astrocytes in subthalamic nucleus deep brain stimulation in a Parkinson's disease rat model. Cell Mol Neurobiol. 2020;40(6):939–54.
15. Lopes PSS, Campos ACP, Fonoff ET, Britto LRG, Pagano RL. Motor cortex and pain control: exploring the descending relay analgesic pathways and spinal nociceptive neurons in healthy conscious rats. Behav Brain Funct. 2019;15(1):5. https://doi.org/10.1186/s12993-019-0156-0. PMID: 30909927; PMCID: PMC6432755.
16. de Andrade EM, Martinez RCR, Pagano RL, Lopes PSS, Auada AVV, Gouveia FV, Antunes GF, Assis DV, Lebrun I, Fonoff ET. Neurochemical effects of motor cortex stimulation in the periaqueductal gray during neuropathic pain. J Neurosurg. 2019;132(1):239–51. https://doi.org/10.3171/2018.7.JNS173239. PMID: 30611141.
17. Fonoff ET, Pereira JF Jr, Camargo LV, Dale CS, Pagano RL, Ballester G, Teixeira MJ. Functional mapping of the motor cortex of the rat using transdural electrical stimulation. Behav Brain Res. 2009;202(1):138–41. https://doi.org/10.1016/j.bbr.2009.03.018. Epub 2009 Mar 24. PMID: 19447290.
18. Fonoff ET, Dale CS, Pagano RL, Paccola CC, Ballester G, Teixeira MJ, Giorgi R. Antinociception induced by epidural motor cortex stimulation in naive conscious rats is mediated by the opioid system. Behav Brain Res. 2009;196(1):63–70. https://doi.org/10.1016/j.bbr.2008.07.027. Epub 2008 Jul 31. PMID: 18718490.
19. Heinsen H, Arzberger T, Schmitz C. Celloidin mounting (embedding without infiltration) – a new, simple and reliable method for producing serial sections of high thickness through complete human brains and its application to stereological and immunohistochemical investigations. J Chem Neuroanat. 2000;20:49–59.
20. Alho EJL, Alho ATDL, Grinberg L, Amaro E Jr, Dos Santos GAB, da Silva RE, Neves RC, Alegro M, Coelho DB, Teixeira MJ, Fonoff ET, Heinsen H. High thickness histological sections as alternative to study the three-dimensional microscopic human sub-cortical neuroanatomy. Brain Struct Funct. 2018;223(3):1121–32. https://doi.org/10.1007/s00429-017-1548-2. Epub 2017 Nov 1. PMID: 29094303; PMCID: PMC5899898.
21. Alho ATDL, Hamani C, Alho EJL, da Silva RE, Santos GAB, Neves RC, Carreira LL, Araújo CMM, Magalhães G, Coelho DB, Alegro MC, Martin MGM, Grinberg LT, Pasqualucci CA, Heinsen H, Fonoff ET, Amaro E Jr. Magnetic resonance diffusion tensor imaging for the pedunculopontine nucleus: proof of concept and histological correlation. Brain Struct Funct. 2017;222(6):2547–58.
22. Nieuwenhuys R, Voogd J, van Huijzen C. The human central nervous system. 4th ed. Berlin/Heidelberg/New York: Springer-Verlag; 2008.
23. Andrew D, Krout KE, Craig AD. Differentiation of lamina I spinomedullary and spinothalamic neurons in the cat. J Comp Neurol. 2003;458:257–71.
24. Han ZS, Zhang ET, Craig AD. Nociceptive and thermoceptive lamina I neurons are anatomically distinct. Nat Neurosci. 1998;1:218–25.
25. Zhang ET, Craig AD. Morphology and distribution of spinothalamic lamina I neurons in the monkey. J Neurosci. 1997;17:3274–84.
26. Craig AD, Kniffki KD. Spinothalamic lumbosacral lamina I cells responsive to skin and muscle stimulation in the cat. J Physiol. 1985;365:197–221.
27. Fang P-C, Stepniewska I, Kaas JH. The thalamic connections of motor, premotor, and prefrontal areas of cortex in a prosimian primate (*Otolemur garnetti*). Neuroscience. 2006;143(4):987–1020.

28. Lima MC, Fregni F. Motor cortex stimulation for chronic pain: systematic review and meta-analysis of the literature. Neurology. 2008;70:2329–37.
29. Canedo A. Primary motor cortex influences on the descending and ascending systems. Prog Neurobiol. 1997;51:287–335.
30. Adams JE. Naloxone reversal of analgesia produced by brain stimulation in the human. Pain. 1976;2:161–6.
31. Sillery E, Bittar RG, Robson MD, Behrens TEJ, Stein J, Aziz FRCS, Johansen-Berg H. Connectivity of the human periventricular–periaqueductal gray region. J Neurosurg. 2005;103:1030–4.
32. Hermann DM, Luppi PH, Peyron C, Hinckel P, Jouvet M. Afferent projections to the rat nuclei raphe magnus, raphe pallidus and reticularis gigantocellularis pars alpha demonstrated by iontophoretic application of choleratoxin (subunit b). J Chem Neuroanat. 1997;13(1):1–21.
33. Mason P. Central mechanisms of pain modulation. Curr Opin Neurobiol. 1999;9:436–41.
34. Melzack R, Wall PD. Pain mechanisms: a new theory. Science. 1965;150:971–9.
35. Mayer DJ, Wolfle TL, Akil H, Carder B, Liebeskind JC. Analgesia from electrical stimulation in the brainstem of the rat. Science. 1971;174:1351–4.
36. Budai D, Howard L. Fields endogenous opioid peptides acting at m-opioid receptors in the dorsal horn contribute to midbrain modulation of spinal nociceptive neurons. J Neurophysiol. 1998;79:677–87.
37. Yousry TA, Schmid UD, Alkadhi H, Schmidt D, Peraud A, Buettner A, Winkler P. Localization of the motor hand area to a knob on the precentral gyrus. A new landmark. Brain. 1997;120:141–57.
38. Teixeira MJ, de Andrade DC, Fonoff ET. Intra-operative transdural electric stimulation in awake patient: target refining for motor cortex stimulation. Acta Neurochir Suppl. 2013;117:73–8.

Index

T. d. S. Freitas et al. (eds.), *Neuromodulation Techniques for Pain Treatment*,
https://doi.org/10.1007/978-3-030-84778-4

Printed by Printforce, the Netherlands